D0938475

EMOTIONS

EMOTIONS AND SOCIAL BEHAVIOR

Series Editor: Peter Salovey, Yale University

EMOTIONS

Current Issues and Future Directions

Edited by
TRACY J. MAYNE and GEORGE A. BONANNO

Series Editor's Note by Peter Salovey
Foreword by Klaus R. Scherer

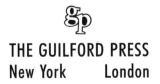

THE GUILFORD PRESS
New York   London

© 2001 The Guilford Press
A Division of Guilford Publications, Inc.
72 Spring Street, New York, NY 10012
www.guilford.com

Printed in the United States of America

This book is printed on acid-free paper.

Last digit is print number: 9   8   7   6   5   4   3   2   1

Library of Congress Cataloging-in-Publication Data

Emotions : current issues and future directions / edited by Tracy J. Mayne,
  George A. Bonanno.
        p.   cm. — (Emotions and social behavior)
    Includes bibliographical references and index.
    ISBN 1-57230-622-X
        1. Emotions.   2. Affect (Psychology).   3. Mood (Psychology).
    I. Mayne, Tracy.   II. Bonanno, George A.   III. Series.
  BF531.E514 2001
  154.4—dc21   00-061689

*To Paul Ekman—Thank you for the warmth,
friendship, and guidance you've shown us
over the years. These pages wouldn't exist
if it weren't for you.*

*And to Jonathan Schlesinger and Paulette Roberts—
Your love and support, as with all else
in our lives, made this possible.*

About the Editors

Tracy J. Mayne, PhD, is the Director of HIV Epidemiology and Surveillance for Prevention Planning at the New York City Department of Health and an Adjunct Associate Professor in the Department of Psychology at New York University. He received his PhD from Rutgers University in 1993. His research includes the epidemiology of HIV/AIDS in New York City, with a special focus on gay men working in close collaboration with the Gay Men's Health Crisis. His interests also include the relationships between emotion and health and the history and development of the field of clinical psychology.

George A. Bonanno, PhD, is Assistant Professor of Psychology in the Clinical Psychology Program at Teachers College, Columbia University. He received his PhD from Yale University in 1991. His research and scholarly interests center on emotion and self-deception and the role they play in coping with extreme adversity. Dr. Bonanno is also an avid painter of portraits.

Contributors

Jo-Anne Bachorowski, PhD, Department of Psychology, Vanderbilt University, Nashville, Tennessee

George A. Bonnano, PhD, Department of Counseling and Clinical Psychology, Teachers College, Columbia University, New York, New York

Christine Branigan, PhD, Department of Psychology, University of Michigan, Ann Arbor, Michigan

Lisa Feldman Barrett, PhD, Department of Psychology, Boston College, Boston, Massachusetts

Barbara L. Fredrickson, PhD, Department of Psychology, University of Michigan, Ann Arbor, Michigan

Jonathan Haidt, PhD, Department of Psychology, University of Virginia, Charlottesville, Virginia

James J. Gross, PhD, Department of Psychology, Stanford University, Stanford, California

Dacher Keltner, PhD, Department of Psychology, University of California, Berkeley, California

Ann M. Kring, PhD, Department of Psychology, University of California, Berkeley, California

Tracy J. Mayne, PhD, Disease Prevention Intervention, New York City Department of Health, New York, New York

Batja Mesquita, PhD, Department of Psychology, Wake Forest University, Winston-Salem, North Carolina

Judith Tedlie Moskowitz, PhD, Center for AIDS Prevention Studies, University of California, San Francisco, California

Kevin N. Ochsner, PhD, Department of Psychology, Harvard University, Cambridge, Massachusetts

Michael J. Owren, PhD, Department of Psychology, Cornell University, Ithaca, New York

Pierre Philippot, PhD, Faculté de Psychologie, Université de Louvain, Louvain-la-Neuve, Belgium

James Ramsey, PhD, Department of Economics, New York University, New York, New York

Alexandre Schaefer, PhD, Faculté de Psychologie, Université de Louvain, Louvain-la-Neuve, Belgium

Series Editor's Note

I am delighted to introduce *Emotions: Current Issues and Future Directions* as the first multicontributor volume included in Guilford's Emotions and Social Behavior series. Although we originally conceptualized this series to feature "authored" books, Tracy Mayne and George Bonanno's collective effort is unusually well conceived and coherent, and thus warrants inclusion. Many of the contributors represent the "new age" of emotion researchers. Trained by the founders of this field of study, they are pushing it in new directions—from dynamical systems theory to neuroscience to culture.

The broad, integrative, and multidisciplinary approach reflected in the contributions to this volume herald the emergence of a new field called, variously, affect science or affective science. This field focuses its research on the emotions at multiple levels of analysis (from neurons to societies). Less dependent on traditional modes of inquiry, it is likely that, in the coming decade, affective scientists will discover and rely on new paradigms for studying feelings. Nonetheless, unlike other emerging fields of study, affective scientists are not ahistorical, but, rather, seem quite willing to build on the excellence of their teachers.

Emotions: Current Issues and Future Directions is a fascinating, stimulating, and even entertaining volume that I look forward to assigning to the undergraduates and graduate students in my Psychology of Emotion seminar.

PETER SALOVEY, PHD
Professor of Epidemiology and Public Health
Yale University

Foreword

Emotion psychology has come of age. If one needed further evidence for this claim—in addition to the tremendous increase in publications in this area over the past 30 years—this book provides it. The volume consists of chapters by a group of emotion researchers who are likely to make important contributions to this field in the next decades. In addition to reviewing the state of the art in a number of major research areas on the topic of emotion, many of which had been given somewhat short shrift in the past, the authors focus squarely on the future of emotion research—an issue that is taken up at the end of each chapter as well as, in an integrative fashion, in the concluding chapter by the editors. In this fashion, the reader obtains a clear view of the research agendas that motivate the work of the scientists contributing to this volume. This, in itself, is a major achievement, allowing for critical examination not only of current theoretical proposals and empirical data but also of the blueprints for further work. Quite apart from the intrinsic interest of such attempts at extrapolation, this may serve as an important frame of reference for the next generation of young emotion psychologists. In addition, it may help to bring about something that has often been absent from emotion research: a certain cumulativeness of theory and research findings.

For someone who has lived through the establishment of emotion psychology as a field in its own right, after decades of not always benign neglect, the present volume is refreshing in more than one sense. Most importantly, the battles of the past are finally abandoned: little attention is given to the issues that have dominated many of the debates in this field in the past, such as the relative merit of classic theories, the role of cognition in emotion, or the issue of the biological versus cultural nature of emotion. The members of this new cohort of emotion researchers take an uncomplicated, constructive approach to these issues. They turn to the phenomenon and attempt to design pragmatic approaches, both in theory and research design, that allow better understanding of the underlying processes. In fact, the insistence on the dynamic nature of emotion and the need to adopt theoretical models and research strategies that do justice to this essential characteristic of the phenomenon pervades the discussions in the book, giving rise to hopes that the days when emotion psychologists paid mostly lip service to the idea of emotion as a process are over.

It is interesting to examine the areas that constitute the foci of the current volume. One center of gravity is the interest in positive emotions, a welcome change from the predominance of concern with negative emotions in the past. The evolution, the functions, and the consequences of positive emotions are touched upon in nearly every chapter, making this book a good introduction to this new way of thinking about emotion (which may well change our general outlook on the phenomenon). Another important issue that is addressed in several chapters is the role of regulation, acknowledging the fact that in the process of emotion generation and unfolding there is virtually never a "pure emotional state"—regulation and control enters in from the very start, changing the process through multiple recursive effects at any one moment. As one might expect, this very fluidity is likely to produce major headaches for theorizing and designing experimental studies. Yet, it is essential to invest in appropriate research strategies if we are to move to more ecologically valid models of the emotion process in everyday life. Another strong point of the current volume, linked to the interest in emotions in real-life and concrete situational settings, is the emphasis on the interactional functions of emotion and their embedding in social and cultural contexts. Again, while past work has mentioned this aspect of emotional life in passing, it is only now that the issues are directly addressed. Finally, it is interesting to note the strong emphasis on health and coping as one of the major areas of application of emotion research. While this may in part reflect the specialization of some of the contributors, it also testifies to the fruitfulness of looking at health functions and health behavior from an affective point of view.

This last focus, above all others, also brings out the need for reaching beyond the confines of emotion psychology into other areas of psychology (cognition, motivation, personality, psychopathology, and development, to mention but a few of the most obvious ones) and to other disciplines (ranging from the neurosciences to cultural anthropology). Again, the current volume is refreshing in that one immediately notes that the contributors have a great facility in looking "over the fence," using models and methods from other sciences as required by the issues at hand. It is this fundamental readiness to treat emotion as a complex, multifaceted phenomenon that makes one most hopeful that the vision of a truly interdisciplinary affective science is more than a pious wish.

KLAUS R. SCHERER, PHD
University of Geneva

Preface

Emotions. Passions. Humors. From Lao-Tsu and Galen to René Descartes and William Shakespeare, emotions have been the province of physicians, philosophers, poets, and priests through the ages. It was only in the latter half of the 19th century, however, that emotions became the focus of scientific inquiry and research. G. B. Duchenne de Bologne, Charles Darwin, William James, and Walter B. Cannon used experimentation and systematic observation to define what emotions are and understand how they are structured and function. Despite these seminal contributions, affect science as a field of study did not begin to coalesce until halfway through the 20th century. Within psychology, psychoanalytic thought, then behaviorism, then cognitive theory overshadowed emotion and relegated it to a secondary status. But emotion research was not dead. In fact, a small handful of scholars in the 1960s and 1970s kept the light of emotion research alive in the midst of the cognitive revolution. These individuals sowed the seeds of the future of affect science by developing the basic tools for measuring emotion, founding a literature of emotion theory, and (perhaps most importantly) training students to carry on and advance work in this field. The individuals who shepherded the development of affect science include Silvan S. Tomkins, Magda B. Arnold, Paul Ekman, Carroll E. Izard, Klaus Scherer, and Nico H. Frijda.

These are the scientists who served, and continue to serve, as our mentors and colleagues. Many of us writing chapters for this volume have studied directly under these men and women, and even when we didn't work in their laboratories, they influenced us through their teachings and writings. Indeed, thanks to their efforts, affect science is in the midst of a renaissance. Questions of emotion now pervade many natural and social science disciplines. Neuroscience is focused on the ways in which emotion is processed in the brain. Medicine and health are delving into the ways that emotion directly affects the body (from immune function to cardiovascular disease), as well as the health consequences of emotion-related behaviors. Education has adopted the works of scientists on emotional intelligence, integrating these constructs into primary school curricula concerned with socioemotional development. Perhaps G. Terence Wilson voiced this zeitgeist best when he prophesied, "Emotion will be to the turn of the century what the cognitive revolution was to the 1960s and 70s."

In the midst of this revolution are the authors of this volume. What distinguishes this group of scientists, at this important juncture, is their background and training. This cohort represents the first emotion researchers trained primarily as affect scientists. Instead of applying theories, models, and techniques from other disciplines to understand emotion, these researchers use emotion theory to shed light on research in other disciplines, to further develop models within our own discipline, and to treat and prevent problems of individual and social concern. When this group came of age (academically speaking), there was only one professional organization for emotion researchers: the International Society for Research on Emotions (ISRE). At the time, ISRE was open only to senior scientists who had already made a significant contribution to affect science. There were several journals that focused on emotion research, but always in the context of another discipline. There was one NIH-funded postdoctoral program, created by Paul Ekman and Richard Davidson, through which many of the authors in this volume have passed. We knew of each other, but there were no ongoing mechanisms for bringing us together.

In 1994 Tracy J. Mayne, James J. Gross, and Tamara Newton took the initiative to connect young emotion researchers, and in 1995 oversaw the first meeting of the Emotion Research Group (ERG) in San Francisco. The mission of the ERG is to foster the development of young affect scientists and in so doing support the growth of our field. The group has continued to meet yearly, working toward its mission. In 1998, ISRE voted to open its doors to junior researchers, and many of us are now working within ISRE toward these same goals. One area in which we have seen clear success is the integration of courses on emotion into the curricula at our respective university departments. In part, this book grew from our need to present advanced affect theory to our students and the lack of an existing text of the appropriate level.

This book looks to bring advanced emotion theory not only to students but to a wider audience, with chapters that reflect the cutting edge of emotion research. It is intended as an advanced undergraduate/graduate-level text on emotion theory and research that will also be of interest to professionals and researchers in emotion and other disciplines. The chapter topics cover the broad subfields of emotion research and are ordered to move from basic to more applied areas. We start with the structure and function of emotion, and next address the neuroscience of emotion and emotion memory. From there we explore positive emotions, including a chapter on the evolution of positive affect. We then move from individual to social and cultural approaches to affect. We end with chapters that address applied and clinical aspects of emotion theory: emotional regulation, intelligence, and coping, and finally psychopathology and physical health.

The chapters do not endorse a single emotion perspective (e.g., social emotion, dimensional structure). Instead, they adopt a unified "affect science" approach that is able to incorporate emotion's many aspects without making one function dominant. Within each chapter, the authors first review the historic development of the field, defining basic terms and helping readers to understand the evolution of concepts, as well as revolutionary changes that have resulted in functional leaps in our understanding of emotion. In many places, it will be clear that we stand upon the shoulders of those who came before us. In other places, you will find departures from current emotion theory and innovations in the field. The authors discuss current theoretical and research issues, research methods and measurements, and ongoing debates, up to and including the cutting-edge work in their own specialty area. The chapters end by looking ahead to the important questions yet to be answered and laying out the paths likely to be taken by future researchers. Though this is an edited volume, we have attempted to bring to it a uniform voice by standardizing chapter style and language. The book can work as a "stand-alone" text for professors teaching a seminar on emotions, or it can be used in conjunction with other emotions books (e.g., Ekman & Davidson, 1994; Lewis & Haviland-Jones, 2000; Oatley & Jenkins, 1996). Our hope is that this book may help inspire others to teach affect science courses at their own universities.

We hope also that this book will foster the development of students in emotion research and thus itself become a chapter in the unfolding story of the development of affect science. We believe it is important to share with students the cultural and historic contexts of the field, which this preface and the concluding chapter begin to address. With that in mind, we would like to thank the mentors who have so generously taken us under their wings and fostered our own development. Paul Ekman, perhaps more than anyone else in the field, has touched each of our lives in very personal ways. His work continues to spur controversy and debate, never failing to inspire! Along with Paul, many of us look to Carroll E. Izard as the father of modern emotion theory. Perhaps Silvan S. Tomkins, in mentoring these two scientists, consciously planned for there to be bastions of emotion research on both coasts. Klaus Scherer, who with Paul Ekman cofounded ISRE, continues to push the envelope of emotion research. This year, he took on the coeditorship of the American Psychological Association's journal *Emotion*, the first exclusively devoted to affect science. His work will continue to pave the way for the next generation of affect scientists. Magda B. Arnold was prescient in her vision of emotion research, and her theories of cognition and emotion were decades ahead of their time. She continues to provide us with words to live by: "Emotion is to be used and to help one grow: spiritually, intellectually, in every way!" Finally, Nico Frijda is (for many of us) our favorite European uncle! His warmth as a dinner companion belies the keen intellect that makes his work both insightful and a pleasure to read. These six individuals have done more for the field of emotion research than can be touted in these pages. As we reiterate in the final chapter of this volume, our intent is not to fill their shoes but to walk a mile in them, carrying emotion research into the new millennium!

TRACY J. MAYNE
GEORGE A. BONANNO

REFERENCES

Ekman, P., & Davidson, R. J. (Eds.). (1994). *Questions about emotions*. New York: Oxford University Press.
Lewis, M., & Haviland-Jones, J. M. (2000). *Handbook of emotions* (2nd ed.). New York: Guilford Press.
Oatley, K., & Jenkins, J. M. (1996). *Understanding emotions*. Oxford: Blackwell.

Contents

EMOTIONS

1

The Structure of Emotion
A Nonlinear Dynamic Systems Approach

TRACY J. MAYNE
JAMES RAMSEY

I (TJM) recently saw a Broadway show that several reviewers had described as exceptionally moving and poignant. Half way through the second act, the leading man was killed—there were French horns soaring in a minor key, the lighting dimmed and turned blue, and the actors on stage were weeping and hugging each other. To my left, I heard the woman sniffling and immediately knew that she was feeling very sad. I didn't consciously think about it, but I knew it just the same.

Thinking back on that night, I wonder several things. How did I know what her emotion was at that time? Was I right in that assumption? If I asked, would she have told me she was feeling sad (and would I have believed her if she told me she wasn't)? How did I know that *I* was sad, and *why* was I feeling sad (especially since I was well aware that no one had really died)? How did the composer and director know how to induce this emotion in me and most of the audience? Why did I choose that musical, given that I knew it was likely to make me sad? And why is it the person in front of me *didn't* feel sad—or at least I don't think he did, since while I was crying he let out an audible sigh, looked at his watch, and shuffled restlessly in his seat?

I can easily construct answers to many of these questions. I knew the woman to my left was sad because I recognized a universal display of emotion—or at least a display that is common among people within my culture. This same cultural knowledge guided the composer and director to choose

1

sights and sounds and themes likely to invoke sadness in others; they also counted on the emotional contagion of sadness to be transmitted from the actors on stage to the audience. I knew I was sad because that's how I label that particular pattern of physiological arousal I felt (tight throat, tears, anergy). And I felt sad because of the thoughts I was thinking as I watched the performance and the memory of past losses that it evoked. I'm certain some of this occurred that night, but I'm also quite sure I wasn't consciously aware of or thinking any of these things.

Supreme Court Associate Justice Potter Stewart (1967) said this about obscenity: "I can't define [it], but I know it when I see it." For most of written history, this definition could easily have been applied to emotion. Without any specialized training, nearly everyone is capable of recognizing an emotion and having a good idea about what it means. Quantifying and measuring emotion, on the other hand, is much more difficult. The scientific study of emotion has led to progress in this area, but much of this research has focused on one or two specific components of affect, with the lion's share of research using self-report. Bernard Rimé (1997) has likened emotion research to "the Lilliputian investigators studying the elephant. We are all there with our magnifying glasses, exploring some particular body part—specialists of the eye, the tail, the neck or the nail" (p. 1). It is important to study and understand the components of emotion, but in doing so we lose track of the fact that emotion is truly more than the sum of its parts.

Emotion manifests across physiological, cognitive, behavioral, social, and cultural systems; thus it is no surprise that specialists in each domain have constructed definitions, measures, and theories of function as they relate to that specific domain. But the result of this, in the words of one prominent affect scientist, is that "we don't agree, as a discipline, on the nature of what we are studying" (Feldman Barrett, 1998, p. 6). It is crucial that we step back and view emotion in its gestalt. Add to this the fact that we all come to affect science with firsthand experience of emotion, as well as many cultural biases, and it's a wonder that there is a field of affect science at all!

Specialization and bias are one reason for some of the basic disagreements in the field of emotion research. Another is that emotion research has been reliant on linear statistics and static models. Agrarian-based statistics were not developed for phenomena as complex as emotion and do not have the capacity to adequately model and predict them. This is not to say that they are not useful and have not advanced the study of emotion, but their limits impede a more complete understanding of emotion as a complex process. Emotion includes physiological arousal and behavioral displays; it includes self-awareness and verbal report; it has innate and cultural influences—but none of these things comes close to adequately capturing what an emotion is. Real understanding comes from seeing these myriad pieces fit together and observing how they interact together over time. The premise of this chapter is that a fuller understanding and prediction of emotion requires the use of nonlinear dynamic theory, models, and equations. Our goal is to help readers understand the basic tenets of nonlinear dynamic theory and see why they are appropriate to studying and understanding complex emotional phenomena.

In this chapter, we define what nonlinear dynamic systems are and show how emotions possess the characteristics of such systems. We then discuss the shortcomings of linear models and how nonlinear dynamic models are better equipped to answer basic questions about the nature of emotion. Throughout the chapter, we have attempted to avoid some obvious pitfalls. There is a tendency for new and unfamiliar techniques to generate articles and chapters that argue by loose analogy, using the language of the new techniques without elucidating the fundamental principles underlying them. We attempt to avoid these mistakes by providing concrete examples and graphic representations throughout the text. For mathematicians and statisticians, we also provide equations. However, we discuss these equations in a way that should allow all readers to grasp the major concepts, even if the exact mathematics underlying them is not accessible. In the end, we hope that this approach will provide more insight into the structure and function of emotion than other approaches do, and pique the interests of affect scientists to learn and apply these models.

THE STRUCTURE OF EMOTION: BEYOND DISCRETE AND DIMENSIONAL

Perhaps one of the hottest current debates in the emotion field is whether there are discrete, basic, universal emotions, or whether emotions are best characterized as points within a two-dimensional space (Ekman, 1992a; Ortony & Turner, 1992; Russell & Feldman Barrett, 1999). One school of thought (Russell, 1980), using self-report data, has found that emotions can be plotted in a two-dimensional space, with one axis representing level of arousal (high and low) and the other hedonic value (positive vs. negative; see Figure 1.1). When arousal is high and positivity is high, one experiences happiness. When arousal is low and negativity is high, one experiences sadness. The circumplex model is attractive for a number of reasons. The model is orderly and logical, has a certain aesthetic appeal, and mirrors factoral models of personality allowing it to integrate well into other theories in psychology (Plutchik & Conte, 1997). This dimensional structure has been replicated in numerous studies, supporting the validity of this theory (Feldman Barrett & Russell, 1999). And there is neuropsychological evidence pointing to the existence of separate brain structures for processing

HIGH AROUSAL

tense	alert
nervous	excited
stressed	elated
upset	happy

NEGATIVE ———————————————— **POSITIVE**

sad	contented
depressed	serene
lethargic	relaxed
fatigued	calm

LOW AROUSAL

FIGURE 1.1. The emotion circumplex. From Feldman Barrett and Russell (1988). Copyright by the American Psychological Association. Adapted by permission.

positive and negative emotional valence (see K. N. Ochsner & L. Feldman Barrett, Chapter 2, this volume). The major criticism of this theory is that it may simply reflect the underlying structure of self-reported emotion, or emotion language, and not emotion itself (Izard, 1994). Recent research has suggested that dimensionality may even be a matter of individual differences: Some people may experience and report their emotions as the circumplex dictates, whereas others may experience emotions discretely (Feldman, 1995). As we discuss later, the experience and report of emotion should not be confused with emotion itself, and the circumplex model may well characterize the structure of self-reported affect.

The opposing argument is that there are discrete, basic, universal emotions (Ekman, 1992b). Each of these emotions has unique physiological arousal patterns, behavioral display patterns, motivational value, etc. The theory of discrete emotions fits well with evolutionary theory, in that unique emotional patterns developed to meet unique challenges in our early environments (for a current discussion on evolutionary theory and emotion see Ekman's introduction and commentary to Darwin, 1872/1999; also M. J. Owren & J. A. Bachorowski, Chapter 5, this volume). Those animals that had inherent and adaptive patterns for fighting a rival, fleeing a predator, coping with familial loss, etc. may have had a survival advantage. In this vein, there is ample evidence that different emotions do have unique arousal patterns that do not exist along a single continuum (Ekman, Levenson, & Friesen, 1983; Schwartz, Weinberger, & Singer, 1981). There is also evidence that different neural structures, or different areas within neural structures, may be responsible for the basic processing of different negative emotions, though clearly emotion involves multiple neurological structures (see Ochsner & Feldman Barrett, Chapter 2, this volume). But criticisms include the fact that the model does not differentiate or explain positive emotions as well as it does negative emotions. Others have argued that the distinctions between emotions are the product of social construction and are not inherent in the emotions themselves.

We will not presume to resolve this debate in these pages but, in fact, hope to supersede it. Let us start by using a very simple analogy and then begin to consider nonlinear dynamic theory in a more sophisticated way. The analogy we'll use here (and in other places) is *weather*. If I ask 10 people to describe the weather outside, several of them would look around and pronounce, "The weather's good" or "It's bad outside." Others might say, "It's partially cloudy, and kind of windy" or "It's foggy and rainy, and those clouds look like a thunderstorm is coming." Someone with greater sophistication might say, "Those are cumulus clouds over there, probably marking the edge of a cold front, and there's probably a 75% chance of rain later today."

Compare these analyses to what an expert weatherman might say: "It's currently 70° F in Central Park, the wind is out of the north–northwest at 25 miles per hour with gusts up to 35. The humidity is at 50%, and the barometer is at 98 mmHg and falling. There's a low pressure cold front moving in from Canada, and the leading edge of thunderstorms will arrive in this area bringing heavy rain at approximately 10 o'clock tonight, lasting through approximately 8:00 A.M." In this example, how one perceives and reports the weather depends on one's level of sophistication and knowledge: specialized knowledge of the parameters that define and determine weather allows one to describe it in more exact terms and predict its course. No one would confuse a layman's report of weather with actual meteorology, and when weather is important to us we inevitably turn to experts to describe and predict it.

This is not to say that laymen's reports don't have value. If you are going to the beach, knowing that the weather will be "gorgeous today" or "yucky this afternoon" may give you just the information you need. And this information may well be easily and reliably plotted on a two-dimensional scale: cloudy versus sunny, warm versus cold. It's not that self-report isn't useful; it may give us important information on how people perceive weather. But this is not to be confused with a scientific understanding of meteorology.

Weather also falls into very discrete patterns. A foggy day is quite easy to differentiate from a clear and sunny day, and it would be difficult to confuse a hurricane with light snow showers. But identifying the pattern is far easier than scientifically quantifying it. Anyone who has seen a satellite map of a hurricane can readily identify one. However, understanding the dynamics of the storm, and even more important the path that it will take, means not just identifying the pattern but also understanding its evolution over time. Discrete patterns are the starting point, but defining the patterns necessary to characterize it and to understand how the parameters unfold over time is the key to understanding weather.

We suspect that readers have already made the connection between the weather analogy and emotion. Many individuals may experience and report their emotions in dimensional ways, but this is a measure of experience and report, not actual emotion. There are clearly discrete patterns that signal discrete emotions, and though they may be easily observable to the layperson, accurately describing them takes a high level of sophistication. And to truly understand emotion, one must define its basic parameters and then understand how those parameters interact and unfold over time. It's not enough to identify the discrete emotion—one must understand how that emotion will influence an individual or a group. Let us now begin to consider some basic concepts of nonlinear and dynamic systems and then examine their application to emotion.

DEFINING NONLINEAR DYNAMIC SYSTEMS

The literature on nonlinear dynamic systems is vast and includes several subareas, such as chaos theory. Readers with greater interest are referred to introductory texts (see, e.g., Bergé, Pomeau, & Vidal, 1984; Nicolis & Prigogine, 1989) and specialized texts on the application of nonlinear dynamics to biological systems (Duke & Pritchard, 1991; Glass & Mackey, 1988).

Systems

Let us start with some basic definitions. First, what is a system? Quite simply, systems are multidimensional phenomena. Weather includes temperature, pressure, humidity, wind speed, etc. A system requires that you use multiple probes to assess their diverse parameters: a thermometer, a barometer, a wind gauge, etc. In a system, each variable provides essential information about weather. However, no one variable, no matter how reliably and validly measured, gives a complete description of the weather. At this point, there is widespread agreement that emotions are multidimensional systems (Mayne, 2000). Emotion researchers use a wide array of probes to measure emotion: neurohormonal arousal (Cannon, 1911), facial action (Ekman & Rosenberg, 1998), self-report (Feldman, 1995), behavior (Kaloupek & Levis, 1983; Kern, 1984), localized central nervous system (CNS) activity (LeDoux, 1998) and even precipitating stimulus characteristics (Scherer, 1993). There is, however, disagreement over which of these parameters are necessary and sufficient components of emotion.

An irony of complex systems is that they are often easier for naive observers to identify qualitatively than for specialists to quantify. As mentioned earlier, it is easy for nonmeteorologists to identify a hurricane from a satellite photo. It is far more difficult for meteorologists to quantify the complex atmospheric conditions that define a hurricane and to predict its path. Similarly, naive observers can readily identify emotions in themselves and others, whereas scientifically quantifying the phenomena is far more difficult.

Dynamic Systems

In the simplest terms, dynamic systems are multidimensional phenomena in which "time matters." This is deceptively simple for scientists who may be accustomed to measuring variables over time. Here the definition of "time" is somewhat different. Time in dynamic systems is not just an index or an ordering of events, like the concentration of blood alcohol each hour after a research subject has taken a drink. Events in dynamic systems are time-linked. The future evolves from the past. Current activity is influenced by reactions to past events. For example, learning is a dynamic process, a process that does more than just unfold over time: Rather, understanding calculus depends upon first learning trigonometry, which itself depends upon learning algebra. Past events determine future ones.

Emotional systems are dynamic. For example, pairing a noxious stimulus with an object can produce a conditioned fear response (Watson & Rayner, 1920). However, that fear response can itself *generate* hypervigilance, increasing sensitivity to related objects, producing more fear, and eventually leading to phobic avoidance and diagnosable phobia (Barlow, 1988). As the fear unfolds in time, what happens on previous occasions influences responses and behaviors later, which themselves influence future reactions.

Time is an essential component of dynamic systems; therefore it is critical that the sequence of events be uncorrupted in nonlinear analysis. The measure of time must be specific and consistent, regardless of whether it is measured in milliseconds, days, or decades.

Nonlinear Dynamic Systems

Defining the *nonlinear* aspects of dynamic systems is a more difficult task than the definitions in the previous two subsections. Describing something that is defined by a negative, that nonlinear dynamics is "not" linear dynamics, does not tell us very much. Let us start by providing examples of linear systems and analysis, and then point out the inherent limitations of linear analysis, as well as the potential richness encompassed by nonlinear functions.

Linear Equations

There are three basic types of linear equations that high school and college graduates are likely to be familiar with. These are point-slope, differential, and difference equations. Point-slope equations are simply linear regressions, and in their most basic form are represented by the algebraic formula $y_t = \alpha + \beta x_t$. In this equation, y_t is the outcome variable, α represents an additive constant (or intercept), β is the "slope" coefficient, and x_t is the predictor variable. If two variables are linearly related, say, education and income, we can use this formula to predict income if we know an individual's educational level and the relationship between income and education.

Simple relationships are rare in psychology, and most phenomena of interest have multiple predictors. Therefore, multiple linear regression equations have been developed to predict an outcome with multiple predictors. Though more complex, these equations use the same basic format:

$$y_t = \alpha + \beta_1 x_1 + \beta_2 x_2 + \beta_3 x_3 + \varepsilon$$

In this case the outcome variable (y_t), let's say someone's score on an anxiety scale, can be predicted from a combination of their heart rate (x_1), the degree of facial display of fear (x_2), the proximity to a feared object (x_3), plus a constant (α) and an error term (ε). The constant can be thought of as the base level of anxiety, and the error a combination of factors not measured (e.g., epinephrine in the blood, parental history of phobia) and errors in measurement.

The second type of linear equation is a differential equation, represented by the formula $dy_t = \alpha + \beta y_t$. In this case dy_t is a differential, or an "instantaneous rate of change" in the outcome variable, as a linear function of the existing level (y_t). This type of equation is closely related to the third kind of linear equation: the difference equation (and in practice the difference equation is most likely to be used). Difference equations are very similar to differential equations, in that they measure changes in an outcome variable over time. However, where differential equations measure instantaneous change, difference equations measure discrete change over a given period. It's the difference between saying that the car's speed is 60 miles per hour (differential) and saying that the car traveled 120 miles in 2 hours (difference). Difference equations are represented by the formula: $\Delta y_t = \alpha + \beta y_{t-1}$.

There are both simple and complex reasons why none of these linear equations adequately model emotion. Let us begin with point-slope and multiple regression equations. If emotion could be defined as a single variable, these sorts of equations might serve to model emotion well. However, at the moment there is no agreed-upon scale for emotion, no rating system whereby we researchers can agree: "At this moment he has anxiety level 12" and reliably differentiate between that and anxiety level 8, or anger level 2. We can agree that his blood pressure was 142/95. We can agree that he manifests high action unit 4 (a way of measuring emotion on the face). We can agree that there was a 20% increase in activity in the amygdala using a functional MRI (magnetic resonance imaging) scan or specify a level of epinephrine in the blood, or ascertain sympathetic neural arousal. But to date, no one has put together an agreed-upon metric for combining these into a single measure, which is necessary for a point-slope equation. Such metrics have been developed in other areas: H. Saffir and R. Simpson developed a 5-point scale for categorizing hurricanes (or, more specifically, the expected damage therefrom) based on the wind speed, barometric pressure, and storm surge. However, meteorologists are as concerned about the path the level-5 hurricane will take as whether it is a category-5 or category-4 storm.

Multiple regression might be helpful in designing an emotion metric. We could weight and combine multiple variables (tension of specific facial muscles, blood pressure, serum epinephrine, amygdala activation, etc.) in order to develop a regression equation that would produce a single measure of affect at a specific instant in time. But, like a hurricane, there is limited utility in describing an emotion at a single moment—it is more interesting to understand and even to predict how it will unfold over time, and how the individual components interact over time. At best, linear regressions may be able to show that one component of emotion (fearful thoughts) is related to other components (blood pressure and behavior). But when the phenomena of interest is a complex system, the logic of linear regression becomes circular: self-report predicts blood pressure, which predicts facial expression, which predicts proximity to feared object, which predicts self-report, and so on. Thus, linear equations cannot model a system, though they may be useful in modeling individual components of a system.

Another shortcoming of multiple regression is the underlying assumption that predictors not be highly correlated. High correlations between predictors, known as colinearity, cause myriad problems in regression models. The components of a dynamic system are, by definition, correlated. If we again use the example of weather: temperature and barometric pressure in part determine how much moisture the air can hold (humidity); humidity also affects heat absorption and retention (temperature), and so on. In the same way, the components of emotion tend to be correlated, if not perfectly (Lang, 1979; Lang, Levin, Miller, & Kozak, 1983), limiting the ability to apply linear regression models in studying relationships between components.

The advantage of difference equations over point-slope equations is that the former can model change in a variable over time. Differential equations are similar, but in practical applications only discrete differences can be measured. As such, difference and differential equations can be used to map much more complex relationships between variables, and increasingly so by using the first, second, third, . . . derivatives of the equations. Let us cite three simple examples utilized in most first-year physics classes (Equations D, E, and F in Figure 1.2). The symbols y' and y'' represent the first and second differentials of the variable y that is evolving through time t.

Equation D represents a variable that shows steady exponential growth and could represent the increase in a bacterial colony multiplying without population pressure. Equation E represents a simple oscillation, like the reaction of pulling and releasing a spring *without* friction. The term y'' represents "acceleration," and the equation indicates that a system displaced by the amount y accelerates in the opposite direction (i.e., a reaction equation). Equation F is also a reaction equation, representing the reaction of a spring *with* friction. Thus, it includes a "dampening" term, $0.5y'$, which decreases the strength of the system's reaction to displacement. In Figure 1.2, the solution path to Equation D is given by the solid line; the solution path to Equation E, the dotted line; and the solution path to Equation F, by the dashed line.

Though each of these equations models more complex relationships than a linear slope, they are still by and large simple models predicting the path of a single variable. Even if we could compute a composite emotion score that could be modeled using these equations, no emotion would have the unlimited exponential growth modeled by Equation D. Emotion is also not an undampened reaction shown in Equation E: there are clearly internal and external forces that act to regulate and limit emotional responding (see, e.g., Gross, 1998). Of the three equations, F may come closest to modeling the wavelike form of emotion episodes, but emotion does not have the fixed period, amplitude, or frequency of a regular oscillation. If it did, predicting emotional responses would be a relatively easy task. Thus, neither simple difference equations nor differential equations are likely to adequately model the complexity of emotion.

Another advantage of difference and differential equations is their

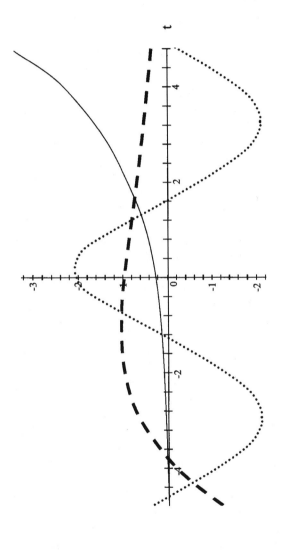

—— Equation D: $y' - .05y = 0$: *solution* $y(t) = C\exp(0.5t)$; $C = .025$

••••••• Equation E: $y'' + y = 0$: *solution* $C_1\sin(t) + C_2\cos(t)$; $C_1 = 0.5$, $C_2 = 2$

— — Equation F: $y'' + 0.5\,y + y = 0$: *solution* $\exp(-0.25t) * (C_1\cos(0.968 * 0.25t) + C_2\cos(0.968 * 0.25t))$; $C_1 = 1.0$, $C_2 = 2$

FIGURE 1.2. Illustrations of the solutions to three differential equations.

11

ability to model "steady states," which are essentially states of homeostasis. For both differential equations and difference equations, if all the roots imply convergence as time t approaches infinity, then the point to which the system converges is a steady state. Let us explain that in simpler terms: "Convergent roots" simply indicate that the system is dissipative, or that energy is lost over time. A spinning top is a system with convergent roots, and when it stops it is in a steady state. The top will not spin again unless energy is added to the system.

As noted at length by Glass and Mackey (1988), the behavior of living organisms is dominated by such "cycles" of varying periods and varying degrees of regularity. In a very real sense, human and animal behavior is characterized by oscillations of many types, where energy or a stimulus increases activation of a system, which then returns to a steady "resting" state until another stimulus is applied. As we discuss below, on one level emotions can be seen in this way: A stimulus produces an emotional response, and a number of systems (physiological, cognitive, behavioral, social) become activated; eventually the emotion dissipates, and these systems return to baseline levels.

Though difference and differential equations can model steady states, they do so in a very limited way. A steady state means that the system is at least temporarily stable, and stability indicates that small perturbations of the system will not change the solutions to it in any significant manner. Move the top from your desk to the kitchen table and it is still in a steady state. "Local stability" indicates that small perturbations do not alter the overall stability of the system. "Global stability" means that stability is robust even in the face of very large perturbations. And herein lies a shortcoming of linear equations in modeling steady states: In linear systems, local stability implies global stability. In other words, if small perturbations do not affect the system, large ones do not either. While these properties of linear systems are of great analytical convenience, they seriously limit the types of behavior and systems that could be usefully analyzed in linear terms.

In the real world, any stimulus, if maintained at a high enough intensity, will inhibit a system from returning to a steady state in the subsequent absence of the stimulus. Schacter and Singer (1962) and Marshall and Zimbardo (1979) showed that injecting subjects with epinephrine can induce a temporary emotional steady state. However, if one injects a subject with enough epinephrine, it will cause cardiac arrest, after which no amount of epinephrine will produce any emotion ever again. In most real-world systems, local stability *does not* imply global stability. Though there may be stable patterns to individual emotions, and even patterns between different emotions over time, they do not have the global stability of linear models.

In summary, emotions are multidimensional phenomena that evolve over time and in a way that cannot be modeled linearly. This, however, does not necessarily argue for the application of nonlinear dynamic theories and models. Let us therefore examine some of the characteristics of emotions that might lend themselves to such analysis.

THE APPLICATION OF NONLINEAR DYNAMICS TO THE STUDY OF EMOTION

Nonlinear dynamic systems analysis has the ability to describe and model complex phenomena, and there are a vast number of questions that might be answered by applying such equations to emotion research. We have selected a series of fundamental areas and questions that we believe most readily lend themselves to nonlinear dynamic analyses and the answers to which are essential for the evolution of the field. We have organized these areas/questions in order of mathematical and theoretical complexity. We begin by discussing the concepts of noise and feedback, with special reference to consciousness and the self-report of emotion. We next discuss the coupling of emotional subsystems and the self-organization of emotion. We then consider the importance of initial conditions for the development of nonlinear dynamic systems, and their utility in elucidating the relationship between emotion and mood. Finally, we discuss the organization of different emotional systems and their interactions with each other, and we conclude with a discussion of the possible application of nonlinear dynamic theory to the understanding of pathological emotions.

Noise and Feedback

Let us begin with a relatively easy application of nonlinear dynamics by addressing an area already familiar to psychologists. Noise, or error, is a part of all systems. The terms "noise" and "error," however, refer confusingly to a broad spectrum of notions. Noise can be induced by the measurement process (as in Heidegger's theorem). Noise can also be produced by the system itself, such as the resonating noise produced by speakers coupled with microphones that quickly produce a very high pitched tone.

There is a critical difference between nonlinear and linear systems as to how noise can be handled and its implications for analysis. In linear systems, noise (ε) can almost always be treated as an additive component, or an "error term," as in the standard linear regression equation

$$y_t = \alpha + \beta_1 x_1 + \beta_2 x_2 + \varepsilon$$

The noise is the unexplained and measurement error. In nonlinear systems, the situation is quite different. As an example, let us use the differential equation $dy_t = \beta dt + \sigma(y_t)\zeta_t$. (Readers unfamiliar with the actual mathematics can still easily grasp the basic concepts underlying the terms in the equations.) The outcome (dy_t) depends on the time interval of observation of the flow (βdt) and on the error term (ζ_t). But the error itself is dependent on the state of the system $(\sigma(y_t))$, which measures the degree to which the system responds to the noise. In other words, the outcome $(dy_t,$ on the left side of the equation) is in part self-determined (appearing as dt and y_t on the right side of the equation)

In this case, we have "resonating" noise, which is noise that interacts with the dynamics of the system itself. Thus, both the dynamics and the distribution of the noise change with the interaction. In other words, the error becomes part of the system, interacts with the system, and that interaction produces change in both the system and the error term. The usual linear models cannot analyze such systems, even approximately. There are many everyday examples of resonating noise, with important real-world implications. "Noise traders" on Wall Street trade stocks in reaction to random variations in prices, acting as if they represented changes in information about the value of the stock. The noise is not a simple static error term—it was quite likely such noise trading that produced the U.S. stock market crash of 1987!

A concept related to resonating noise is "feedback." Feedback is critical for the operation of biological mechanisms and allows organisms to adapt to signals generated by their own actions. Glucose regulation is a ready example of a feedback system: when an animal's blood glucose falls, its brain is signaled to increase the sensation of hunger. Upon eating, the animal's blood glucose increases, the brain is signaled to diminish feelings of hunger, and feeding stops. Feedback itself introduces elements of nonlinearity into systems. In other words, the reaction of the system depends on the current state of the system as measured by the feedback mechanism. The modeling of the reaction can no longer be made independent of the state of the system. Some feedback mechanisms lead to stability of the system, some lead to gross instability. The outcome depends on the type and timing of the feedback mechanism.

An excellent example of noise and feedback in emotional systems is the prevalence of panic disorder in people with mitral valve prolapse (Kantor, Zitrin, & Zeldis, 1980). Mitral valve prolapse is a condition that can cause the heart to beat hard and fast for no apparent reason. Though the sudden, rapid pounding heart is literally an error (noise), the person perceives this sudden physiological change (feedback). This unexpected arousal mimics the arousal associated with fear. In addition, the unexplained and uncontrollable arousal signal can generate fearful cognitions. The synchrony of these fear components can then recruit other components, such as fearful facial affect and actual fear-associated physiological arousal, which then evolves into frank panic. Though the original physiological signal may be noise, that noise is perceived (feedback) and the system *reacts* to that noise and it becomes a part of the system. A fear system is generated.

In this example, it is the conscious perception of arousal and emotion that defines feedback. This has obvious implications for the measurement of emotion. The majority of research studies use self-report as a direct measure of emotion, a practice that has come under recent scrutiny and question (Ekman, 1997; Feldman Barrett, 1998; Scherer, 1998). In nonlinear dynamic systems, self-perceived/reported emotion is not emotion per se but a form of feedback. This does not imply that self-perception is unimportant. On the contrary, it can be concretely measured and it influences and is influenced by the emotional system. But self-perception is a predictor of emotion, not an outcome, and belongs on the right side of the equation. Nonlinear dynamics provide us the opportunity to begin to understand the role of consciousness and feeling in the emotion system not as a direct measure of emotion but as feedback that interacts with the system as it evolves. Nonlinear dynamic analysis is capable of providing us a more sophisticated understanding of the role of consciousness and perception play in the process of emotion.

Coupling and Self-Organization

The application of nonlinear dynamic theory to emotions requires a fundamental reconceptualization of emotion. Many affect scientists have defined emotion in essentially stimulus–response terms. For example, Fridja (1987, p. 477) has defined emotion as an "ever ready monitoring of event relevance and concomitant adjustment readiness." Levenson (1994, p. 123) has defined emotions as "short-lived psychological–physiological phenomena that represent efficient modes of adaptation to changing environmental demands." Scherer (1994, p. 128) has defined emotion as a "relevance detection and response preparation system." In each definition, emotion entails surveillance of and response to the environment. Nonlinear dynamics can be used to inform scientists about the organization of emotion as a system, and not merely as a response system with physiological and psychological components. Let us first consider the coupling of the components of the emotion system, and then the organization of the emotion system itself.

To begin, let us examine the seminal example of coupling between components. In the 17th century, Christian Huygens made a discovery regarding the behavior of two pendulum clocks that were both attached to a board. Initially, both clocks had different but close frequencies in their operation. Huygens noticed that after a short period of time, the two clocks had the same frequency and were in phase with each other. This is an example of "phase locking," a phenomenon in which separate but proximal systems become synchronized. Phase locking is common in biological systems. For example, Strogatz and Stewart (1993) discuss the case of fireflies that flash in synchronization during their nocturnal mating display. Lest we think that this is limited to more primitive life-forms, Grammer, Fink, Kruck, and Magnusson (1998) have described how repetitive behavioral patterns form and synchronize between pairs of humans when they are attracted.

Certainly, many of the components of emotion may be definable through relatively simple functions exhibiting oscillations, like those shown by Equations E and F. These are shown graphically in Figure 1.3, a multichannel measure of fear following exposure to a large snake. Figure 1.3A is a sample of blood pressure following exposure. Figure 1.3C is the coalescence of facial affect, measured as number of fear action units multiplied by the intensity of those units. Figure 1.3B represents self-reported fear. In isolation, each measure shows an oscillation, followed by return to a steady state (though the timescale for each aspect of emotion differs). But these reactions do *not* occur in isolation. There is "coupling" between measures—they occur together and influence each other. In fact, these aspects of emotion may be thought of as linked in such a way that, given adequate intensity, one subsystem can begin to *recruit* the others. As Marshall and Zimbardo (1979) demonstrated, physiological activation can lead to thoughts and attributions of fear. Behavioral (specifically facial) displays of emotion can induce both emotion-specific physiological arousal and self-report (Ekman et al., 1983; Levenson, Ekman, & Friesen, 1990). Emotional displays in one person can stimulate congruent displays and physiological arousal in others (Hatfield, Cacioppo, & Rapson, 1994). Cognitive theory is based upon the assumption that thoughts can induce emotion-associated behavior and arousal (Barlow, 1988; Beck, Rush, Shaw, & Emery, 1979). And more recently it has been shown that emotion even influences individuals to choose/precipitate emotion-congruent environments/events (Bolger & Schilling, 1991; Bolger & Zuckerman, 1995). These systems are coupled, and conscious awareness may well function specifically to enhance coupling between these systems.

In a very real way, emotion *is* the synchronization of physiological, cognitive, behavioral, and social systems. Conceptually, it may be useful to think of emotion episodes in the same way one thinks of a hurricane. Let's go back to the weather metaphor. If the initial conditions are right, a low-pressure system off the African coast begins to organize into a tropical storm. Ongoing conditions, as well as the storm's own dynamics, either augment or dissipate the system's energy, with greater energy leading to a higher degree of systemic organization. The storm system then follows a globally predictable (though sometimes locally unpredictable) path. Even-

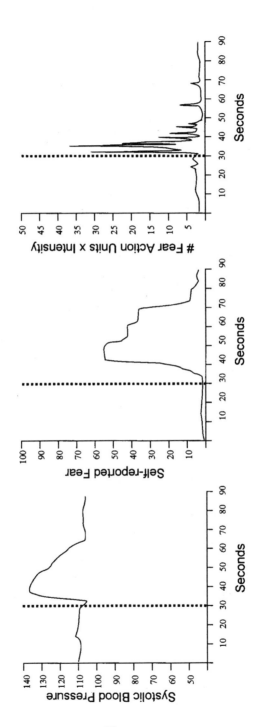

FIGURE 1.3. Simultaneous measures of blood pressure, self-reported fear, and fear facial affect in response to a fear-eliciting stimulus.

tually the system will decay and cease to exist as a unified entity (the roots converge to a steady state of low energy).

In fairness, some of the previously mentioned affect scientists have moved beyond response-based models of emotion to a more nonlinear dynamic view. Levenson (1994) has gone so far as to propose that "the essential function of emotion is organization" (p. 123), with organization entailing the coupling of the biological and psychological systems. Scherer has been at the forefront of proposing that nonlinear dynamic analysis be used to model emotion. In the arena of coupling, Scherer (1998) has suggested conceptualizing emotional states as "attractor spaces in the ongoing coupling and uncoupling of the oscillating activities of different organismic subsystems" (p. 4). This concept of emotions as organizing systems has been most closely embraced by the affective neurosciences (see, e.g., Damasio, 1994).

Thus, emotions may be seen, literally, as the coupling of various organismic subsystems. In defining emotions this way, two important questions are raised: What are the necessary and sufficient subsystems that can be used to define emotions? And how do these systems become organized, and what does the resulting "organization" look like? Let us turn our attention to the latter concept first.

Nicolis and Prigogine (1989) discuss in detail the concept of "self-organization," an important but still imperfectly understood concept. The basic idea arose out of thermodynamics, where physicists observed that complex large systems often evolve a striking degree of organization. At the time, these scientists attempted to link this "ordered structure" of the macro state (defined by thermodynamic equilibrium) to the microdynamics of individual molecular paths. In the end, it became apparent that the equilibrium and organization of the macro state could not be predicted by the individual dynamics of the micro system. In other words, the macro state, or the state of the whole system, has structure or organization that cannot be directly explained by our understanding of the behavior of the individual molecules.

Most real systems exhibit this form of self-organization to varying degrees. A good example comes from economics. Consider an economy of only a few thousand individuals. Each of them has his/her own initial conditions and special circumstances. Each individual will, over the course of a year, make millions of decisions (from buying cheese to selling stocks) based on a relative paucity of information about everyone else's decisions. And yet the macro system is far more structured than this microanalysis would indicate is possible. What this suggests for emotion is that there may be extremely stable (though complex) patterns of emotional responding that *cannot be predicted from knowledge of the individual dynamics of neurology, physiology, cognition, behavior, social interaction, and so on*!

This point bears elucidation. Emotion may have a macro level of organization that cannot be explained simply by knowing about its individual components (sympathetic arousal, amygdala activity, facial affect, etc.).

There may be stable community, national, and even global patterns of affect that cannot be predicted from the affect of individuals. Cases of mass hysteria suggest such a pattern, where a structured group emotional response occurs that cannot be predicted from the emotional history of the constituents. The emotional response takes on a "life of its own." An understanding of nonlinear dynamics is a first step toward discovering the potential role of self-organization in both individual- and community-level affective phenomena. In other words, even combining our knowledge of the components of emotion may not be sufficient—there may be ways of examining emotional systems where the whole is not only greater than the sum of its parts but also qualitatively distinct!

Initial Conditions: The Importance of Mood

Though emotional systems may be self-organizing, and the resulting organization may not be understandable simply in terms of the dynamics of its components, there is also ample evidence that specific stimuli can precipitate an emotion episode. For many individuals, being cut off on a freeway when you are late for work produces anger. However, that precipitating event can have radically different effects on the anger system depending upon the state of that system when the event occurs. This mathematically important phenomenon is called "sensitivity to initial conditions."

In linear systems, the degree of sensitivity to the initial conditions for a differential or difference equation is constant. In other words, regardless of the initial variables input into the equation, the same waveform will be produced in the outcome variable. But in non-linear dynamic systems, the degree of sensitivity may vary depending on the state of the system. In other words, how the system forms and what it does may vary widely if the initial conditions differ slightly. An example of this is initial birth weight in human beings. In full-term babies within a normal range of birth weights, the difference of 1 or 2 ounces has little long-term effect on the child's growth and development. But if the baby's birth weight is low, the difference of a few ounces can have profound and long-term repercussions. The system is said to be highly sensitive to the initial conditions, and in some cases the sensitivity may be so severe that the system essentially "explodes," at least locally. An important initial condition for an emotional episode is preexisting mood.

Several theorists hypothesize that the main function of moods is to "alter the threshold for excitation of particular emotions" (Ekman, 1994; Panksepp, 1994). This indicates that the dynamics of emotions are dependent on the initial state of the system (i.e., the underlying mood). Such dependencies are clear indicators of the need for nonlinear dynamic analysis. Many studies fail to differentiate between mood and emotion, and mood is a less well-understood phenomenon, though moods appear to show an oscillating structure of longer duration than emotion (Ekman, 1994).

If moods alter the threshold for emotion, then the effect of an emotional stimulus will depend upon where it occurs in the mood cycle. An example of this is shown in Figure 1.4. In Figure 1.4A, the thick line represents an angry mood over time, and the stimulus (being accidentally shoved when entering a subway car) by the vertical dashed line. When the stimulus occurs during a low angry mood, there is no sustained or synchronized activation of the emotional subsystems. However, the same stimulus applied during a high angry mood produces sustained synchronized activation (emotion, shown by the thin line). Figure 1.4B shows a stimulus of greater intensity, perhaps being deliberately pushed aside when trying to enter the subway train and missing the train because the doors have closed. In this case, the amplitude and duration of both emotion and mood are influenced by where in the angry mood cycle the stimulus occurs. Once again, the elements in a dynamic system are coupled, in this case mood (an initial condition) and emotion, such that the mood can foster the emotion, which in turn can increase the duration of the angry mood.

We have discussed error terms and feedback within nonlinear equations, phase locking between components, and the potential global stability of the system. We have also touched upon the importance of initial conditions in determining the formation of an emotion system. But if we define emotion literally as the coupling or organization of myriad subsystems, an important unanswered question remains: What are the dimensions of this system? In other words, how many components are necessary to model an emotion system, and what are those components?

Emotional Dimensions

The route to answering the above question is mathematically complex, and there is no way to address this issue without introducing advanced mathematical concepts and equations. Readers less interested in the technical aspects of nonlinear dynamics may wish to skip to the concluding paragraph, though we encourage you to at least skim the major concepts underlying the mathematical models.

A major qualitative change in the analysis of nonlinear systems relative to linear systems is the capacity to generate stable limit cycles. An example of an equation that gives rise to such limit cycles is Van der Pol's equation:

$$\ddot{y}_t - \gamma \left(k - y_t^2 \right) \dot{y}_t + y_t = 0$$

In this equation, $\ddot{y}_t$ and $\dot{y}_t$ represent the second and first differentials, respectively, and y_t is the state of the system. This equation indicates a relationship between the rate of acceleration $(\ddot{y}_t)$, the rate of change in state

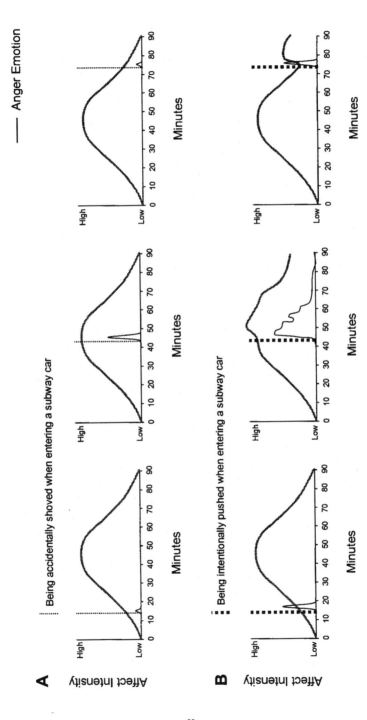

FIGURE 1.4. Angry mood and emotion over time and in response to a weak and strong stimulus.

21

$(\ddot{y}_t)$, and the state of the system (y_t). In comparing this equation to Equation F, the sole difference in formulation that makes all the difference in behavior is that in Van der Pol's equation the dampening term $(\dot{y}_t)$ is now a nonlinear function of y_t. When the value of y_t is smaller than k, the oscillation is explosive and the values of y_t increase. But when the value of y_t is greater than k, the oscillation is contractive and the value of y_t diminishes. The result is to produce a stable limit cycle wherein the velocity and the acceleration oscillate as a pair and endlessly repeat their cycle of values. The limit cycle is stable, for if the path is perturbed off the limit cycle path, it will soon return to that limit path. Oscillations in sleep and wakefulness illustrate this kind of a limit cycle: Isolated perturbations of the limit cycle, say, a single late night, enable the cycle to return to its steady-state periodic oscillation. The move to a different time zone results only in a change in the phase of the limit cycle to accommodate the new time zone.

An illustration of a solution to the Van der Pol equation is shown in Figure 1.5A,B. For the particular example plotted, we have chosen the values $\gamma = 1$, $k = 1$, and initial conditions of $y_0 = 0$, $y'_0 = -0.1$. That is, the system starts at a state of zero but is declining, as is indicated by the value of y'_0. From Figure 1.5A,B it is easy to see that the dynamic path expands out toward the limit cycle. We could also have shown the time path converging to the limit cycle from a positive origin.

The existence of limit cycles led to the idea of plotting phase space in order to investigate the dimensions and dynamics of a system. In other words, the same "lasso" pattern that this equation produces in Figure 1.5B can exist in many places on these two-dimensional axes without the pattern itself being corrupted. This is not simply a mathematical ascetic: Hurricanes form a well-defined system (not unlike the one shown in Figure 1.5B), but that system then travels through a two-dimensional phase space. The path of that system is separate from the system itself and can make the difference between light showers and a devastating storm!

Let us demonstrate this concept in concrete mathematical terms. For example, let us reexpress Van der Pol's equation as

$$\text{G.1: } \dot{z}_t = \frac{\partial z_t}{\partial t} = f(y, z)$$

$$\text{G.2: } \dot{y}_t = \frac{\partial y_t}{\partial t} = g(y, z)$$

where $z_t = \dot{y}_t$. What we have done is merely to reexpress a single second-order equation as a pair of first-order equations. This process simplifies our

A

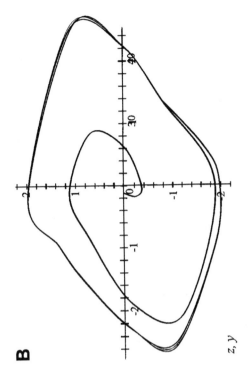

$y'' - (1 - y^2) * y' + y = 0$

$y'(0) = -0.1$

Functions defined: $y(0) = 0$

B

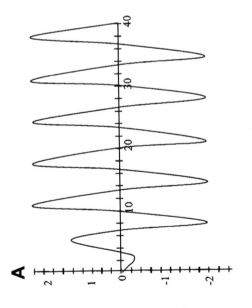

z, y

$z' = (1 - y^2) z - y$

$z' = y'$

Functions defined: $y(0) = 0, z(0) = -0.1$

FIGURE 1.5. Two solutions to the Van der Pol equation: (A) a time series plot; (B) a phase space diagram.

23

calculations: $\dot{y}_t$ is as before; $\dot{z}_t$ represents $\ddot{y}_t$ in the original equation. By considering the ratio of these two equations, we can eliminate the parameter "time." We obtain

$$\text{G.3:} \quad \frac{\dfrac{\partial z_t}{\partial t}}{\dfrac{\partial y_t}{\partial t}} = \frac{\partial z_t}{\partial y_t} = \frac{f(y,z)}{g(y,z)} = h(y,z)$$

This equation defines the phase space. Phase space is the space of the variation of the coordinates of the system and can be used to analyze the long-term dynamics of a nonlinear system. The phase space for the Van der Pol equation is shown in Figure 1.5B.

We can generalize this idea. Imagine that we are observing the behavior of a dynamic system over a long time period and that the system is in some form of enduring steady state. For example, Lorenz (1963) postulated a model of the dynamics of weather as generated by surface heating and cooling. He simplified his system down to three essential variables, that is, a three-dimensional system. If we were able to examine a graph of the path of the system in a high enough dimension when in its steady state, we would observe that it would eventually trace out a path that would be endlessly repeated, if not exactly, at least approximately. This is the phase portrait of the system. This is not simply a theoretical construct: Atlantic hurricanes always originate from westward tropical depressions off the coast of Africa, and the path they take is actually narrowly defined (from west to north–northeast).

A first key question in nonlinear dynamics is "What is the dimension of this subspace?"—or, alternatively stated, "How many variables are needed to model the system?" We are looking for the smallest dimension into which the path of the dynamics can be placed without giving the impression that the dynamic paths cross. The importance of "noncrossing" is simply this: If two paths crossed, then the point of crossing could be regarded as an initial condition and we would observe two *different* paths emanating from the same initial condition. This result violates the uniqueness of the solutions to the differential equations. We therefore conclude that in the correct number of dimensions the solution paths of dynamic systems do not cross.

Suppose for the sake of argument that the dimension is three. We need three axes to represent the phase portrait without observing intersections of the time path. That indicates that we need three variables to describe the system: x_t, y_t, z_t. As an example, let's consider Lorenz's equation modeling the weather. The system of differential equations is:

H1: $x'_t = \sigma(y_t - x_t)$

H2: $y'_t = rx_t - y_t - x_t z_t$

H3: $z'_t = x_t y_t - b z_t$

where x_t measures the rate of convective overturning, y_t measures the horizontal temperature variation, and z_t measures the vertical temperature variation. We recognize that we can plot out the trimplet (x_t, y_t, z_t), by solving the differential equation system given in Equation G.3 as a function of time. We could also rewrite the path in terms of the parametric equations in time, namely, the triplet $\{x\{t\}, y\{t\}, z\{t\}\}$, but where each of the three variables is a parametric function of time. Taken's innovation was to realize that the shape of the path in the phase portrait could be reproduced by plotting $\{x\{t\}, x\{t - \tau\}, x\{t - 2\tau\}\}$ for some suitable choice of delay τ. In short, by observing only a time sequence on one of the variables, say, $\{x\{t\}\}$, we could reproduce the shape in the phase portrait that we would obtain by plotting the triplet, $\{x\{t\}, y\{t\}, z\{t\}\}$. This result is what underpins the reconstruction of phase space from observations on a single probe.

Ironically, from investigating the phase space, we have gained information about the long-term dynamics by eliminating the parameter "time." In our simple example using the Van der Pol equation, the dimension is one and it is embedded in a two-dimensional space. In effect, we observe a single loop within the plane as a description of the path of the pair (y_t, z_t), or equivalently of the pair $(\dot{y}_t, \dot{z}_t)$. In the Lorenz system the dimension is three. Dimension is important in empirical analysis because we often do not know a priori what the dimensions of a dynamic system are and our first task is to discover this very important fact. We can consider examining even higher-dimensional spaces using ever more delays in the reconstruction of phase space.

The importance of this point cannot be overstated. In the introductory remarks to this chapter, we mentioned that affect scientists do not agree on what are the necessary and sufficient components of emotion. By using this technique, which relies on one probe measured over time, *it is possible to determine the number of essential components in an emotion system!* Once the number is known, it would then be possible to add and subtract components from a model to determine which are the essential dimensions. We can postulate an example of this procedure in terms of the interaction between physiological arousal (x_t), cognition (y_t), and facial affect (z_t). In short, we have here at least a three-dimension system. For a probe, we might consider systolic blood pressure and measure change over time. If our hypothesis about the relationship between physiology, cognition, and facial affect is approximately correct, and if systolic blood pressure is an appropriate probe in the circumstances, then a plot of the time path of a "delay reconstruction" will yield information on the properties of the phase space generated by observing the triplet (x_t, y_t, z_t) itself. That is a plot of $\{\xi\{t\}, \xi\{t - \tau\}, \xi\{t - 2\tau\}\}$, where $\xi\{t\}$ represents measures on the probe over time during emotive episodes. Alternatively, we might investigate a four-dimensional system that is represented by $\{\xi\{t, \xi\{t - \tau\}, \xi\{t - 2\tau\}, \xi\{t - 3\tau\}\}$, where $\xi\{t\}$ is our systolic pressure probe. In other words, by using nonlinear dynamic equations, we should be able to determine first the number of necessary and sufficient components of emotion, and subsequently what those dimensions are. However, it should be noted that it is only relatively low-dimensional systems that we can handle effectively in this way. These techniques will not be applicable if, in the end, emotion is a 12-dimensional system.

Organization between Emotions

"Human systems do not exist in isolation. Rather, they have multiple interactions among themselves as well as with the external and internal environment" (Glass & Mackey, 1988, p. 10).

Up to this point, we have been discussing single emotions and emotion episodes. But emotions are not "islands unto themselves." The are sensitive to and interact with other emotions, as well as biological, environmental, and social systems. Farley and Clark (1961), in discussing neural networks, indicate that at a given time the state of each cell in the network is a function of the states of neighboring cells at preceding times. So, too, individual emotions exist as part of an emotion network, and they are likely influenced by the emotions that precede them, and influence those that follow.

Nonlinear dynamic theory provides statistical approaches to analyzing relationships between different states that can be readily applied to emotional states. Let's begin by considering patterns of emotions, and the transitions from one emotion to another over a period of time. We will continue our conceit of imagining there is a single index for each discrete emotion, so that we can definitely say whether person A is currently in a specific emotional state or not. Let's look at five basic emotional states: F(ear), A(nger), Dg(isgust), E(lation), and D(istress). Others could be easily added to the list, but this set of five will provide a rich enough set of alternatives. In this schema, an individual, over time, represents a dynamic system subject to a sequence of external stimuli that we label as "random shocks." These are events that impact the system, though in truth such events are hardly random in human beings, who actively self-select their environment to favor certain emotional responses and to disfavor others (see the works of Diener, Larsen, & Emmons, 1984; Emmons & Diener, 1986a,

1986b; Emmons, Diener, & Larsen, 1986). In our example, there will be a sequence of episodes of discrete emotional states (ignoring for now the varying intensity of these states). We will measure the duration of time in each emotional state and mark the transitions from one emotion state to another.

The statistical approach we will use to examine this multiemotion system is known as a Markov process. A Markov process assumes that the probability of transiting from any one state to another depends only the current state of the system. In other words, only proximal emotional states, not those that occurred long before, influence whether one transitions from one emotion to another. To begin, the situation can be viewed in terms of a probability transition matrix as illustrated in Table 1.1.

The entries in each cell $\{a_{ij}\}$ indicate the probability of transiting from state $\{i\}$ to state $\{j\}$ in a specific period of time—let's say 15 minutes. The sum of any row is 1. We label this matrix of probabilities as $\mathbf{A}$; here $\mathbf{A}$ gives the transition probability of transiting from one emotion state $\{i\}$ to another emotion state $\{j\}$ in 15 minutes, while $\{a_{ii}\}$ represents the probability of staying in the same emotion state $\{i\}$. Next we construct a matrix to represent a second 15-minute interval. The entries in the matrix $\mathbf{A}^2 = A'A$ represent the transition probabilities of moving from state $\{i\}$ to state $\{j\}$, or staying in a state $\{a_{ii}\}$, in two 15-minute periods. We could construct a series of these matrices: $\mathbf{A}^3, \mathbf{A}^4, \mathbf{A}^5, \ldots \mathbf{A}^n$. Finally, let the vector p_0 represent the initial probabilities of being in each state: p_0 could have a 1 in one element and 0's elsewhere.

A first question is whether the vector $\mathbf{A}^n p_0$ converges to a vector π, which represents a steady state for the relative occurrence of each emotional state after a long period of transitions from an arbitrary initial probability distribution p_0. In concrete terms, do individuals tend to return to a specific emotion, an emotional steady state? After going from elation to fear to anger to fear to disgust to fear, does an individual tend to return to elation, or to a state of vacillation between fear and distress? It may be the case that convergence does not occur for all p_0 but only for a subset of all

TABLE 1.1. Transition Probabilities across Five Emotions

	Fear	Anger	Disgust	Elation	Distress
Fear	a_{11}	a_{12}	a_{13}	a_{14}	a_{15}
Anger	a_{21}	a_{22}	a_{23}	a_{24}	a_{25}
Disgust	a_{31}	a_{32}	a_{33}	a_{34}	a_{35}
Elation	a_{41}	a_{42}	a_{43}	a_{44}	a_{45}
Distress	a_{51}	a_{52}	a_{53}	a_{54}	a_{55}

possible p_0. The existence of such a state is of critical importance for emotion researchers, since it suggests that emotional states may reflect a stable personality characteristic. Consistently returning to a state of disgust is likely to have broad implications for cognition, behavior, social interaction, etc.

The entries in the matrix **A** are, in principle, easily estimated if one can reliably and validly define each distinct emotional state. Given the matrix **A**, it is possible to determine if there are—

- States that can never be reached: Someone who never feels angry.
- Absorbing states, that is, once reached the probability of leaving the state is zero: A possible characteristic of depressive episodes.
- The average duration for each state.
- The probabilities of first return to each state: Once you've stopped being afraid, how soon will you likely feel that way again?
- An equilibrium, or stationary probability distribution of states, that is π and its values: Do we tend to cycle through emotions in a predictable order over a predictable period of time?

It is possible that some individuals exist who never experience a particular state, so that the probability of reaching that state is indeed zero. This is likely to have profound implications for psychosocial functioning. Few states, except death, are absorbing, but some states may tend to be of longer duration. It is possible that, across individuals, distress may well have a longer duration than fear or anger. The average duration of a state is very important, and so is the existence of a stationary distribution of states. Once we can measure the average duration of an emotional state, we can begin to look for individual differences to discover what factors determine duration. Furthermore, the existence of a stationary distribution indicates that there exists an "equilibrium" situation: People spend time in every state with positive probability, but people differ in their distribution of probabilities across states. In other words, people develop affective traits, or have preferential affective states they are more likely to return to, that is, affective personality traits.

As mentioned earlier, frequency locking describes the tendency for oscillations to become locked together, and it may explain differential transition probabilities. In emotion terms, there may be characteristics that allow for the flow from one emotion to another. For example, the sympathetic arousal characteristic of anxiety may facilitate the flow to anger, which shares some underlying neurohormonal substrates. Or the stimulus characteristics for anxiety (a stimulus that cannot be overcome by effort) may facilitate the flow to distress (a stimulus that is overwhelming). In fact, dimensional views of emotion may be the result of frequency locking between emotions on common characteristics (positive or negative valence; high or low arousal). Thus, there may be specific shared characteristics of emotion that define the probable transition from one to another.

Let us examine how this construct might be expressed in terms of mood and emotion. In Figure 1.6, we see three moods and emotions as they unfold over a day. In the morning, the clock radio blares loud music and awakens you, after only 7 hours of slumber. Thus starts an irritable mood that acts as a sensitizing initial condition. Your drive into work provides several "random shocks" (being cut off, or a slow driver in the passing lane) that, given an already irritable mood, result in anger episodes. Upon your arrival at work, this angry mood precipitates a fight with the manager (i.e., noise from random shocks becomes incorporated into the system). This fight leads you to believe you've ruined your chances for an upcoming promotion, and you transition to a distressed mood (a new sensitizing initial condition). Over the course of the day, minor stimulus events occur: The copier breaks down, the boss gives you another large assignment, a colleague is "downsized," and the like. The distressed mood allows these shocks to produce a distressed emotion state. However, your administrative assistant notices your mood and sends you a funny e-mail to cheer you up, so that you transit to elation. Later, you read the e-mail again and laugh. Awareness that this makes you happy feeds back into the system and allows you to regulate it. As the day comes to a close, the happy mood intensifies. Several stimulus events occur to produce joy (a beer after work with friends, a rerun of your favorite television sitcom).

It is possible, indeed probable, that an approximate affective pattern repeats during the week. The "random shocks" are not random at all—you wake to the same loud clock radio every day; you take the same route to work every day. You see the same individuals, who manifest approximately the same emotional patterns every day. Thus, emotions and events are coupled in a relatively bounded system during the week, with dynamics changes on the weekend (given the different stimuli likely to be encountered then). In fact, analyses of moods over the week do show stable patterning, with changes on the weekend (Kennedy-Moore, Greenberg, Newman, & Stone, 1992; Stone, Hedges, Neal, & Satin, 1985; Stone, Neal, & Shiffman, 1993). The concept of coupling could be applied here on a macro level. There is some relative stability to the aspects of our daily lives: social support systems (family, close friends), daily activities, and environmental stimuli are more stable than random day to day. Given a constant home, work, and social system, as well as stable mood traits (both our own and others), our patterns of affect may unfold in globally predictable and stable patterns, with pronounced coupling between all factors. Tomkins (1978) described this concept in his exposition of script theory. Family systems theory is based on this premise—that family systems are

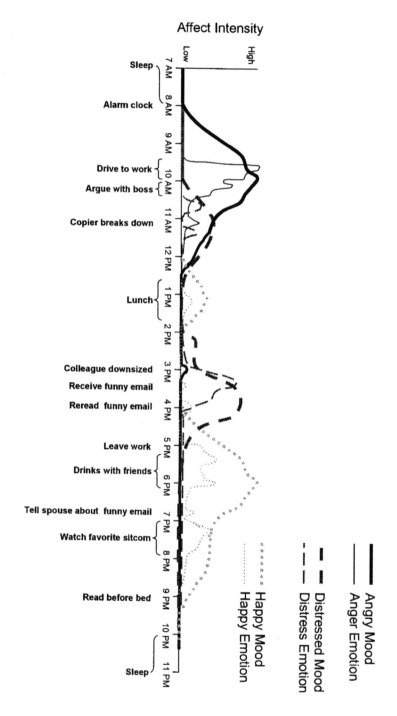

FIGURE 1.6. Mood, emotion, and eliciting events over the course of a day.

30

self-organizing and self-perpetuating, and often highly resistant to change (for an overview, see Becvar & Becvar, 1998). The ramifications of this cannot be understated. Many professions would seem to have dominant affects: trial lawyers need to be able to experience, express, and tolerate high levels of anger; academics need to sustain high levels of interest; professional food tasters must tolerate high levels of disgust. Professions may well bring together people with similar affective traits and tolerances, and provide affect congruent experiences that become self-perpetuating. *Affect may well be the central organizing principle of individuals, groups, and society as a whole, with a stability that cannot be ascertained by a knowledge of individual affect components.*

Dysfunctional Moods and Emotions

Finally, let us turn our attention to emotional pathology, or some possible ways in which we can define dysfunctional moods and emotions. We have proposed that within emotions and between emotions, there may be discernable and stable patterns/steady states that are relatively resistant to perturbations. But what happens when that stability, that limit cycle, is interrupted?

The interruption of a steady state is known as a "bifurcation." A bifurcation is said to occur when varying a parameter of a dynamic system produces change in the qualitative dynamics of the system. Remember, steady states within linear systems are extremely resistant to even large shocks. In contrast, nonlinear dynamic systems can at times be extremely sensitive to small variations in some parameters. This marks the sharpest contrast between the properties of linear systems and nonlinear systems.

If the qualitative behavior of a dynamic system is sensitive to the value of some parameter, then intervening in the operation of such a system can be very dangerous, especially if the actual parameter value is near a critical value for a bifurcation. Consider a very simple example: The U.S. Army has long known that bridges have a fundamental frequency of oscillation, so that if troops were to march over a bridge at a pace that resonated with that fundamental frequency, the bridge would collapse. In this example, the critical parameter is the fundamental frequency. If troops marching over the bridge produce a periodic forcing that resonates with the fundamental frequency, the bridge collapses. This has, in fact, happened on more than one occasion.

In emotion terms, there may be periods in an affective cycle when normally innocuous stimuli produce disproportionate or unpredictable emotional reactions. One example may be road rage, where a common incident suddenly provokes rageful emotion and behaviors otherwise uncharacteristic of an individual. Studies on mob behavior show a similar pattern, where emotion and environment converge, and people engage in uncharacteristic acts of violence and destruction. It may be possible for nonlinear dynamic equations to discover which emotion parameters display such sensitivity and when in the cycle they are most sensitive.

Bifurcations, then, may be established through stimulus events that are either large in scale or occur at a critical point in the oscillation phase, disrupting the stable flow of the system. Nonlinear dynamics may also shed light on the solutions to such disruptions. For example, most low-intensity shocks that occur at noncritical periods allow the individual to return to an equilibrium. A minor auto accident that results in a dented fender does not throw most individuals into serious emotional disequilibrium most of the time. Alternatively, a higher-level shock, or one administered when the system is more sensitive, may cause the system into a different steady state. A moderately serious auto accident with some physical injury might lead someone to be regularly more fearful and vigilant. Yet again, a higher-intensity shock, or one given at a sensitive period in the limit cycle, may lead to a vast number of different resolutions. Imagine that the accident was serious and led to the loss of life of a passenger. The driver's emotional system could change dramatically and in a number of unforeseeable ways.

Bifurcations can take a nearly limitless number of quantitative forms, but qualitatively they tend to fall into a small number of discernable categories. In other words, there may be a relatively bounded set of emotional changes that take place after trauma, resulting in a relatively bounded set of possible psychopathologies. In fact, multicultural studies suggest that there are a limited set of psychopathologies that appear to occur in all cultures, with similar ramifications for functioning and quality of life (Ormel et al., 1994; Verhulst & Achenbach, 1995). One set of bifurcation solutions leads to periods of oscillation with increasing amplitude, breaking down into turbulent motion over time, and eventually reverting to the oscillatory motion. This concept is termed "intermittency" in the mathematical literature. In this construct, turbulence is defined as reactions that exhibit very little autocorrelation, even over very short time periods. Thus, reactions to stimuli can lead to a cascade of short-time-period erratic actions that are "spun off" by the major reaction. Other common resolutions include increasing frequency of oscillation leading to chaos; also, seemingly no reaction followed by the sudden occurrence of turbulence. In the end, any qualitative leap in a system (jumps in the learning curve, movement from one developmental stage to another) may represent bifurcation points. The emotional, or personality, steady state is interrupted. The resolution might result in a return to the same emotion/personality steady state, to a new and differently organized steady state, or to a bounded set of solutions comprising "psychopathology." Modeling this mathematically may give us insight as to how to return an individual to his/her emotional equilibrium before the trauma occurred. The social value that would come of understanding, predicting, and preventing or diffusing such situations cannot be overstated!

CONCLUSIONS

Given our current knowledge of emotional phenomena, nonlinear dynamics are clearly a viable and potentially enlightening tool of analysis. Simple linear systems cannot capture or address the complexity of affect, though the works of Gottman and Levenson on emotion and marital relationships (Gottman & Levenson, 1985, 1992; Levenson & Gottman, 1985), Dunn and colleagues on children's emotional development (Dunn, 1995; Dunn, Brown, & Maguire, 1995; Dunn, Creps, & Brown, 1996), and Bolger and colleagues on person–environment transactions (Bolger & Schilling, 1991; Bolger & Zuckerman, 1995) have pushed the envelopes of such analysis to their probable limits.

There are some key questions regarding emotion to which non-linear dynamic analyses can be applied:

- How many and what are the essential dimensions of emotion?
- Are dimensions constant across affects? Across individuals? Within individuals?
- What does the phase space of emotion look like?
- Does the phase space vary across affects? Across individuals? Within individuals?
- Is there a global stability to emotions that cannot be predicted from the dynamics of their component parts?
- What are the transition probabilities between affects? What are their determinants?
- What are the characteristics of a stimulus, and where in the affective oscillation must it occur, to produce different bifurcations?
- How can the above concepts be applied to the understanding of emotional pathology?

The contribution of nonlinear dynamics is not only that complex emotional phenomena can be qualitatively described but that they can now be expressed as mathematical functions. The challenge for psychologists is to design experiments and studies in which nonlinear models can be applied and tested. Nonlinear dynamics can then be incorporated into affective models and theories that further our ability to understand and influence affective processes. As stated by Scherer (2000), there is a need for a paradigm shift in affective science. Ultimately such models will inform us not only about emotion but about personality, development, social interaction, and the corrective therapeutic process.

ACKNOWLEDGMENTS

We would like to thank Wes Hawfield and George A. Bonanno for their careful reading and suggestions.

REFERENCES

Barlow, D. H. (1988). *Anxiety and its disorders.* New York: Guilford Press.

Beck, A. T., Rush, A. J., Shaw, B. F., & Emery, G. (1979). *Cognitive therapy of depression.* New York: Guilford Press.

Becvar, D. S., & Becvar, B. J. (1998). *Systems theory and family therapy: A primer* (2nd ed.). Blue Ridge Summit, PA: University Press of America.

Bergé, P., Pomeau, Y., & Vidal, C. (1984). *Order within chaos.* New York: Wiley.

Bolger, N., & Schilling, E. A. (1991). Personality and the problems of everyday life: The role of neuroticism in exposure and reactivity to daily stressors. *Journal of Personality, 59,* 355–386.

Bolger, N., & Zuckerman, A., (1995). A framework for studying personality in stress process. *Journal of Personality and Social Psychology, 69,* 890–902.

Cannon, W. B. (1911). Emotional stimulation of adrenal gland secretion. *American Journal of Physiology, 28,* 64–70.

Damasio, A. R. (1994). *Descartes' error: Emotion, reason, and the human brain.* New York: Grosset/Putnam.

Darwin, C. (1999). *The expression of the emotions in man and animals* (Introduction by P. Ekman). London: HarperCollins. (Original work published 1872)

Diener, E., Larsen, R. J., & Emmons, R. A. (1984). Person–situation interactions: Choice of situations and congruence response models. *Journal of Personality and Social Psychology, 47,* 580–592.

Duke, D. W., & Pritchard, W. S. (1991). *Measuring chaos in the brain.* London: World Scientific Publishing.

Dunn, J. (1995). Children as psychologists: The later correlates of individual differences in understanding of emotions and other minds. *Cognition and Emotion, 9,* 187–201.

Dunn, J., Brown, J. R., & Maguire, M. (1995). The development of children's moral sensibility: Individual differences and emotion understanding. *Developmental Psychology, 31,* 649–659.

Dunn, J., Creps, C., & Brown, J. (1996). Children's family relationships between two and five: Developmental changes and individual differences. *Social Development, 5,* 230–250.

Ekman, P. (1992a). Are there basic emotions? *Psychological Review, 99,* 550–553.

Ekman, P. (1992b). An argument for basic emotions. *Cognition and Emotion, 6,* 169–200.

Ekman, P. (1994). Moods, emotions, and traits. In P. Ekman & R. J. Davidson (Eds.), *The nature of emotions* (pp. 56–58). New York: Oxford University Press.

Ekman, P. (1997). The future of emotion research. *Affect Scientist, 11*, 4–5.

Ekman, P., Levenson, R. W., & Friesen, W. V. (1983). Autonomic nervous system activity distinguishes among emotions. *Science, 221*, 1208–1210.

Ekman, P., & Rosenberg, E. (1998). *What the face reveals: Basic and applied studies of spontaneous expression using the facial action coding system.* Oxford, UK: Oxford University Press.

Emmons, R. A., & Diener, E. (1986a). An interactional approach to the study of personality and emotion. *Journal of Personality, 54*, 371–384.

Emmons, R. A., & Diener, E. (1986b). Situation selection as a moderator of response consistency and stability. *Journal of Personality and Social Psychology, 51*, 1013–1019.

Emmons, R. A., Diener, E., & Larsen, R. J. (1986). Choice and avoidance of everyday situations and affect congruence: Two models of reciprocal interactionism. *Journal of Personality and Social Psychology, 51*, 815–826.

Farley, B. G., & Clark, W. A. (1961). Activity in networks of neuron-like elements. In C. Cheery (Ed.), *Information theory.* London: Butterworths.

Feldman, L. A. (1995). Valence focus and arousal focus: Individual differences in the structure of affective experience. *Journal of Personality and Social Psychology, 69*, 153–166.

Feldman Barrett, L. (1998). The future of emotion research. *Affect Scientist, 12*, 6–8.

Feldman Barrett, L., & Russell, J. A. (1998). Independence and bipolarity in the structure of current affect. *Journal of Personality and Social Psychology, 74*, 967–984.

Feldman Barrett, L., & Russell, J. A. (1999). Structure of current affect. *Current Directions in Psychological Science, 8*, 10–14.

Frijda, N. H. (1987). *The emotions.* Cambridge, UK: Cambridge University Press.

Glass, L., & Mackey, M. C. (1988). *From clocks to chaos.* Princeton, NJ: Princeton University Press.

Gottman, J. M., & Levenson, R. W. (1986). Assessing the role of emotion in marriage. *Behavioral Assessment, 8*, 31–48.

Gottman, J. M., & Levenson, R. W. (1992). Marital processes predictive of later dissolution: Behavior, physiology and health. *Journal of Personality and Social Psychology, 63*, 221–233.

Grammer, K., Fink, B., Kruck, K. B., & Magnusson, M. S. (1998, August). *Automated detection of hidden patterns of nonverbal synchronization in opposite-sex encounters.* Paper presented at the 10th annual meeting of the International Society for Research on Emotions, Wuerzberg, Germany.

Gross, J. J. (1998). Antecedent- and response-focused emotion regulation: Divergent consequences for experience, expression, and physiology. *Journal of Personality and Social Psychology, 74*, 224–237.

Gump, B. B., & Kulik, J. A. (1997). Stress, affiliation, and emotional contagion. *Journal of Personality and Social Psychology, 72*, 305–319.

Hatfield, E., Cacioppo, J. T., & Rapson, R. L. (1994). *Emotional contagion.* New York: Cambridge University Press.

Izard, C. E. (1994). Innate and universal facial expressions: Evidence from developmental and cross-cultural research. *Psychological Bulletin, 115,* 288–299.

Kaloupek, D. G., & Levis, D. J. (1983). Issues in the assessment of fear: Response concordance and prediction of avoidance behavior. *Journal of Behavioral Assessment, 5,* 239–260.

Kantor, J. S., Zitrin, C. M., & Zeldis, S. M. (1980). Mitral valve prolapse syndrome in agoraphobic patients. *American Journal of Psychiatry, 137,* 467–469.

Kennedy-Moore, E., Greenberg, M. A., Newman, M. C., & Stone, A. A. (1992). The relationship between daily events and mood: The mood measure may matter. *Motivation and Emotion, 16,* 143–155.

Kern, J. M. (1984). Relationships between obtrusive laboratory and unobtrusive naturalistic behavioral fear assessments: Treated and untreated subjects. *Behavioral Assessment, 6,* 45–60.

Lang, P. J. (1979). A bio-informational theory of emotional. *Psychophysiology, 16,* 495–512.

Lang, P. J., Levin, D. N., Miller, G. A., & Kozak, M. J. (1983). Fear behavior, fear imagery, and the psychophysiology of emotion: The problem of affective response integration. *Journal of Abnormal Psychology, 92,* 276–306.

LeDoux, J. (1998). *The emotional brain.* New York. Simon & Schuster.

Levenson, R. W. (1994). Human emotion: A functional view. In P. Ekman & R. J. Davidson (Eds.), *The nature of emotions* (pp. 123–126). New York: Oxford University Press.

Levenson, R. W., Ekman, P., & Friesen, W. V. (1990). Voluntary facial action generates emotion-specific nervous system activity. *Psychophysiology, 27,* 363–384.

Levenson, R. W., & Gottman, J. M. (1985). Physiological and affective predictors of change in relationship status. *Journal of Personality and Social Psychology, 49,* 85–94.

Lorenz, E. N. (1963). Deterministic non-periodic flow. *Journal of Atmospheric Science, 20,* 282–293.

Marshall, G., & Zimbardo, P. G. (1979). The affective consequence of inadequately explained physiological arousal. *Journal of Personality and Social Psychology, 37,* 970–988.

Mayne, T. J. (2000). The future of emotion research. *The Emotion Researcher, 14,* 6–7.

Nicolis, G., & Prigogine, I. (1989). *Exploring complexity.* New York: Freeman.

Ormel, J., Von Korff, M., Ustun, T. B., Pini, S., Korten, A., & Oldehinkel, T. (1994). Common mental disorders and disability across cultures: Results from the WHO Collaborative Study on Psychological Problems in General Health Care. *Journal of the American Medical Association, 272,* 1741–1748.

Ortony, A., & Turner, T. J. (1992). What's basic about basic emotions? *Psychological Review, 97,* 315–331.

Panksepp, J. (1994). Basic emotions ramify widely in the brain, yielding many concepts that cannot be distinguished unambiguously . . . yet. In P. Ekman & R. J. Davidson (Eds.), *The nature of emotion* (pp. 86–88). New York: Oxford University Press.

Plutchik, R., & Conte, H. R. (Eds.). (1997). *Circumplex models of personality and emotions.* Washington, DC: American Psychological Association.

Rimé, B. (1997). President's column. *Affect Scientist, 11,* 1–6.

Russell, J. A. (1980). A circumplex model of affect. *Journal of Personality and Social Psychology, 39,* 1161–1178.

Russell, J. A., & Feldman Barrett, L. F. (1999). Core affect, prototypical emotional episodes, and other things called emotion: Dissecting the elephant. *Journal of Personality and Social Psychology, 76,* 805–819.

Schacter, S., & Singer, J. (1962). Cognitive, social and physiological determinants of emotional state. *Psychological Review, 69,* 379–399.

Scherer, K. R. (1993). Studying the emotion-antecedent appraisal process: An expert system. *Cognition and Emotion, 3,* 325–355.

Scherer, K. R. (1994). Emotion serves to decouple stimulus and response. In P. Ekman & R. J. Davidson (Eds.), *The nature of emotion* (pp. 127–130). New York: Oxford University Press.

Scherer, K. R. (1998). The future of emotion research. *Affect Scientist, 12,* 6–8.

Scherer, K. R. (2000). Emotions as episodes of subsystem synchronization driven by nonlinear appraisal processes. In M. D. Lewis & I. Granic (Eds.), *Emotion, development, and self-organization: Dynamic systems approaches to emotional development* (pp. 70–99). New York: Cambridge University Press.

Schwartz, G. E., Weinberger, D. A., & Singer, J. A. (1981). Cardiovascular differentiation of happiness, sadness, anger and fear following imagery and exercise. *Psychosomatic Medicine, 43,* 343–364.

Stewart, P. (1967). Redrup v. State of N.Y., U.S. Supreme Court 386 U.S. 767.

Stone, A. A., Hedges, S. M., Neal, J. M., & Satin, M. S. (1985). Prospective and cross-sectional mood reports offer no indication of a "blue Monday" phenomenon. *Journal of Personality and Social Psychology, 49,* 129–134.

Stone, A. A., Neal, J. M., & Shiffman, S. (1993). Daily assessments of stress and coping and their association with mood. *Annals of Behavioral Medicine, 15,* 8–16.

Strogatz, S. H., & Stewart, I. (1993, December). Coupled oscillators and biological synchronization. *Scientific American, 269,* 102–109.

Tomkins, S. S. (1978). Script theory: Differential magnification of affects. In *Nebraska Symposium on Motivation: Vol. 26* (pp. 201–236). Lincoln: University of Nebraska Press.

Verhulst, F. C., & Achenbach, T. M. (1995). Empirically based assessment and taxonomy of psychopathology: Cross-cultural applications. A review. *European Child and Adolescent Psychiatry, 4,* 61–76.

Watson, J. B., & Rayner, R. (1920). Conditioned emotional responses. *Journal of Experimental Psychology, 3,* 1–14.

2

A Multiprocess Perspective on the Neuroscience of Emotion

KEVIN N. OCHSNER
LISA FELDMAN BARRETT

During the past century, neuroscientists and psychologists have viewed emotion through different lenses. According to many contemporary psychologists our emotions are a product of the way in which we interpret the world. In this view, the way we think about, or appraise, the significance of an event determines whether it will make us happy or sad, angry or glad. The same stimulus, such as your brother punching you in the arm, will have an entirely different meaning depending upon whether his action seems deliberately harmful or playfully affectionate. How you respond to his punch will be determined by how you interpret its meaning. The goal of this research is to identify how appraisal patterns give rise to complexities of emotional experience, expression, and regulation (see, e.g., Frijda, 1986; Lazarus, 1991).

In contrast, neuroscientists have viewed emotions as expressions of inherited programs for action in specific situations that have been of importance to humans and related species for millions of years (see, e.g., Panksepp, 1998). In this view, complex emotions are learned responses to primary reinforcers that have been built on top of these simple and prepotent response tendencies (see, e.g., Rolls, 1999). The goal of research is to identify the neural systems responsible for the basic responses of fear, rage, disgust, affiliation, and so on. Although some researchers acknowledge that neural systems carry out some simple forms of appraisal (e.g., for fear, see LeDoux, 1996), by and large, neuroscience theories simply do not speak to the issue of how complex person–situation relationships determine what feelings will be elicited.

Which view is correct? Are emotions the product of complex cognitive appraisals, or are they the product of simple programs embedded in our genes and brains? This is the crux of the conflict between psychology and neuroscience as it traditionally has been understood, and debates over this and related issues have been the source of much consideration (for discussion, see Ekman & Davidson, 1994; LeDoux, 1996). A complete account of emotion, however, should make reference to all levels of analysis, ranging from the feelings and behaviors associated with emotion to how they are computed at the neural level of brain structures and systems.

The purpose of this chapter is to begin sketching a theoretical framework that bridges these levels. We begin with the view that this conflict is more apparent than real by arguing that psychological and neuroscience approaches are asking complementary questions about emotion that are couched at different levels of analysis. In the following section we outline the basic elements of our framework, specifying two kinds of processes that are used to generate and regulate emotions. In this theory, emotion is the product of an interaction between simple, nonconscious, automatic processes and deliberative, conscious, and controlled processes. Then, in subsequent sections we use data from multiple fields to support and develop this theory, describing how the functions of specific brain regions can be understood in terms of their role in automatic or controlled emotion processing. Finally, we briefly consider how our theory can begin to foster a rapprochement between neuroscience and psychological approaches to emotion.[1]

AUTOMATIC AND CONTROLLED PROCESSING IN EMOTION

In recent years there has been an explosion of interest in questions concerning the nature of emotional experience, both in the scientific disciplines (see, e.g., Ekman & Davidson, 1994; Lewis & Haviland, 1993) and in lay domains (see, e.g., Damasio, 1994; Goleman, 1995; LeDoux, 1996). Many studies have been directed at determining what kinds of emotions people generate and when they report feeling them (see, e.g., Feldman, 1995; Feldman Barrett,1998). Studies examining the kinds of emotion regulatory strategies people use are receiving increasing attention as well (see, e.g., Gross & Levenson, 1993). Most of this research has been descriptive rather than causal in its analysis, however, leaving unexplored issues concerning the information processing mechanisms used to generate and regulate the emotional responses in question. Our theory is aimed at specifying the information processing mechanisms involved in emotion generation and regulation, identifying their neural substrates, and seeking to ultimately understand the factors that determine when and how effectively they are used. The present chapter tackles the first two of these three goals.

Many mental phenomena have been well modeled as the product of a quick and automatic process that sets the stage for a slower and more deliberative processes which modify and/or monitor ongoing activity (Chaiken & Trope, 1999). We hypothesize that emotion generation and regulation are no different. Considerable evidence suggests that the automatic processes associated with an emotional response both quickly and effortlessly classify people, objects, and events as positive or negative (Quigley & Feldman Barrett, 1999; Robinson, 1998). This *automatic emotion processing* is consistent with what has been called primary appraisal (Lazarus, 1991). It is also consistent with automatic evaluations of environment features (Bargh, 1990; Bargh, Chaiken, Govender, & Pratto, 1992; Bargh, Chaiken, Raymond, & Hymes, 1996; Chaiken & Bargh, 1993; Chartrand & Bargh, 1996; Fazio, Sanbonmatsu, Powell, & Kardes, 1986), various kinds of affective conditioning (sometimes with subliminally presented stimuli; see, e.g., Ohman, 1988), and the inability to ignore emotionally relevant information (as in the emotional Stroop Task; see MacLeod, 1991). An important aspect of automatic emotion processing is that the rapid detection of potential threats or possible rewards, and the accessing of associated information, can initiate appropriate approach or avoidance behaviors (e.g., fleeing a threat or approaching a reward). More complex emotion knowledge (in the form of discrete emotion scripts or mental representations; see, e.g., Fehr & Russell, 1984; Shaver, Schwartz, Kirson, & O'Connor, 1987) are thought to be deployed during the generation of an emotional response, either because they are chronically accessible or because it is directly primed or preconsciously activated by the mere presence of features in the environment (for a discussion, see G. A. Bonanno, Chapter 8, this volume). Such occurrences also constitute automatic emotion processing.

But emotions are only partly the result of processes that interpret the significance of events in an automatic, or bottom–up, fashion. We also consciously direct attention to internal sensations and thoughts or external people and objects, search for and retrieve information from memory, construct a representation of our experience, and select or inhibit our actions. Collectively, the use of directed, effort-demanding processes in the generation and regulation of emotion can be termed *controlled emotion processing*. Examples of controlled emotion processing abound in the clinical and experimental social psychology literatures and include the following:

- Studies of pain perception demonstrating that deliberately attending to and describing painful physical sensations can lessen the psychological experience of them as painful (Cioffi, 1993)

- Studies relying on self-reports of emotional experience (see, e.g., Feldman Barrett, 1998)
- Studies of emotion disclosure demonstrating that retrieving and recounting past personal traumas can lessen negative affect accompanying their recollection, and even improve one's physical health (see, e.g., Pennebaker, 1997)
- Studies of decision making demonstrating that emotions may sometimes help (see, e.g., Damasio, 1994) or bias judgments (Forgas, 1995)
- Studies of emotion regulation demonstrating our abilities to inhibit or alter ongoing emotional responses (Gross & Levenson, 1993)

By deliberately monitoring, activating, and processing emotions, one may consciously reconstrue the meaning of an experience and respond differently.

Automatic and controlled emotion processing can configure in a number of ways to produce emotional experience and expression. For example, consider the emotion generation process in an individual whose emotional reactions are complex and subtle. On the one hand, the fine texture of her experience could result from the automatic activation of a rich network of semantic and affective schemas (composed of both linguistic labels and organized personal experiences) that are easily accessible due to repeated use. In addition, past painful or rewarding experiences may have stamped in certain action tendencies and physiological responses that also are elicited automatically. In this way, her highly differentiated emotional response is mediated by a complex knowledge base without effort or intent. On the other hand, her automatic and quick responses could have been simple and undifferentiated, with the complexity of her experience and behavior arising only after she attempts to describe and understand her feelings. She might possess a rich and consciously accessible vocabulary specialized for doing so. But, unlike the first case, complex emotional responses would take shape slowly, requiring effort and concentration to apply emotion knowledge in the description and regulation of her feelings. Both of these examples stand in contrast to individuals who do not parse their emotional responses with much granularity or precision and instead rely upon global judgments of hedonic tone. They might simply note, "I feel good" or "I feel bad," either because they lack the knowledge, motivation, or executive capacity to construe their feelings otherwise.

Unfortunately, current understanding of the brain structures involved in emotion is still a long way from providing the precise neural dynamics underlying the complexities of everyday examples of emotion such as these. However, as elaborated in the section that follows, neuroscience data support the general theory that automatic and controlled processes are involved in emotion, and suggest further that each type of processing may be carried out by a number of separate neural systems.

NEURAL SYSTEMS FOR EMOTION GENERATION AND REGULATION

Evidence from multiple domains suggests that automatic and controlled emotion processes are carried out by at least five distinct neural systems. Each system plays a different but essential functional role in the generation and regulation of emotion. Each function is carried out by mechanisms that operate with differing degrees of deliberative control and are identified in the top row of Figure 2.1.

Considerable evidence suggests that the first three systems can operate automatically and comprise three distinct kinds of automatic emotion processing. Separate processes detect potential threats (Function 1) and possible rewards (Function 2), as well as acquire and execute appropriate approach or avoidance behaviors (e.g., fleeing a threat or approaching a reward). A third system (Function 3) adds complexity to these responses through the automatic activation of semantic emotion knowledge. This system oversees retrieval from memory of complex emotion knowledge that is used to form more discrete emotional experiences, attribute an emotional quality to a stimulus, and devise strategies to cope with emotional states and emotionally evocative stimuli.

The extent to which one deliberately differentiates and regulates this initial response is determined by the third, fourth, and fifth functions. The deployment of complex emotion knowledge (Function 3) can also occur under conscious direction. One can deliberately look up information in semantic memory about how to understand or regulate an emotional response, as well as to decide whether to alter that response. The fourth system determines whether it is necessary to seek greater understanding or control over emotional responses (Function 4) by detecting discrepancies between competing response tendencies or consciously held plans. When a discrepancy is detected, one can deliberately use emotion knowledge to alter or regulate the emotional response (i.e., a return to Function 3). In addition, we need to evaluate the current affective meaning of an external stimulus or behavioral response so that one can make the decisions or take the actions necessary to make these changes (Function 5). The distinctions between these different functions and between automatic and controlled emotion processing is supported by various types of neuroscience data, reviewed below.

The Amygdala: Detecting and Responding to Potential Threats

Currently, more is known about the function of the amygdala in emotion than any other brain structure. In the past few years, data from various domains have provided converging evidence that the amygdala might be best characterized as a preattentive analyzer of the environment that looks for

BRAIN STRUCTURE	Amygdala	Basal Ganglia	Lateral Prefrontal and Association Cortices	Anterior Cingulate Cortex	Orbital and Ventromedial Frontal Cortex
FUNCTION	Detecting & Learning about Potential Threats	Registering Rewards & Acquiring Habits	Retrieving and Storing Semantic Emotion Knowledge	Conflict Monitoring	Context-dependent action selection
USE AND APPLICATION	Detect arousing, potentially threatening stimuli and associate them with corresponding physiological responses and appropriate actions	Automatize sequences of behavior and thought that have proved consistently reinforcing	Identify stimuli & differentiate feeling states; attribute emotional qualities to stimuli; repository of regulatory strategies & lay emotion knowledge	Monitor on-going behavior and determine whether change is necessary	Inhibit ongoing emotional responses based on analyses of context; generate affective reactions based on these analyses that guide further regulatory judgments
TYPE OF PROCESS	Automatic	Automatic, but requires attention	Retrieval can be Automatic or Controlled	Conflicts detected automatically, but making changes takes control	Controlled

FIGURE 2.1. Chart showing the brain structures thought to be important for emotion processing, their functional role, how they are used and applied to processing emotional information, and the type of processing they carry out (whether it is automatic, controlled, or both).

significant information that should be encoded into memory (Holland & Gallagher, 1999; LeDoux, 1996; Whalen, 1998). It would make sense for a system performing this function to be biased toward the early detection of ambiguous but evocative stimuli, even though these objects may ultimately prove to be either threatening or rewarding. For both kinds of stimuli, the amygdala would code the association between the appearance of stimulus and the affective response evoked. But if the stimulus proves to be rewarding over time, other areas may be more important for promoting the long-term reinforcement of approach behaviors that the amygdala is not designed to perform (such as the basal ganglia, discussed in the following subsection). In this way, the amygdala would still play a role in encoding the significance of rewarding/positive stimuli but would play a different role in mediating behavior toward those stimuli later on.

The anatomy of the amygdala is consistent with this conclusion (for location see Figure 2.2A). Information about the identity of a stimulus can reach the amygdala by one of two routes: the first is a cortically based system used to recognize stimuli on the basis of distinct perceptual features; the second consists of more direct connections to sensory organs via the thalamus, bypassing the longer cortical route (Aggleton, 1992). In a series of experiments conducted with rats, LeDoux and colleagues have shown that each input pathway supports a different kind of emotional learning. The cortical route allows the discrimination of stimuli on the basis of complex analyses of their distinctive features, as well as the acquisition of differential conditioned responses to them. In contrast, the subcortical pathway by itself can support rapid leaning of conditioned responses to crude, coarsely defined perceptual stimuli (LeDoux, 1996; LeDoux, Romanski, & Xagoraris, 1989). On the basis of these results, LeDoux suggested that the subcortical pathway provides a quick analysis of the affective properties of stimuli that serves as an initial template for subsequent processing.

Some recent results in humans and animals have corroborated LeDoux and colleagues' findings. Neuroimaging studies have shown amygdala activity while subjects are learning to associate aversive noise with neutral tones (LaBar, Gatenby, Gore, LeDoux, & Phelps, 1998), and neuropsychological studies have shown that amygdala lesions block the acquisition of such responses (LaBar, LeDoux, Spencer, & Phelps, 1995). In addition to its role in these implicit forms of memory, the amygdala also has been shown to influence the consolidation of explicitly accessible, episodic memories for emotional events (for further discussion see Chapter 3). For example, recall of the emotional elements of a negative story is correlated with amygdala activity during encoding (Cahill et al., 1996), and degenerative decay of the amygdala due to disease eliminates this memory advantage (Cahill, Babinsky, Markowitsch, & McGaugh, 1995; Markowitsch et al., 1998). Studies in animals have indicated that modulation of

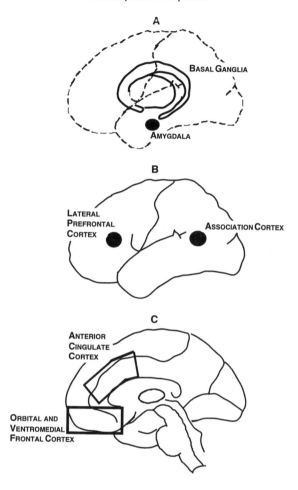

FIGURE 2.2. Anatomical locations of the brain structures discussed in this chapter. Figure 2.2A depicts two subcortical structures shown with dark (solid) lines beneath a transparent (dashed line) lateral view of the left hemisphere. The basal ganglia are important for encoding sequences of thought and behavior that have proved rewarding over time. The amygdala is important for detecting threats and encoding relationships between the sensory characteristics of stimuli and the internal affective states elicited by them. Figure 2.2B depicts two cortical areas superimposed on a lateral view of the left hemisphere. The left prefrontal cortex is important for looking up abstract semantic and associative knowledge in a posterior area that stores semantic information. Figure 2.2C depicts two cortical areas superimposed on a medial view of the right hemisphere. The anterior cingulate cortex (ACC) is used to track the extent to which current behavior is failing to achieve a desired outcome. Signals from the ACC are used to indicate errors, conflicts, pain, uncertainty, anxiety, and violations of expectation. The ventromedial frontal cortex (VMFC) and orbital frontal cortex (OFC) are used to represent the current affective value of a stimulus in the context of current goals. This subsystem enables an individual to alter responses to a stimulus on the basis of its shifting motivational significance.

explicit memory by the amygdala results, at least in part, from enhancing consolidation of memories by a hippocampus-based system that is specialized for encoding nonemotional information about episodes (McGaugh et al., 1995). This has been corroborated in humans by demonstrating that amygdala lesions eliminate improved memory for negatively arousing words, which emerges some time after encoding and is attributed to enhanced consolidation of memory for emotional stimuli (LaBar & Phelps, 1998). Drugs that block release of the neurotransmitter norepinephrine (NE) within the amygdala eliminate both the explicit memory advantage for negative events in humans (Cahill, Prins, Weber, & McGaugh, 1994; van Stegeren, Everaerd, Cahill, McGaugh, & Gooren, 1998) and conditioning effects in animals (Cahill et al., 1995). This suggests that NE release is a key component of the amydala's affect-encoding and memory modulatory mechanism.

A pair of recent studies also has supported LeDoux's conclusions concerning the role of the subcortical pathway in the quick analysis of stimuli. Whalen, Rauch, and colleagues (1998) found that brief, backward-masked presentations of fearful but not happy faces activated the amygdala even though participants were unaware that either type of face had been presented. Morris, Ohman, and Dolan (1999) conducted a similar experiment and found that the pathway of activation passed through the thalamus and amygdala but bypassed the cortex.

Intriguingly, it appears that the amygdala's response decreases to stimuli that signal a safe, nonthreatening environment. This is true both for stimuli whose value as a safety signal already has been learned before the study begins (such as happy faces; Whalen, Rauch, et al., 1998), or for stimuli that initially seemed threatening but proved not to be so during the course of an experiment. Conditioning studies have found that the amygdala response to negative faces (Breiter, Etcoff, & Whalen, 1996; Morris et al., 1996) or aversive conditioned stimuli (LaBar et al., 1998) decreases and habituates with repeated presentation, although activity in other cortical areas does not decrease. An important question for future research will be to determine whether these decreases in amygdala activity are due to passive habituation or active inhibition by other areas.

A system sensitive to potential threats[2] should be activated by positive stimuli that are relatively unfamiliar or novel. This was demonstrated recently by a neuroimaging study investigating perception of unfamiliar faces of black and white individuals by African American and European American participants (Hart, Whalen, Shin, McInerney, & Rauch, 1999). For African American individuals, black faces should presumably be more positive and less threatening than are white faces, whereas the opposite should be true for European American participants. However, during an initial block of trials, amygdala activation was observed for both types of faces in both groups of participants. This suggests that novel same-race faces, although presumably more positive and less threatening than are other-race faces, are still sufficiently ambiguous that they elicit an initial amygdala response. This view was confirmed by results from a second block of trials in which amygdala activation to same-race faces habituated but activation to different-race faces did not.

More generally, evaluating the role of the amygdala in coding the affective significance of positive stimuli is somewhat difficult at present because roughly 10 times as many studies have investigated perception and memory for negative information as for positive information (based on a *PsycINFO* search in February 1999). And the handful of studies that have used positive stimuli have produced mixed results. One neuroimaging study has related memory of both positive and negative stimuli to amygdala activity at encoding and found significant correlations for both stimulus types (Hamann, Ely, Grafton, & Kilts, 1998). This study also included a control condition in which interesting and unusual but not emotional stimuli were presented. Memory for these stimuli was not correlated with amygdala activity. Other studies have not found amygdala activation when participants view positive and negative photos (Canli, Desmond, Zhao, Glover, & Gabrieli, 1998) or experience an induced elated mood (Baker, Frith, & Dolan, 1997). Two studies have reported amygdala activation when averaging responses to perception of positive and negative films (Lane, Reiman, Ahern, & Schwartz, 1997) or during induction of positive and negative moods (Schneider et al., 1997), which precludes determining which stimulus type is responsible for the observed activity.

Studies of appetitive conditioning in rats have obtained more consistent results. The connection between the amygdala and portions of the basal ganglia (called the ventral striatum) appears to play a key role in these animals learning to associate neutral stimuli with appetitive (e.g., food or sex) rewards (Everitt & Robbins, 1992; Schultz, 1998). Lesions of the basal ganglia impair the acquisition of such associations, whereas lesions to the striatum impair the transformation of such associations into habitual responses to the reinforced stimulus (Everitt & Robbins, 1992; MacDonald & White, 1993). Single-unit recording studies in animals show that once learned, cells in the basal ganglia can signal the positive or negative reward value of a stimulus (Rolls, 1999). Although the amygdala may store associations between the appearance of a rewarding stimulus and the physiological responses it elicits, other brain regions such as the ventral striatum or medial and orbital frontal cortex seem to be more important than the amygdala for the perception of stimuli that already have acquired positive/reward value (see Adolphs, 1999; Lane, Reiman, Bradley, et al., 1997; Rolls, 1999). These brain regions are discussed in the subsections that follow.

Summary

Animal and human studies are generally consistent with the claim that the amygdala functions to determine whether incoming stimuli are threatening and, if so, to rapidly associate perception of those stimuli with the appropriate responses. Any novel or ambiguous stimulus may initially seem threatening and thus warrant a response from the amygdala.

The Basal Ganglia: Learning to Skillfully Attain Rewards

Situations that elicit positive and negative affect seem to require very different kinds of responses. On the one hand, it behooves us to learn very quickly and rapidly that something (or someone) engenders fear, anger, or disgust so that we can respond immediately and appropriately the next time we encounter it. On the other hand, it makes sense to stamp in behaviors and thoughts that have led to a desirable end only if they continue to do so reliably. The old aphorism, "Fool me once, shame on you, fool me twice, shame on me," suggests that it is advisable to be sure that rewards are due neither to chance nor deception. Whereas the amygdala is especially well suited for the former function (as discussed above), the basal ganglia are especially well suited for the latter. The basal ganglia are designed to slowly encode sequences of behavior that, over time, have been repeated and rewarded—or at least not punished (Lieberman, 2000). The representations thus encoded support not only the execution of habitual behaviors but the prediction of what comes next in a sequence of thoughts or actions.[3]

Anatomically, the basal ganglia are well suited for making habitual the patterns of action or thought that repeatedly have led to a desired or positive outcome. They lie in the center of the brain underneath the cortex, receive inputs from areas of the parietal and temporal lobes that code the spatial and physical characteristics of a stimulus, and send outputs to various motor control centers (see Figure 2.2A). The basal ganglia also participate in a number of functional control circuits that link it with areas of the frontal lobe and other cortical regions (Alexander, Crutcher, & DeLong, 1990). Each circuit has a specific functional domain, including spatial and object working memory, and motor control. One of these circuits connects four of the structures for emotion discussed in this chapter: the amygdala, ventral portions of the basal ganglia, the anterior cingulate cortex, and the orbital frontal cortex.

The basal ganglia are composed of two main parts, the caudate and putamen, which are involved with habitual cognition and action, respectively (Alexander et al., 1990; Houk, Davis, & Beiser, 1995; Lieberman, 2000). Lesions to the caudate, either as a result of stroke or degenerative disease (e.g., Huntington's chorea) impair perception of emotion conveyed through facial expression and tone of voice (see, e.g., Cohen, Riccio, & Flannery, 1994; Speedie, Wertman, Ta'ir, & Heilman, 1993). Importantly, the perception of vocal prosody, which requires integration of changes in vocal tone across time, is impaired by damage to the basal ganglia but not to the amygdala (Anderson & Phelps, 1998). In contrast, damage to the putamen impairs the production of nonverbal behavior, including emotional intonation and the production of voluntary facial expressions (see, e.g., Van Lancker & Pachana, 1995).

Many streams of animal and human research demonstrate that the sequencing and habit-forming function of the basal ganglia play a special role in positive emotion. For example, basal ganglia damage in rats eliminates the potentiation or rapid repetition of responses to rewards that increases with repeated receipt of them (Everitt & Robbins, 1992) and eliminates the ability to learn simple stimulus–reward associations that are repeated over time (Mishkin & Appenzeller, 1987; Packard, Hirsh & White, 1989). In humans, selective left basal ganglia lesions often cause depression, as do left prefrontal lesions (Robinson & Paradiso, 1996), and depression is common among patients with either Huntingtons's chorea (Hopkins, 1994) or Parkinson's disease (McPherson & Cummings, 1996), both of which involve basal ganglia degeneration. Neuroimaging results dovetail with and extend these neuropsychological findings. Basal ganglia activation has been found during the subconscious registration of positive faces (Morris et al., 1996), during the experience of positive but not negative emotion elicited by films or recall of personal experiences (Lane, Reiman, Bradley, et al., 1997), and during cocaine-induced euphoria (London et al., 1990). Selective caudate activation has been observed during the presentation of emotional words (Beauregard et al., 1997) and positive pictures (Canli et al., 1998). Some investigators have found basal ganglia activation during recall of sad but not happy memories (George et al., 1995; Lane, Reiman, Ahern, & Schwartz, 1997); however, the exact reason for these findings is unclear at present.

A problem with many of these studies is that they do not make clear whether basal ganglia involvement in positive affect is associated with the experience of positive affect per se, with the activation of learned response sequences that promote movement toward a reward, or both. Some other evidence suggests that the basal ganglia may be especially important for the approach-related behaviors associated with various kinds of emotions (but are particularly characteristic of positive emotional states). Berridge and Robinson (1998) have dissociated the processes involved in approach-related behaviors and the experience of reward. Their studies show that dopamine release in the basal ganglia changes how much a rat works to get a reward but not how it responds once that reward is received. They suggest that dopamine in the basal ganglia mediates "wanting," or the motivation to seek out and approach a reward or outcome, but not the phenomenal "liking" of that reward as it is experienced (see Breiter & Rosen, 1999).

Summary

The basal ganglia are important for encoding the temporally patterned stimulus–stimulus and stimulus–response relationships that underlie implicit cognitive and motor skills. These implicit skills are essential because they allow us to make automatic the sequences of thought and action that lead to the attainment of goals and receipt of rewards of various kinds.

The Lateral Prefrontal and Association Cortex: Using Complex Emotion Knowledge

Much of the knowledge that we use to assess the emotional relevance of stimuli and events is stored in the form of organized knowledge structures that specify the meaningful relationships among different stimuli (Fiske & Taylor, 1991). These emotion concepts or schemas may represent several things (Fehr & Russell, 1984; Mesquita & Fridja, 1992; Shaver et al., 1987; Shweder, 1993) including:

- The abstract cause of an experience
- The meaning of a situation to the individual and his or her immediate goals
- Bodily sensations
- Expressive modes (i.e., display rules for expression)
- How the emotion functions interpersonally
- Sequences of action to take to enhance or reduce the experience (i.e., plans of emotion management)

These kinds of emotion knowledge may function like culturally constructed internal guides or working models of emotional episodes (Saarni, 1993). This knowledge may be learned episodically, through experience. For example, children rapidly learn the type of psychological events and abstract situations that are associated with particular emotion labels (fear, sadness, happiness, anger, guilt, and so forth; see, e.g., Harris, Olthof, Meerum, Terwogt, & Hardman, 1987). They are also aware of the typical actions and expressions that are supposed to accompany a particular emotional state (Trabasso, Stein, & Johnson, 1981). Over time and repeated use, however, this episodic knowledge may become instantiated as semantic representations of the possible objects that can cause an emotional experience, the relational contexts associated with the experience, and the behavioral repertoire that exists for dealing with the experience and the larger situation.

Currently, we know much more about the structure and function of semantic memory than we do about its neural locus. Classic models of semantic memory depicted it as a system of linked information nodes, where the number of links between nodes corresponds to the conceptual distance between two pieces of information in the associative network (Bower & Forgas, 2000). Thus, the concept "doctor" and "nurse" are separated by fewer links than are "doctor" and "horse." The system of associations for a given concept has links or pointers to visual, auditory, and other representations of that concept in separate, modality-specific processing/memory systems (Kosslyn & Koenig, 1992; Ochsner & Kosslyn, 1999). More recent connectionist models of semantic memory describe sets of subsymbolic or subconceptual nodes, which become active in different combinations to represent higher-order conceptual information (Rumelhart, 1989). These models readily explain how existing schematic knowledge can automatically facilitate encoding and retrieval by filling in missing information and guiding the interpretation of ambiguous stimuli (see, e.g., McClelland, 1995).

Although semantic memory involves widespread connections throughout the entire brain, neuropsychological and neuroimaging studies suggest that the left temporal–parietal–occipital junction may play a special role in storing semantic information. Such studies also suggest that the left inferior prefrontal cortex may be important for retrieving semantic (especially verbal) information (see Figure 2.2B; see also Kosslyn & Koenig, 1992; Tulving, Kapur, Craik, Moscovitch, & Houle, 1994). Storage and access to semantic information about the emotional connotations of verbal material might well depend more on these structures in the right than in the left hemisphere (Borod, 1992). Both areas receive highly processed information from all sensory modalities.

Semantic memory plays a role in emotion in several different ways: First, semantic memory is a repository of schematized knowledge about the origins, evolution, and sequelae of our emotions. It includes our implicit or explicit theories about what emotions are, when we feel them, why we feel them, and what we should do when we feel them. People may differ in their degree of emotion knowledge and the way they use it to cope, and such differences can have a profound impact on the emotions they experience and their ability to cope with them (Lane & Schwartz, 1987). When semantic knowledge is activated without accompanying activation of the amygdala or basal ganglia, it can be used to tell us something about an emotion. But when semantic knowledge is activated in conjunction with either or both of these systems, the activated knowledge becomes part of an emotion. That is, a discrete emotional episode can emerge in the context of complex emotion knowledge that allows us to differentiate, label, and even draw inferences about our emotional states.

Second, repeated use of semantic knowledge "greases the wheels" of accessibility and over time can lead to the automatic activation of chronically accessed knowledge in the presence of appropriate cues. For instance, depressives tend to evaluate themselves negatively and view the future with great pessimism. Repetition of these thoughts over time may make access to them so automatic that it is not impeded by performing another task at the same time this information is being retrieved (Andersen, Spielman, & Bargh, 1992; Bargh & Tota, 1988). Highly accessible and schematized emotion knowledge also can guide the construal of ambiguous events. For example, depressives will interpret neutral sentences as negative and remember them that way later on (Williams, Watts, MacLeod, & Mathews, 1990). Interestingly, depressives show decreased activation of the left inferior prefrontal cortex, an area important for effortfully retrieving semantic information (Drevets & Raichle, 1998). The hypofunctionality of this area could belie depressives' tendencies to rely on automatically accessible negative information.

A third way in which semantic memory plays a role in emotion is by providing a link between stimuli with similar valence. This role was advocated strongly by Bower (see Bower & Forgas, 2000; see also Bradley, 1994), who proposed that there are nodes for different emotions in semantic memory. In this model, words, objects, visual images, and so on, gain emotional meaning through their common connections with these emotion nodes. This model can account for many of the effects of moods or affective states on judgment and memory, in terms of the spread of activation between items that share links with a given emotion node (for a review, see Bower & Forgas, 2000, although this model has been heavily criticized and supplanted by more elaborate views of emotion and memory—see Chapter 3). Repeated use of these affective associations can also make the activation and spread among them automatic. Similarly valenced concepts will thus tend to activate each other by virtue of their semantic, emotional association (Bargh et al., 1992; Fazio et al., 1986; Hermans, De Houwer, & Eelen, 1994).

A fourth and final point about semantic emotion knowledge concerns its relationship with the associations stored by the amygdala and the amygdala's role in consolidating episodic memories that become the basis for semantic memory. Semantic knowledge is derived from regularities in our daily episodic experience, and many different kinds of experience contribute to the emotional meaning of people, places, events, and so on. Undoubtedly, much of this knowledge comes from the norms for emotional expression specified by our familial and national cultures (see, e.g., Markus & Kitayama, 1991). Importantly, this emotion knowledge is stored separately from the affective associations stored by the amygdala, and it can influence behavior in different ways. Recent research has shown that patients with amygdala lesions can rate the emotional valence and the degree of arousal elicited by photos (see, e.g., van Stegneer et al., 1998) in the same way as control subjects do. This is despite the fact that they fail to show the boost in episodic recall for the emotionally evocative information that controls exhibit (Cahill et al., 1994). Similarly, patients with amygdala lesions may fail to show fear conditioning, even though they possess explicit knowledge about the relationship between the conditioned and unconditioned stimuli (see, e.g., Bechara, Tranel, Damasio, & Adolphs, 1995). Data such as these suggest that explicit judgments of the emotional meaning of stimuli may be guided by explicitly accessible semantic knowledge independent of the associations coded by the amygdala. Furthermore, these data support the division between processes that automatically detect potential threats (Function 1) and processes that learn more complex semantic information about them.

Although each type of knowledge is accessed in different ways, the systems do interact. Their interaction allows the amygdalar response to significant and arousing stimuli to influence the development and consolidation of semantic knowledge. This has been shown strikingly by the contrast between patients who have suffered amygdala damage in adulthood and patients who suffered amygdala damage early in life. The former judge emotional faces to be as arousing as controls do (Adolphs, Russell, & Tranel, 1999, cited in Adolphs, 1999), whereas the latter judge the faces to be much less arousing (Adolphs, Lee, Tranel, & Damasio, 1997). It is possible that loss of the amygdala early in life keeps an individual from learning the significance of certain facial expressions because they could not become aroused when seeing them.

Summary

Semantic emotion knowledge is intimately involved with the generation of distinct emotional experiences. It is the repository of emotion concepts and theories, and links diverse and discrete memories together that share a common emotional association. We can draw upon this database automatically during the generation of an emotional state, or when we consciously represent or label emotional states to draw inferences about the emotions we are experiencing. Although it is not yet known exactly which brain structures mediate automatic use of this knowledge, it is clear that effortful access involves areas of the lateral prefrontal cortex specialized for this function (Tulving et al., 1994). It also is not yet determined definitively whether these lateral prefrontal brain regions alone are responsible for the labeling and attribution of emotional states. The emotional contents of semantic memory have been influenced by the amygdala, which facilitates consolidation of episodic memories for significant, arousing events. Research on the relationship between episodic and semantic memory has shown that over time the important regularities of our episodic memories slowly become incorporated into our database of semantic knowledge. This suggests that the amygdala contributes to the development of semantic knowledge by influencing what information is incorporated into long-term semantic memory.

Anterior Cingulate Cortex: Evaluating the Need for Controlled Processing

Regulation or conscious modification of emotional responses requires that one know such intervention might be necessary. Evaluating the need for regulation is the function of the anterior cingulate cortex (ACC), and this evaluative function is an essential part of many types of controlled processing. At a broad level, the ACC can be seen as part of an executive system used to regulate behavior in many domains (Ochsner et al., 2000; Posner & DiGirolamo, 1998; Shallice, 1994; Stuss, Eskes, & Foster, 1994).

The evaluative role of the ACC is supported by its rich connectivity with many brain areas. The ACC is a large heterogeneous area on the medial wall of each hemisphere just behind the frontal lobes (see Figure 2.2C), and different subregions within the ACC have connections with different parts of the brain. Like the orbital frontal cortex (OFC) and ventromedial frontal cortex (VMFC), the more anterior parts of the ACC have connections with other frontal areas as well as with subcortical areas involved in emotion, such as the amygdala, hypothalamus, and striatum. More posterior areas of the ACC have interconnections with frontal, parietal, and subcortical areas involved in attention. Separate middle and posterior subregions of the ACC have connections with cortical and subcortical areas involved in motor control and pain, respectively (Devinsky, Morrell, & Vogt, 1995; Dum & Strick, 1993). A large fiber tract, the cingulum bundle, courses through the center of the cingulate gyrus connecting the different subregions and may facilitate communication between them and functional integration among them (Ballantine, Flanagan, Cassidy, & Marino, 1967).

Data from animal and human studies has implicated the ACC in various kinds of behaviors that involve monitoring and evaluation of one's behavioral performance, one's internal state, or the presence of external rewards. The ACC also monitors for the occurrence of events (such as uncertainty, conflict, or expectancy violation) that signal the need for a deliberate change in behavior. A clear example of such monitoring comes from neuroimaging and event-related-potential studies in humans (Carter et al., 1998; Deheane, Posner, & Tucker, 1994; Gehring, Goss, Coles, Meyer, & Donhin, 1993) and single-unit recording studies in monkeys (Brooks, 1986). These studies have shown that the ACC emits a signal whenever participants make errors in simple reaction time tasks. Importantly, this signal is larger when participants are more motivated to respond correctly. The signal occurs whether participants become aware that they have responded incorrectly on their own (Gehring et al., 1993) or when error feedback has been provided (Badgaiyan & Posner, 1997). The signal also occurs when the correct response has been made but an expected reward is withheld (Brooks, 1986).

More generally, the ability to monitor both for errors and for the correct execution of desired responses is necessary whenever sensory input or behavioral performance is being closely monitored to ensure optimal performance.[4] Such monitoring is necessary during the learning of new skills, when uncertainty regarding performance parameters is high. Neuroimaging studies have shown that the ACC is active during the learning of motor sequences (Rauch, Savage, Brown, et al., 1995) or word pairs (Raichle, 1997), but this activity drops away when such tasks have been well learned, performance has become habitual, and monitoring is no longer necessary. Physical pain is another important signal that current behavior is not meeting desired ends. Neuroimaging studies have shown that ACC activity is correlated with the degree of painful stimulation experienced (Davis, Taylor, Crawley, Wood, & Mikulis, 1997; Porro, Cettolo, Francescato, & Baraldi, 1998; Rainville, Duncan, Price, Carrier, & Bushnell, 1997; Talbot et al., 1991) even if it is illusory (i.e., not due to direct physical stimulation; see Craig, Reiman, Evans, & Bushnell, 1996). ACC lesions (for cingulotomy) lessen the psychological experience of pain but not the ability to discriminate differences in the amount of painful stimulation (Hebben, 1985).

The evaluative process sensitive to uncertainty, conflict, pain, or expectancy violation may play an important role in both the generation and regulation of emotion. For example, an ACC signal may be involved with the transformation of an initial affective response into a discrete emotional episode. When a response is initiated, the affective feeling can be attributed to an object via the deliberate use of emotion knowledge, resulting in the initiation of an emotional episode. ACC activation is probably a necessary component of this emotion generation process. After an emotion is generated, an ACC signal that the current course of behavior is in need of change could also initiate searches for more appropriate responses and the causes of conflict. The experience of conflict or pain accompanying ACC activation may thus be part of more complex emotional responses that emerge as other emotion systems become activated. In this way ACC activation can be the trigger for a cascade of responses that brings experience and behavior in line with expectations or situational requirements.

These speculations are supported by recent studies showing that monitoring one's current emotional state while viewing emotionally evocative photographs activates portions of the very same region of the ACC responsive to pain (Lane, Fink, Chau, & Dolan, 1997; Lane et al., 1998). Moreover, studies with both animals and humans have shown that monitoring the affective states elicited by painful and rewarding stimuli is important for learning about their significance. In rabbits ACC lesions impair the ability to discriminate reinforced from unreinforced stimuli (Gabriel, 1993), and in humans ACC activity is correlated with the acquisition and expression of conditioned skin conductance responses (Fredrikson, Wik, Fischer, & Andersson, 1995; Fredrikson et al., 1998). Interestingly, ACC lesions eliminate the distress call emitted by infant monkeys when separated from their mothers, which also could be due to an inability to evaluate and experience the pain associated with separation (von Cramon & Jurgens, 1983).

The ACC also seems important for mediating some of the physiological changes associated with monitoring and learning about significant stimuli. ACC lesions eliminate both the anticipatory slowing of the heart rate that precedes presentation of a conditioned stimulus in rabbits (Buchanan & Powell, 1993), as well as the gastrointestinal distress produced by learned helplessness in monkeys (Henke, 1982). And electrical stimulation of the ACC causes changes in the heart rate and respiration in both animals and humans (Buchanan & Powell, 1993; Pool & Ransohoff, 1949).

A final and important point is that it is not yet clear whether ACC activation is associated merely with the occurrence of events over which control should be exerted or whether it plays a direct role in implementing this control as well. The data reviewed above suggest that the ACC represents the conscious correlates of pain, uncertainty, conflict, emotional experience, and expectancy violation, signaling that behavioral change and reorientation of attention may be necessary. But the data necessary to indicate that the ACC helps implement these changes is somewhat ambiguous. Lesion studies of ACC function sometimes show deficits in emotional behavior (see, e.g., Damasio & Van Hoesen, 1986) or executive control (see, e.g., Cohen, Kaplan, Moser, Jenkins, & Wilkinson, 1998; Ochsner et al., 2000) but not always (see, e.g., Corkin, 1980). Part of the reason for these discrepancies may be that the patients studied often have lesions in other brain areas as well (see, e.g., Damasio & Van Hoesen, 1986) or that the studies have involved psychiatric populations whose brain function may have been abnormal before ACC damage occurred (see, e.g., Corkin, 1980).

Studies of psychiatric populations may shed unexpected light on ACC function, however. Psychosurgical lesions to the ACC have been used as a treatment for mood-related disorders such as obsessive–compulsive disorder (OCD), chronic pain syndrome, and depression (Baer et al., 1995; Ballantine, Bouckons, Thomas, & Giriunas, 1987; Ballantine et al., 1967). When such cingulotomies are effective, patients report a lessening of the anxiety associated with their symptoms even though the frequency of symptoms does not immediately decline. The conflict and uncertainty signaled by the ACC may be an essential ingredient of anxiety, which would explain the efficacy of cingulotomy for treating anxiety disorders.

However, cingulotomy results in either no deficit or minor and short-lived deficits in performance of various cognitive tasks, including many that activate precisely the ACC area that has been surgically removed (Cohen, Kaplan, Meadows, & Wilkinson, 1994; Corkin, 1980; Janer & Pardo, 1991; Ochsner et al., 2000). If the ACC is necessary for implementing regulatory behavioral changes, then deficits in task performance should have been observed. But if the ACC is only responsible for signaling the need for control, then we would expect performance deficits only if one is trying to use this conscious signal but is unable to do so. Thus it is possible that cingulotomy patients, who experience a great deal of uncertainty and conflict before the operation is performed, have become quite skilled at *ignoring* the signal that the ACC generates. Because they are quite good at performing tasks without using their anxiety as an indicator of performance accuracy, when the ACC is lesioned they suffer no performance decrement whatsoever.

Summary

The ACC has many subregions that together seem to serve a similar function in different domains. Together they enable the ACC to evaluate the "congruence" of feelings that one is experiencing by signaling uncertainty, conflict, or pain. The ACC also may be important for determining whether a stimulus will generate threat or pain in the future. This evaluation is represented in consciousness and can be used by other components of an executive system responsible for self-monitoring and regulation.

The Orbital and Ventromedial Frontal Cortex: Selecting and Implementing Regulatory Actions

Our bottom–up emotional responses are not always appropriate for every situation, and effective emotion regulation involves the active modification of these prepotent responses as well as the active use of emotional responses to guide judgment and decision making. Data from both animal and human studies indicate that the OFC and VMFC (see Figure 2.2C) are important for selecting and implementing these regulatory actions (Rolls, 1999; Stuss et al., 1993). The ability to deliberatively deploy regulatory responses based on an analysis of the current context requires integrating many different kinds of information, including bottom–up analyses of the affective value of a stimulus and information about situational factors that might indicate a change in those values. Anatomically, these areas are well suited to integrate these kinds of information: they receive input from every sensory modality, have reciprocal connections with subcortical and brainstem nuclei involved in emotion, and receive input from other areas of the frontal and temporal lobes that integrate and associate information from many modalities (Vogt, 1986).

Selecting and implementing the appropriate means of regulation requires the ability to determine the motivational relevance of an object (be it a person, place, thing, or thought), and studies in humans and animals suggest that OFC/VMFC is involved in this process. Neurophysiological recording studies in monkeys have shown that OFC areas are sensitive to stimuli with reward value, including faces, tastes, and smells only if such stimuli are relevant to current goals or needs. Thus, food-sensitive neurons will respond only when an animal is hungry (Rolls, 1999). OFC neurons also are capable of rapidly learning to associate a novel stimulus with a reward, firing whenever the newly reinforced stimulus is presented. Importantly, these neurons will cease firing to that stimulus soon after its presentation is no longer reinforced, even though neurons in subcortical areas (such as the amygdala or basal ganglia) may continue to fire when that stimulus is shown (Rolls, 1999). This suggests that whereas subcortical areas continue to represent information about the past reinforcement properties of a stimulus, the OFC/VMFC tracks the current affective value stimuli. And, when necessary, the OFC/VMFC changes their value when a stimulus–reward pairing changes (see Bouton, 1994).

Neuroimaging experiments in humans also support the OFC/VMFC's role in computing the motivational value of external stimuli. OFC activation has been found during the perception of both primary reinforcers, including pleasantly experienced touches, odors, and tastes (Francis et al., 1999), and secondary reinforcers including happy or fearful faces (Morris et al., 1998), negatively valenced words (Beauregard et al., 1997), and visual mental images of aversive scenes (Shin et al., 1997). Similarly, VMFC activation has been found for negative photos (Canli et al., 1998), anxiety elicited by anticipation of painful electric shock (Drevets, Videen, Price, & Preskorn, 1992), and the experience of sadness elicited by the combined recollection of sad personal memories and viewing of photos of sad faces (Drevets et al., 1992). A limitation of these studies is that they have not been designed to test whether OFC activity is due to the experience of emotion, the learning, inhibition, or remapping of affect–response relationships, or some other reason.

Beyond computing the significance of external stimuli based on the current context, the OFC/VMFC is important for acting on the basis of these computations. In general, OFC/VMFC lesions in animals impair the ability to change stimulus–reinforcement associations and cause responses to perseverate in old patterns (Bechara, Damasio, Tranel, & Damasio, 1996; Stuss et al., 1994). Thus VMFC lesions in rats increase the time it takes to extinguish conditioned fear responses (Morgan & LeDoux, 1995).

OFC lesions also can lead to feeding, drinking, and sexual behavior that is no longer sensitive to external cues indicating the availability of food, water, or sexual partners (Rolls, 1999).

Data from human studies generally support the findings from animal research: OFC/VMFC lesions impair the ability to change stimulus–reward relationships and cause perseveration of previously learned or prepotent responses (Freedman, Black, Ebert, & Binns, 1998; Rolls, Hornak, Wade, & McGrath, 1994). This inability to use information about the current value of stimuli to control the expression of previously learned behavioral or experiential responses can have serious social and interpersonal consequences.[5] Various kinds of personality and emotional changes have been reported following OFC and VMFC lesions, including apathy, violence, and the exhibition of socially inappropriate behavior and language (Damasio, 1994; Saver & Damasio, 1991; Rolls, 1999). To an observer, some patients may seem to lack affect and can speak without passion about experiences that should evoke emotion (Damasio, 1994). Other patients might seem unpredictable, suddenly violent, exhibiting outbursts of sudden anger or sexual attraction, punctuated by periods of apathy and indifference (Rolls, 1999). Although the experience and expression of emotion clearly seems to be dysregulated in these patients,[6] at least some of these problems may be due to impairments in understanding the emotions conveyed through the facial and vocal expressions of others, which also is impaired by OFC lesions (Hornak, Rolls, & Wade, 1996). This apparent perceptual deficit could reflect an inability to evaluate the meaning of external cues that normally provide regulatory feedback.

In everyday life, the OFC/VMFC may help encode and represent information about the shifts and changes in affective or emotional responses that are part and parcel of complex human social life. When we reason using our feelings, we may feel that we are "guessing" which response might be correct because we can't explicitly verbalize the criteria that guide our decisions. Such guessing has recently been shown to activate the VMFC (Elliott, Rees, & Dolan, 1999). Without the OFC/VMFC, the ability to represent affective/emotional responses that constrain the application of social knowledge is missing, leaving an individual adrift in a sea of knowledge without his emotions to anchor him.

Finally, it is important to note that the affective representations mediating OFC/VMFC function are distinct from those stored in semantic memory in that semantic memory is important for knowing how to behave but OFC/VMFC is important for being able to act accordingly. This has been demonstrated most clearly in studies of stimulus–reward reversal in patients with OFC/VMFC lesions. On these tasks patients often report knowing that the stimulus–reward relationship has changed but are unable to alter their behavior accordingly (Rolls et al., 1994; Saver & Damasio, 1991).

Similarly, Damasio (1994) has described a patient with OFC/VMFC lesions who performed normally on laboratory tasks tapping explicit knowledge of appropriate emotional responses to a variety of simple and complex social cues, but was completely unable to make use of this knowledge to make decisions or guide behavior in his everyday life. In both of these cases, the failure to represent the current affective value of a stimulus or choice is necessary to constrain the application of semantic knowledge. This fact was demonstrated elegantly by means of a simple laboratory-based gambling task. Patients with OFC/VMFC lesions didn't win money because they failed to generate anticipatory changes in skin conductance that signaled an impending choice would likely result in monetary loss (Bechara et al., 1996). In essence, these patients could not generate affective reactions to analyses of their response options, and were unable to judge which actions would be most appropriate to take.

Summary

Taken together, the human and animal data suggest that the OFC and VMFC (a) represent the current, contextually specified, emotional/motivational value of an external stimulus and (b) bring response tendencies (whether learned or innate) and the judgment process under the control of this emotional/motivational information. Together, these functions allow us both to alter our emotional responses based on analyses of the current context and to generate affective responses based on these analyses. These two functions form the foundation for the active regulation of emotion and emotion-guided behavior.

SUMMARY AND FUTURE APPLICATIONS OF THE THEORY

Based on our brief review, there is evidence that the distinction between automatic and controlled emotion processing is useful for understanding the way in which different brain systems contribute to the generation and regulation of emotion. In most cases, as depicted in Figure 2.3, automatic emotion processing starts the ball rolling as the amygdala and basal ganglia analyze internal and external inputs for the presence of threats and rewards. If a stimulus is threatening, the amygdala quickly associates the stimulus's perceptual characteristics (shape, sound, etc.) with appropriate (e.g., avoidance) responses. If a stimulus proves rewarding, the basal ganglia is essential for encoding and storing the sequences of thought and action that made that reward possible. These types of activation are likely ongoing and ubiquitous within an individual, constituting the core affective life of that individual (Russell & Feldman Barrett, 1999). Core affect varies in intensity, and a person is always in some state of core affect. Core affect becomes directed into an emotional episode when the automatic activation of semantic emotion knowledge attributes this affect to an object. In a bottom–up fashion, complex emotion knowledge stored in semantic memory provides information about the identity of the attributed object, its meaning, its associates, and other possible responses to it.

Controlled emotion processing begins when the anterior cingulate signals the presence of a discrepancy (e.g., between competing approach and avoidance tendencies), a degree of uncertainty, or a violated expectancy. These signals indicate that emotion knowledge may need to be deployed to consciously transform core affect into an emotion or that the trajectory of an ongoing emotional response (initiated via automatic knowledge activation) may be in need of regulation or alteration. The OFC and VMFC are essential for computing the current affective value of an external stimulus, taking into account changing reinforcement contingencies and situational contexts that may dictate that the affective meaning of that stimulus has changed (e.g., what once was positive may now be aversive). These compu-

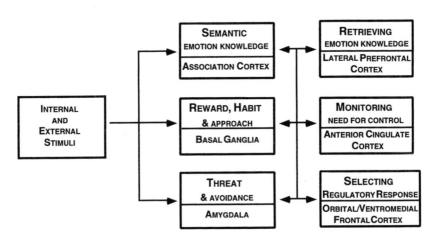

FIGURE 2.3. Flowchart showing the flow of information between different brain structures used for emotion processing. Internal (e.g., body sensations, images, and thoughts) and external (faces, tones of voice, words, actions, etc.) stimuli are processed by three systems that each process a specific type of emotion-related information. Once representations in each system are activated they can influence behavior and experience automatically. The responses generated by these activated representations can influence deliberative, consciously guided behavior through the ACC, OFC, and VMFC. These systems enable an individual to guide choices or direct attention using his or her current feelings about an object or stimulus. See text for details.

tations are essential for guiding decision making, inhibiting prepotent emotional responses, and activating appropriate physiological responses.

Also important for controlled emotion processing is deliberate access to semantic memory and searches of it. Retrieval of emotion knowledge aids in labeling and redirecting emotional responses, making it easier to select emotion regulatory strategies. The effortful application of emotion knowledge may thus serve a regulatory function because the way in which we interpret and draw inferences about the meaning of our current affective responses may change them. Although areas of lateral prefrontal cortex are used to retrieve and manipulate semantic information online, it is not yet clear how those brain regions or others mediate the application of this knowledge to the understanding of affective states. Recent studies have suggested that related regions on the medial surface of the frontal lobes may be important for making such attributions about internal states (Lane, Fink, et al., 1997; Lane, Reiman, Ahern, & Schwartz, 1997).

It is important to note that controlled emotion processing influences both emotion generation and regulation. Any act of regulation necessarily generates a new emotional response. Each time an emotion is inhibited, labeled, or reappraised, the input to the network of emotion processing systems changes and the emotional response that emerges therefore also is changed (i.e., knowledge and its associated language does not just represent the emotion but can also transform it). The term controlled emotion processing intentionally blurs the distinction between generation and regulation partly because we believe the line often is difficult to draw.

NEW DIRECTIONS FOR EMOTION RESEARCH

This chapter began by contrasting neuroscience and psychological perspectives on emotion, and highlighted the different questions that each discipline traditionally has asked about what emotions are and how they operate. Whereas neuroscience research has studied simple and universal forms of emotional behavior so that they may be related to brain function, social psychologists have sought to identify how and why we experience and express more complex blends of emotions in situations more like those we encounter every day. The primary aim of this chapter has been to show how the gap between these two approaches can be bridged by a theory that focuses on the processes that give rise to emotion. The level of information processing is a natural bridging point for low-level analyses of neural systems and high-level analyses of emotional experience and behavior.

We believe that currently available neuroscience data support our account of emotion generation and regulation in terms of the interaction between automatic and controlled processing. However, our review falls short of explaining exactly how the neural systems that instantiate these processes interact to produce many of the phenomena that interest psychologists the most. Indeed, our theory posits that automatic and controlled processes give rise to phenomena such as emotion suppression and reappraisal, the differentiation of blends of emotion, and the interaction of emotion and cognition (Forgas, 1995; Schwarz & Clore, 1988). Unfortunately, we provide little hard data that the neural systems we identify as automatic or controlled emotion processors are involved in these behaviors. The reason for this shortcoming is clear: until very recently, investigations of the brain bases for emotion have been conducted exclusively by neuroscientists pursuing a research agenda that does not cater directly to the tastes of psychologists.

A consequence of the neuroscience approach is that the vast majority of research on the neural basis of emotion has employed simple stimuli (e.g., affective pictures and words or pleasant or unpleasant physical stimulation) in carefully controlled situations. In these studies the appraisal of emotional significance is predetermined and controlled by the experimenter and does not model the way in which emotion appraisals are determined and modulated by context and the meaning of a stimulus to an individual. By limiting the range and kinds of motivational and social relevance of the stimuli used to study emotion, this research has provided information about only a limited class of emotion appraisals that involve clearly positive or negative and arousing stimuli. In essence, this research treats emotion as a property of stimuli that is perceived by individuals, rather than as an interactive process determined by the significance of that stimulus to an individual at a given moment.

Our message is that future neuroscience research on emotion should be guided by theories of the processes used to encode and represent emotional information and the neural systems that instantiate them. Although this may seem obvious to some, it is important to emphasize that this has not been the approach guiding past research. On the one hand, neurologists and neuropsychologists typically correlate locations of brain lesions with deficits in the identification or expression of verbal or nonverbal emotional stimuli (see, e.g., Borod, 1992). On the other hand, neuroimagers correlate areas of metabolic activation with either the presentation of similar stimuli or the presence of emotion disorders (see, e.g., George et al., 1995; Rauch et al., 1996). The problem with this approach is that these correlations don't tell us very much about *why* particular systems are active and what this activation means.

Testing and Applying Theory

We propose that the distinction between automatic and controlled processes used here can serve as a foundation for research with a strong theoretical orientation. From this perspective, research should investigate not just what kinds of stimuli activate different brain systems but what processes each system carries out, in what situations those processes are used, and how different processes interact. To illustrate the way in which our theory can facilitate this process and be tested at the same time, we now consider the way in which it can illuminate four domains of emotion research.

Emotion Generation

An enduring question about the generation of emotional responses is why different individuals experience different emotions. Our theory suggests that this question can be addressed at multiple levels of analysis. As discussed earlier, one could determine whether individuals who experience complex blends of emotions do so because of automatic processes that effortlessly initiate a nuanced response, controlled processes that deliberatively build a complex response, or some combination of the two. By knowing which types of processing are associated with which neural systems, neuroscience data can be used to address this question. Neuroimaging studies could, for example, indicate whether the amygdala and basal ganglia or the anterior cingulate and prefrontal cortices are activated when individuals report emotional experiences of differing complexity. Such studies could also address related questions, such as determining whether individual differences in the ability to articulate emotions are characterized by dysfunction in one or more brain systems.

A first step in this direction was taken in a recent study that showed the ability to complexly express and understand emotional states verbally is correlated with activation of a rostral region of the ACC (Lane et al., 1998). The ACC-based evaluation system likely interacts with other prefrontal brain areas to control the conscious use of information about our emotional states, but the exact way in which this happens remains to be elucidated. By designing studies to test theoretical predictions about the neural systems used to generate emotion, research offers a twofold benefit: it simultaneously allows us to test theories about the processes involved in emotion and informs us about the behaviors in which particular neural systems participate.

Emotion Regulation

The study of emotion regulation is concerned with how, why, and when we change what we do and think in order to change the way we feel. Current interest centers on the efficacy and consequences of adopting particular regulatory strategies, such as emotion suppression, reappraisal, or the retrieval of mood-congruent or -incongruent memories (for a review, see Gross,

1998). From our perspective, research on the neurofunctional bases of these processes should not be limited to drawing inferences based on studies of related phenomena such as extinction or reversal learning. Rather, studies should directly investigate the neural systems involved in these phenomena, taking into account the theoretical perspective advanced here.

For example, neuroimaging studies or studies of lesion patients could determine whether emotion suppression involves the ACC, OFC, and VMFC, as our theory would predict. Other regulatory strategies, such as reappraising the meaning of an emotionally evocative stimulus, should involve lateral frontal areas used to access information in semantic memory. The study of emotion regulation also brings to the fore the question of how controlled emotion processing influences automatic emotion processing. Suppression and reappraisal might exert their effects at a low level by "turning off" automatic processing systems such as those involving the amygdala and basal ganglia, or they might exert their effects at a high level, without influencing automatic processing systems at all. Future work will undoubtedly address these issues.

Relation between Emotion and Cognition

Many contemporary theorists make a distinction between emotion and cognition. From our perspective, the separation of cognition and emotion may depend upon one's level of analysis. The emotion–cognition distinction seems quite useful for understanding high-level phenomena that involve descriptions of phenomenal experience or behavior that can be clearly labeled as emotional (e.g., feeling and acting afraid) or nonemotional (e.g., giving the meaning of a word). But as we move down levels of analysis, the distinction begins to blur. At the level of information processing mechanisms, it often is not clear whether a given process serves a purely emotional or cognitive function because it may be involved in phenomena that may be labeled emotional or cognitive at a higher level. The evaluative/monitoring function carried out by the ACC is a good example: whether one is retrieving a word meaning or running from a bear, it is important to determine whether the current course of action needs to be changed. The blurring and separation of affect and cognition continues at the neural level of analysis. Some brain structures, such as the ACC, carry out computational processes that may be important for all forms of behavior, whereas others, such as the amygdala, seem to be important only for analyzing affective stimuli.

This discussion highlights the crux of the problem: what criteria do we use to distinguish emotion and cognition? Is the distinction experiential, behavioral, computational, or neural? Is the presence of affective feelings or behavior enough even though activity of putatively emotion processing brain systems cannot be detected? Alternatively, should the activation of the amygdala be sufficient to indicate emotion even if the individual is not consciously experiencing emotional feelings? These questions may not have clear answers, and many definitions of emotion resolve the issue by describing a set of criteria all or some of which are necessary constituents of an affective state or emotion episode. It is interesting to note that psychologists seldom debate definitions of cognition, which may be similarly difficult to provide. Indeed, definitions of cognition often turn upon the use of mental representations to mediate the link between responses and behavior. By that definition, many instances of emotion are also instances of cognition.

Definitions of Emotion

Our theoretical approach also may speak to controversies about the proper way to distinguish emotions and moods, or between different kinds of emotional states. The two most prominent proposals posit either a discrete set of distinct, universal affects that are innate, language free, and defined by physiology (see, e.g., Ekman, 1993; Izard, 1977) or a constructed set of social categories that are culturally relative (see, e.g., Averill, 1980; Shweder, 1993). The apparent conflict in this distinction, which has roiled emotion research for decades, may come from the fact that most psychologists formulate emotion from one level of analysis while failing to take the others into consideration. It seems likely that a given neural structure may be involved in more than one kind of emotional response, and it is unlikely that there will be simple one-to-one mappings between a single brain system and any one emotion or component of emotion (i.e., there are no centers for happiness, sadness, or anger in the brain). Furthermore, while emotion concepts and their associated semantic knowledge are important, they are probably not sufficient in and of themselves to constitute an emotional response (although it is conceivable that an emotional response could begin with the activation of this knowledge). Core affect associated with the more automatic processes of the amygdala and basal ganglia are probably necessary for the emergence of a true emotional response.

By integrating theory and research across multiple levels of analysis, our theory suggests that neither perspective is precisely correct. In the broadest context, emotional experiences are not just pure cognitive constructions; nor are they biological universals. Rather, they emerge from a constellation of neurophysiological events across different computational systems differing in degrees of automaticity or controlled processing. The phenomena we typically identify as emotions, that is, anger, sadness, fear, guilt, and so on, are mediated by culture in that discrete emotion concepts and associated knowledge are imposed, either automatically or deliberately, on the more basic elements of pleasant or unpleasant core affect.

A Social Cognitive Neuroscience Approach

In closing, we note that the integration of the neural, information-processing, and behavioral–phenomenological levels of analysis in the study of emotion is an example of an emerging *social cognitive neuroscience approach*. This approach emphasizes that information about the structure and function of the brain systems used for emotion is particularly useful for constraining theories about the relationships between the cognitive/process and behavioral/phenomenological levels of analysis (see Lieberman, 2000; Lieberman, Ochsner, Gilbert, & Schacter, in press; Ochsner & Kosslyn, 1999; Ochsner & Lieberman, 2000; Ochsner & Schacter, 2000). Any theory of emotion should make sense of the complexity of experience and expression observed at the social–interpersonal level in terms of the neural information-processing mechanisms that give rise to these behaviors and experiences. This approach has been our implicit guide throughout this chapter.

CONCLUSIONS

The interaction of automatic and deliberative processing can account for a wide range of emotional phenomena. We humans experience emotion and alter our behavior not only in the pursuit of basic needs to eat, have sex, make friends, or avoid pain. We use our feelings en route to making all kinds of decisions never faced by our ancestors or biological cousins, and perhaps more importantly, we have the ability to deliberately reason about the nature and meaning of our feelings as we make each choice. Because our feelings don't come with explanations, the outcome of this controlled process can have profound consequences in the short and long term. Indeed, in many circumstances it behooves us to figure out whether we're angry or guilty, whether we're sad or frightened, and whether we'll continue to feel that way in the future.

It is our contention that neuroscience research on emotion should address these abilities in full. Only by testing hypotheses about the relationships between socially relevant emotion appraisals, their mediating processes, and their neural substrates will future research close the gap between psychological approaches to emotion and neuroscience descriptions of the brain.

ACKNOWLEDGMENTS

Completion of this chapter was supported by Fellowship No. 97-25 from the McDonnell Pew Foundation awarded to Kevin N. Ochsner and Grant No. SBR-9727896 from the National Science Foundation to Lisa Feldman Barrett. We thank Matthew D. Lieberman and Richard D. Lane for their helpful discussion of relevant issues.

NOTES

1. For comprehensive reviews of the neuroscience literature on emotion, see Gray and McNaughton (1995), LeDoux (1996), Panksepp (1998), and Rolls (1999).
2. More generally, studies have shown that a variety of stimuli with acquired threat value activate the amygdala, including presentation of disgust or fear faces (Morris et al., 1996, 1998), vocal expressions of fear and disgust (Phillips et al., 1998), aversive odors (Zald & Pardo, 1997), negatively valenced photos (Irwin et al., 1996; Lane, Fink, et al., 1997; Taylor et al., 1998), and stimuli that evoke symptoms in psychiatric populations (see, e.g., Birbaumer et al., 1998; Rauch et al., 1995; Shin et al., 1997). A few studies have failed to show amygdala activation during perception of negative stimuli, although the reasons why may differ in each case and are not entirely clear (see, e.g., Canli et al., 1998; see also Adolphs, 1999, for a discussion). Neuropsychological studies also support the importance of the amygdala in the perception of threat-related facial expressions by demonstrating that amygdala lesions will disrupt recognition of expressions of disgust, surprise, and especially fear but will not disrupt perception of facial identity (Adolphs et al., 1994; Calder, Young, Rowland, & Perrett, 1996; Young, Aggleton, Hellawell, & Johnson, 1995).
3. For example, damage to basal ganglia can disrupt the normal sequence of grooming in a rat (Berridge & Whishaw, 1992) or the ability to know what comes next when we are making dinner or doing our job (Caine, Hunt, Weingartner, & Ebert, 1978).
4. The evaluative monitoring function of ACC is required any time controlled or executive processing is needed for task performance. This means that ACC activation should be found anytime a task requires (a) withholding a prepotent response or mediating competition between multiple possible responses, (b) selecting novel or difficult cognitive or behavioral responses, (c) planning and decision making, or (d) correcting erroneous responses (Botvinick, Braver, Carter, Barch, & Cohen, 1999; Posner & DiGirolamo, 1998; Shallice & Burgess, 1993). ACC activation has been observed in all of the following situations (Posner & DiGirolamo, 1998): when one's attention must be divided among many stimuli (Corbetta, Miezin, Dobmeyer, Shulman, & Petersen, 1991); when one is deciding if named animals are dangerous (Petersen, Fox, Posner, Mintun, & Raichle, 1988); when one is generating multipart mental images (Kosslyn et al., 1993); when one is generating words from single letter cues (Phelps, Hyder, Blamire, & Shulman, 1997) or word stems (Buckner et al., 1995); when one is generating word meanings (Petersen, Fox, Posner, Mintun, & Raichle, 1990; Tulving et al., 1994); when one is generating hypotheses (Elliott & Dolan, 1998); when one is spontaneously generating random finger or hand movements (Dieber et al., 1991); while one is holding information in mind during working memory tasks (Petit, Courtney, Ungerleider, & Haxby, 1998); during recognition tasks (Taylor et al., 1998); when one is perceiving stimuli that have been degraded perceptually (Barch et al., 1997); and when a prepared response must be withheld, as in the Stroop task (Bench, Frith, Grasby, & Friston, 1993).
5. The sensitivity of OFC to changes in reinforcement contingencies may be quite general: a recent fMRI study showed OFC activity when an expected visual stim-

ulus failed to appear in a cued location (Nobre, Coull, Frith, & Mesulam, 1999). This result suggests that OFC neurons are sensitive not just to the relationship of stimuli to external rewards but to their relationship with internally generated expectations. OFC activation following violations of expectation could be due to the elicitation of a negative affective response to the violation; it could be due to inhibition of a prepared response to the expected target (Krams, Rushworth, Deiber, Frackowiak, & Passingham, 1998), or it could be due to interference tasks that require inhibition of habitual responses (e.g., the Stroop task; Beauregard et al., 1997). Withholding inappropriate responses could also induce activation of lateral parts of the OFC during retrieval of memories of words (Paradiso et al., 1997).

6. OFC/VMFC also has been associated with emotion dysregulation in psychiatric patients. For example, heightened OFC/VMFC activity has been found during symptom provocation in patients with anxiety disorders, including posttraumatic stress disorder (PTSD), obsessive–compulsive disorder (OCD), and simple phobia (Breiter et al., 1996; Rauch, Savage, Alpert, Fischman, & Jenike, 1997; Rauch, Savage, Alpert, Miguel et al., 1995; Rauch, van der Kolk, Fisler, & Alpert, 1996; Shin et al., 1997). Recently, a posterior area of the VMFC immediately inferior to the genu of the corpus callosum has been associated with unipolar and bipolar depression, showing heightened activity during episodes of mania and decreases during bouts of depression (Drevets, Price, Simpson, & Todd, 1997). The abnormal activity normalizes when symptoms remit, and similar findings have been obtained in OCD patients whose elevated OFC activity normalizes following successful drug or behavior therapy (see, e.g., Saxena et al., 1999). Although consistent with the involvement of OFC and VMFC in emotion, the data from just about every one of these studies is ambiguous. It is not clear whether the symptom-related neural activity indicates an abnormal neural system whose dysfunction produces the disorder, on the one hand, or the use of a normally functioning system to regulate abnormal behavior and experience generated by some other system, on the other.

REFERENCES

Adolphs, R. (1999). The human amygdala and emotion. *The Neuroscientist, 5*, 125–137.

Adolphs, R., Lee, G. P., Tranel, D., & Damasio, A. R. (1997). Bilateral damage to the human amygdala early in life impairs knowledge of emotional arousal. *Society for Neuroscience Abstracts, 23*, 1582.

Adolphs, R., Russell, J. A., & Tranel, D. (1999). A role for the human amygdala in recognizing emotional arousal. *Psychological Science, 10*, 167–171.

Adolphs, R., Tranel, D., & Damasio, A. R. (1998). The amygdala in human social judgment. *Nature, 393*, 470–474.

Adolphs, R., Tranel, D., Damasio, H., & Damasio, A. (1994). Impaired recognition of emotion in facial expressions following bilateral damage to the human amygdala. *Nature, 372*, 669–672.

Aggleton, J. P. (Ed.). (1992). *The amygdala: Neurobiological aspects of emotion, memory, and mental dysfunction*. New York: Wiley-Liss.

Alexander, G. E., Crutcher, M. D., & DeLong, M. A. (1990). Basal ganglia-thalamocortical circuits: Parallel substrates for motor, oculomotor, "prefrontal" and "limbic" functions. In H. B. M. Uylings, C. G. Van Eden, J. P. C. De Bruin, M. A. Corner, & M. G. P. Feenstra (Eds.), *Progress in brain research* (Vol. 85, pp. 119–146). New York: Elsevier.

Andersen, S. M., Spielman, L. A., & Bargh, J. A. (1992). Future-event schemas and certainty about the future: Automaticity in depressives' future-event predictions. *Journal of Personality and Social Psychology, 63,* 711–723.

Anderson, A. K., & Phelps, E. A. (1998). Intact recognition of vocal expressions of fear following bilateral lesions of the human amygdala. *Neuroreport, 9,* 3607–3613.

Averill, J. R. (1980). A constructivist view of emotion. In R. Plutchik & H. Kellerman (Eds.), *Theories of emotion* (Vol. 1, pp. 305–340). New York: Academic Press.

Badgaiyan, R. D., & Posner, M. I. (1997). Mapping the cingulate cortex in response selection and monitoring. *Neuroimage, 7,* 255–260.

Baer, L., Rauch, S. L., Ballantine, H. T., Martuza, R., Cosgrove, R., Cassem, E., Giriunas, I., Manzo, P., & Jenike, M. A. (1995). Cingulotomy for intractable obsessive–compulsive disorder: Prospective long-term follow-up of 18 patients. *Archives of General Psychiatry, 52,* 384–392.

Baker, S. C., Frith, C. D., & Dolan, R. J. (1997). The interaction between mood and cognitive function studied with PET. *Psychological Medicine, 27,* 565–578.

Ballantine, H. T., Bouckons, A. J., Thomas, E. K., & Giriunas, I. E. (1987). Treatment of psychiatric illness by stereotactic cingulotomy. *Biological Psychiatry, 22,* 807–819.

Ballantine, H. T., Flanagan, N. B., Cassidy, W. L., & Marino, R. (1967). Stereotaxic anterior cingulotomy for neuropsychiatric illness and intractable pain. *Journal of Neurosurgery, 26,* 488–495.

Barch, D. M., Braver, T. S., Nystrom, L. E., Forman, S. D., Noll, D. C., & Cohen, J. D. (1997). Dissociating working memory from task difficulty in human prefrontal cortex. *Neuropsychologia, 35,* 1373–1380.

Bargh, J. A. (1990). Auto-motives: Preconscious determinants of social interaction. In E. T. Higgins & R. M. Sorrentino (Eds.), *Handbook of motivation and cognition* (Vol. 2, pp. 93–130). New York: Guilford Press.

Bargh, J. A., Chaiken, S., Govender, R., & Pratto, F. (1992). The generality of the automatic attitude activation effect. *Journal of Personality and Social Psychology, 62,* 893–912.

Bargh, J. A., Chaiken, S., Raymond, P., & Hymes, C. (1996). The automatic evaluation effect: Unconditional automatic attitude activation with a pronunciation task. *Journal of Experimental Social Psychology, 32,* 104–128.

Bargh, J. A., & Tota, M. E. (1988). Context-dependent automatic processing in depression: Accessibility of negative constructs with regard to self but not others. *Journal of Personality and Social Psychology, 54,* 925–939.

Beauregard, M., Chertkow, H., Bub, D., Murtha, S., Dixon, R., & Evans, A. (1997). The neural substrate for concrete, abstracts, and emotional word lexica: A positron emission tomography word study. *Journal of Cognitive Neuroscience, 9,* 441–461.

Beauregard, M., Leroux, J.-M., Bergman, S., Arzoumanian, Y., Beaudoin, G., Bourgouin, P., & Stip, E. (1998). The functional neuroanatomy of major depression: An fMRI study using an emotional activation paradigm. *Neuroreport, 9*, 3253–3258.

Bechara, A., Damasio, H., Tranel, D., & Damasio, A. R. (1996). Failure to respond autonomically to anticipated future outcomes following damage to prefrontal cortex. *Cerebral Cortex, 6*, 215–225.

Bechara, A., Tranel, D., Damasio, H., & Adolphs, R. (1995). Double dissociation of conditioning and declarative knowledge relative to the amygdala and hippocampus in humans. *Science, 269*, 1115–1118.

Bench, C. J., Frith, C. D, Grasby, P. M., & Friston, K. J. (1993). Investigations of the functional anatomy of attention using the Stroop test. *Neuropsychologia, 31*, 907–922.

Berridge, K. C., & Robinson, T. E. (1998). What is the role of dopamine in reward: Hedonic impact, reward learning, or incentive salience? *Brain Research Reviews, 28*, 309–369.

Berridge, K. C., & Whishaw, I. Q. (1992). Cortex, striatum and cerebellum: Control of serial order in a grooming sequence. *Experimental Brain Research, 90*, 275–290.

Birbaumer, N., Grodd, W., Diedrich, O., Klose, U., Erb, M., Lotze, M., Schneider, F., Weiss, U., & Flor, H. (1998). fMRI reveals amygdala activation to human faces in social phobics. *Neuroreport, 9*, 1223–1226.

Borod, J. C. (1992). Interhemispheric and intrahemispheric control of emotion: A focus on unilateral brain damage. *Journal of Consulting and Clinical Psychology, 60*, 339–348.

Botvinick, M. M., Braver, T. S., Carter, C. S., Barch, D. M., & Cohen, J. D. (1999). *Evaluating the demand for control: Anterior cingulate cortex and cross-talk monitoring* [Technical report]. Pittsburgh, PA: Carnegie Mellon University.

Bouton, M. E. (1994). Context, ambiguity, and classical conditioning. *Current Directions in Psychological Science, 3*, 49–53.

Bower, G. H., & Forgas, J. P. (2000). Affect, memory, and social cognition. In E. E. Eich (Ed.), *Cognition and emotion*. New York: Oxford University Press.

Bradley, M. M. (1994). Emotional memory: A dimensional analysis. In S. H. M. van Goozen, N. E. Van De Poll, & J. A. Sergeant (Eds.), *Emotions: Essays on emotion theory* (pp. 97–134). Hillsdale, NJ: Erlbaum.

Breiter, H. C., Etcoff, N. L., & Whalen, P. J. (1996). Response and habituation of the human amygdala during visual processing of facial expressions. *Neuron, 17*, 875–887.

Breiter, H. C., & Rosen, B. R. (1999). Functional magnetic resonance imaging of brain reward circuitry in the human. *Annals of the New York Academy of Sciences, 877*, 523–547.

Buchanan, S. L., & Powell, D. A. (1993). Cingulothalamic and prefrontal control of autonomic function. In B. A. Vogt & M. Gabriel (Eds.), *Neurobiology of cingulate cortex and limbic thalamus: A comprehensive handbook* (pp. 381–414). Boston: Birkhaeuser.

Buckner, R. L., Petersen, S. E., Ojemann, J. G., Miezin, F. M., Squire, L. R., & Raichle, M. E. (1995). Functional anatomical studies of explicit and implicit memory retrieval tasks. *Journal of Neuroscience, 15*, 12–29.

Cahill, L., Babinsky, R., Markowitsch, H. J., & McGaugh, J. L. (1995). The amygdala and emotional memory. *Nature, 377*, 295–296.

Cahill, L., Haier, R. J., Fallon, J., Alkire, M., Tang, C., Keator, D., Wu, J., & McGaugh, J. L. (1996). Amygdala activity at encoding correlated with long-term, free recall of emotional information. *Proceedings of the National Academy of Sciences USA, 93*, 8016–8021.

Cahill, L., & McGaugh, J. L. (1990). Amygdaloid complex lesions differentially affect retention of tasks using appetitive and aversive reinforcement. *Behavioral Neuroscience, 104*, 532–543.

Cahill, L., Prins, B., Weber, M., & McGaugh, J. L. (1994). ß-adrenergic activation and memory for emotional events. *Nature, 371*, 702–704.

Caine, E., Hunt, R., Weingartner, H., & Ebert, M. (1978). Huntington's dementia: Clinical and neuropsychological features. *Archives of General Psychiatry, 35*, 377–384.

Calder, A. J., Young, A. W., Rowland, D., & Perrett, D. I. (1996). Facial emotion recognition after bilateral amygdala damage: Differentially severe impairment of fear. *Cognitive Neuropsychology, 13*, 699–745.

Canli, T., Desmond, J. E., Zhao, Z., Glover, G., & Gabrieli, J. D. E. (1998). Hemispheric asymmetry for emotional stimuli detected with fMRI. *Neuroreport, 9*, 3233–3239.

Carter, C. S., Braver, T. S, Barch, D. M., Botvinick, M. M., Noll, D., & Cohen, J. D. (1998). Anterior cingulate cortex, error detection, and the online monitoring of performance. *Science, 280*, 747–749.

Chaiken, S., & Bargh, J. A. (1993). Occurrence versus moderation of the automatic attitude activation effect: Reply to Fazio. *Journal of Personality and Social Psychology, 64*, 759–765.

Chaiken, S., & Trope, Y. (1999). *Dual-process theories in social psychology.* New York: Guilford Press.

Chartrand, T. L., & Bargh, J. A. (1996). Automatic activation of impression formation and memorization goals: Nonconscious goal priming reproduces effects of explicit task instructions. *Journal of Personality and Social Psychology, 71*, 464–478.

Cioffi, D. (1993). Sensate body, directive mind: Physical sensations and mental control. In D. M. Wegner & J. W. Pennebaker (Eds.), *Handbook of mental control* (pp. 410–442). Englewood Cliffs, NJ: Prentice-Hall.

Cohen, M. J., Riccio, C. A., & Flannery, A. M. (1994). Expressive aprosodia following stroke to the right basal ganglia: A case report. *Neuropsychology, 8*, 242–245.

Cohen, R. A., Kaplan, R. F., Meadows, M.-E., & Wilkinson, H. (1994). Habituation and sensitization of the orienting response following bilateral anterior cingulotomy. *Neuropsychologia, 32*, 609–617.

Cohen, R. A., Kaplan, R. F., Moser, D. J., Jenkins, M. A., & Wilkinson, H. (1999). Impairments of attention after cingulotomy. *Neurology, 53*, 819–824.

Corbetta, M., Miezin, F. M., Dobmeyer, S., Shulman, G. L., & Petersen, S. E. (1991). Selective and divided attention during visual discriminations of shape, color, and speed: Functional anatomy by positron emission tomography. *Journal of Neuroscience, 11*, 2383–2402.

Corkin, S. (1980). A prospective study of cingulotomy. In E. Valenstein (Ed.), *The psychosurgery debate* (pp. 164–204). San Francisco: Freeman.

Craig, A. D., Reiman, E. M., Evans, A., & Bushnell, M. C. (1996). Functional imaging of an illusion of pain. *Nature, 384,* 258–260.

Damasio, A. R. (1994). *Descartes' error: Emotion, reason, and the human brain.* New York: Putnam.

Damasio, A. R., Tranel, D., & Damasio, H. (1990). Individuals with sociopathic behavior caused by frontal damage fail to respond autonomically to social stimuli. *Behavioural Brain Research, 41,* 81–94.

Damasio, A. R., & Van Hoesen, G. W. (1986). Emotional disturbances associated with focal lesions of the limbic frontal lobe. In K. H. Heilman & P. Satz (Eds.), *Neuropsychology of human emotion* (pp. 85–110). New York: Guilford Press.

Davis, K. D., Taylor, S. J., Crawley, A. P., Wood, M. L., & Mikulis, D. J. (1997). Functional MRI of pain- and attention-related activations in the human cingulate cortex. *Journal of Neurophysiology, 77,* 3370–3380.

Dehaene, S., Posner, M. I., & Tucker, D. M. (1994). Localization of a neural system for error detection and compensation. *Psychological Science, 5,* 303–305.

Devinsky, O., Morrell, M. J., & Vogt, B. A. (1995). Contributions of anterior cingulate cortex to behaviour. *Brain, 118,* 279–306.

Dieber, M.-P., Passingham, R. E., Colebatch, J. G., Friston, K. J., Nixon, P. D., & Frackowiak, R. S. J. (1991). Cortical areas and the selection of movement: A study with positron emission tomography. *Experimental Brain Research, 84,* 393–402.

Drevets, W. C., Price, J. L., Simpson, J. R., Jr., & Todd, R. D. (1997). Subgenual prefrontal cortex abnormalities in mood disorders. *Nature, 386,* 824–827.

Drevets, W. C., & Raichle, M. E. (1998). Reciprocal suppression of regional cerebral blood flow during emotional versus higher cognitive processes: Implications for interactions between emotion and cognition. *Cognition and Emotion, 12,* 353–385.

Drevets, W. C., Videen, T. O., Price, J. L., & Preskorn, S. H. (1992). A functional anatomical study of unipolar depression. *Journal of Neuroscience, 12,* 3628–3641.

Dum, R. P., & Strick, P. L. (1993). Cingulate motor areas. In B. A. Vogt & M. Gabriel (Eds.), *Neurobiology of cingulate cortex and limbic thalamus: A comprehensive handbook* (pp. 415–444). Boston: Birkhaeuser.

Ekman, P. (1993). Facial expression and emotion. *American Psychologist, 48,* 384–392.

Ekman, P., & Davidson, R. J. (1994). *The nature of emotion: Fundamental questions.* New York: Oxford University Press.

Elliott, R., & Dolan, R. J. (1998). Activation of different anterior cingulate foci in association with hypothesis testing and response selection. *Neuroimage, 8,* 17–29.

Elliott, R., Rees, G., & Dolan, R. J. (1999). Ventromedial prefrontal cortex mediates guessing. *Neuropsychologia, 37,* 403–411.

Everitt, B. J., & Robbins, T. W. (1992). Amygdala–ventral striatal interactions and reward-related processes. In J. P. Aggleton (Ed.), *The amygdala: Neurobiological aspects of emotion, memory, and mental dysfunction* (pp. 401–429). New York: Wiley-Liss.

Fazio, R. H., Sanbonmatsu, D. M., Powell, M. C., & Kardes, F. R. (1986). On the automatic activation of attitudes. *Journal of Personality and Social Psychology, 50,* 229–238.

Fehr, B., & Russell, J. A. (1984). The concept of emotion viewed from a prototype perspective. *Journal of Experimental Psychology: General, 113,* 464–486.

Feldman, L. A. (1995). Valence focus and arousal focus: Individual differences in the structure of affective experience. *Journal of Personality and Social Psychology, 69,* 153–166.

Feldman Barrett, L. (1998). Discrete emotions or dimensions? The role of valence focus and arousal focus. *Cognition and Emotion, 12,* 579–599.

Fiske, S. T., & Taylor, S. E. (1991). *Social cognition* (2nd ed.). New York: McGraw-Hill.

Forgas, J. P. (1995). Mood and judgment: The affect infusion model (AIM). *Psychological Bulletin, 117,* 39–66.

Francis, S., Rolls, E. T., Bowtell, R., McGlone, F., O'Doherty, J., Browning, A., Clare, S., & Smith, E. (1999). The representation of pleasant touch in the brain and its relationship with taste and olfactory areas. *Neuroreport, 10,* 453–459.

Fredrikson, M., Furmark, T., Olsson, M. T., Fischer, H., Andersson, J., & Langstroem, B. (1998). Functional neuroanatomical correlates of electrodermal activity: A positron emission tomographic study. *Psychophysiology, 35,* 179–185.

Fredrikson, M., Wik, G., Fischer, H., & Andersson, J. (1995). Affective and attentive neural networks in humans: A PET study of Pavlovian conditioning. *Neuroreport, 7,* 97–101.

Freedman, M., Black, S., Ebert, P., & Binns, M. (1998). Orbitofrontal function, object alternation and perserveration. *Cerebral Cortex, 8,* 18–27.

Frijda, N. (1986). *The emotions.* Cambridge, UK: Cambridge University Press.

Gabriel, M. (1993) Discriminative avoidance learning: A model system. In B. A. Vogt & M. Gabriel (Eds.), *Neurobiology of cingulate cortex and limbic thalamus: A comprehensive handbook* (pp. 478–526). Boston: Birkhaeuser.

Gehring, W. J., Goss, B., Coles, M. G., Meyer, D. E., & Donhin, E. (1993). A neural system for error detection and compensation. *Psychological Science, 4,* 385–390.

George, M. S., Ketter, T. A., Parekh, B. A., Horowitz, B., Herscovitch, P., & Post, R. M. (1995). Brain activity during transient sadness and happiness in healthy women. *American Journal of Psychiatry, 152,* 341–351.

Goleman, D. (1995). *Emotional intelligence.* New York: Bantam Books.

Gray, J. A., & McNaughton, N. (1995). The neuropsychology of anxiety: Reprise. In D. A. Hope (Ed.), *Nebraska Symposium on Motivation: Vol. 43. Perspectives on anxiety, panic, and fear. Current theory and research in motivation* (pp. 61–134). Lincoln, NE: University of Nebraska Press.

Gross, J. J. (1998). The emerging field of emotion regulation: An integrative review. *Review of General Psychology, 2,* 271–299.

Gross, J. J., & Levenson, R. W. (1993). Emotional suppression: Physiology, self-report, and expressive behavior. *Journal of Personality and Social Psychology, 64,* 970–986.

Hamann, S. B., Ely, T. D., Grafton, S. T., & Kilts, C. D. (1999). Amygdala activity related to enhanced memory for pleasant and aversive stimuli. *Nature Neuroscience, 2,* 289–293.

Harris, P. L., Olthof, T., Terwogt, M., & Hardman, C. E. (1987). Children's understanding of situations that provoke emotion. *International Journal of Behavioral Development, 10,* 319–343.

Hart, A. J., Whalen, P. J., Shin, L. M., McInerney, S. C., & Rauch, S. L. (1999). Differential response in the human amygdala to racial outgroup vs. ingroup stimuli. *Neuroreport, 11,* 563–586.

Hebben, N. (1985). Toward the assessment of clinical pain. In G. M. Aronoff (Ed.), *Evaluation and treatment of chronic pain* (pp. 451–462). Baltimore: Urban & Schwarzenburg.

Henke, P. (1982). The telencephalic limbic system and experimental gastric pathology: A review. *Neuroscience and Biobehavioral Reviews, 6,* 381–390.

Hermans, D., De Houwer, J., & Eelen, P. (1994). The affective priming effect: Automatic activation of evaluative information in memory. *Cognition and Emotion, 8,* 515–533.

Holland, P. C., & Gallagher, M. (1999). Amygdala circuitry in attentional and representational processes. *Trends in Cognitive Sciences, 3,* 65–73.

Hopkins, A. (1994). *Clinical neurology: A modern approach.* New York: Oxford University Press.

Hornak, J., Rolls, E. T., & Wade, D. (1996). Face and voice expression identification in patients with emotional and behavioural changes following ventral frontal lobe damage. *Neuropsychologia, 34,* 247–261.

Houk, J. C., Davis, J. L., & Beiser, D. G. (1995). *Models of information processing in the basal ganglia.* Cambridge, MA: MIT Press.

Irwin, W., Davidson, R. J., Lowe, M. J., Mock, B. J., Sorenson, J. A., & Turski, P. A. (1996). Human amygdala activation detected with echo-planar functional magnetic resonance imaging. *Neuroreport, 7,* 1765–1769.

Izard, C. E. (1977). *Human emotions.* New York: Plenum Press.

Janer, K. W., & Pardo, J. V. (1991). Deficits in selective attention following bilateral anterior cingulotomy. *Journal of Cognitive Neuroscience, 3,* 231–241.

Kosslyn, S. M., Alpert, N. M., Thompson, W. L., Maljkovic, V., Weise, S. B., Chabris, C. F., Hamilton, S. E., & Buonano, F. S. (1993). Visual mental imagery activates topographically organized visual cortex: PET investigations. *Journal of Cognitive Neuroscience, 5,* 263–287.

Kosslyn, S. M., & Koenig, O. (1992). *Wet mind.* New York: Free Press.

Kosslyn, S. M., & Ochsner, K. N. (1994). In search of occipital activation during mental imagery. *Trends in Neurosciences, 17,* 290–292.

Krams, M., Rushworth, M. F., Deiber, M. P., Frackowiak, R. S., & Passingham, R. E. (1998). The preparation, execution and suppression of copied movements in the human brain. *Experimental Brain Research, 120,* 386–398.

LaBar, K. S., Gatenby, J. C., Gore, J. C., LeDoux, J. E., & Phelps, E. A. (1998). Human amygdala activation during conditioned fear acquisition and extinction: A mixed-trial fMRI study. *Neuron, 20,* 937–945.

LaBar, K. S., LeDoux, J. E., Spencer, D. D., & Phelps, E. A. (1995). Impaired fear conditioning following unilateral temporal lobectomy in humans. *Journal of Neuroscience, 15,* 6846–6855.

LaBar, K. S., & Phelps, E. A. (1998). Arousal-mediated memory consolidation. *Psychological Science, 9,* 490–493.

Lane, R. D., Fink, G. R., Chau, P. M.-L., & Dolan, R. J. (1997). Neural activation during selective attention to subjective emotional responses. *Neuroreport, 8,* 3969–3972.

Lane, R. D., Reiman, E. M., Ahern, G. L., & Schwartz, G. E. (1997). Neuroanatomical correlates of happiness, sadness, and disgust. *American Journal of Psychiatry, 154,* 926–933.

Lane, R. D., Reiman, E. M., Axelrod, B., Yun, L.-S., Holmes, A., & Schwartz, G. E. (1998). Neural correlates of levels of emotional awareness: Evidence of an interaction between emotion and attention in the anterior cingulate cortex. *Journal of Cognitive Neuroscience, 10,* 525–535.

Lane, R. D., Reiman, E. M., Bradley, M. M., Lang, P. J., Ahern, G. L., Davidson, R. J., & Schwartz, G. E. (1997). Neuroanatomical correlates of pleasant and unpleasant emotion. *Neuropsychologia, 35,* 1437–1444.

Lane, R. D., & Schwartz, G. E. (1987). Levels of emotional awareness: A cognitive-developmental theory and its application to psychopathology. *American Journal of Psychiatry, 144,* 133–143.

Lazarus, R. S. (1991). *Emotion and adaptation.* New York: Oxford University Press.

LeDoux, J. E. (1996). *The emotional brain: The mysterious underpinnings of emotional life.* New York: Simon & Schuster.

LeDoux, J. E., Romanski, L., & Xagoraris, A. (1989). Indelibility of subcortical emotional memories. *Journal of Cognitive Neuroscience, 1,* 238–243.

Lewis, M., & Haviland, J. M. (Eds.). (1993). *Handbook of emotions.* New York: Guilford Press.

Lieberman, M. D. (2000). Intuition: A social cognitive neuroscience approach. *Psychological Bulletin, 126,* 109–137.

Lieberman, M. D., Ochsner, K. N., Gilbert, D. T., & Schacter, D. L. (in press). Attitude change in amnesia and under cognitive load. *Psychological Science.*

London, E. D., Broussolle, E. P., Links, J. M., Wong, D. F., Cascella, N. G., Dannals, R. F., Sano, M., Herning, R., Snyder, F. R., Rippetoe, L. R., Toung, T. J., Jaffe, J. H., & Wagner, H. N. (1990). Morphine-induced metabolism changes in human brain: Studies with positron emission tomography and [flourine 18] fluorodeoxyglucose. *Archives of General Psychiatry, 47,* 73–81.

MacLeod, C. M. (1991). Half a century of research on the Stroop effect: An integrative review. *Psychological Bulletin, 109,* 163–203.

Markowitsch, H. J., Calabrese, P., Wurker, M., Durwen, H. F., Kessler, J., Babinsky, R., Brechtelsbauer, D., Heuser, L., & Gehlen, W. (1998). The amygdala's contribution to memory: A study of two patients with Urbach-Wiethe disease. *Neuroreport, 5,* 1349–1352.

Markus, H. R., & Kitayama, S. (1991). Culture and the self: Implications for cognition, emotion, and motivation. *Psychological Review, 98,* 224–253.

McClelland, J. L. (1995). Constructive memory and memory distortions: A parallel-distributed processing approach. In D. L. Schacter (Ed.), *Memory distortions: How minds, brains, and societies reconstruct the past* (pp. 69–90). Cambridge, MA: Harvard University Press.

McDonald, R. J., & White, N. M. (1993). A triple dissociation of memory systems: Hippocampus, amygdala, and dorsal striatum. *Behavioral Neuroscience, 107,* 3–22.

McGaugh, J. L., Cahill, L., Parent, M. B., Mesches, M. H., Coleman-Mesches, K., &

Salinas, J. A. (1995). Involvement of the amygdala in the regulation of memory storage. In J. L. McGaugh, F. Bermúdez-Rattoni, & R. A. Prado-Alcalá (Eds.), *Plasticity in the central nervous system: Learning and memory* (pp. 17–39). Mahwah, NJ: Erlbaum.

McPherson, S., & Cummings, J. L. (1996). Neuropsychological aspects of Parkinson's disease and parkinsonism. In I. Grant & K. M. Adams (Eds.), *Neurological assessment of neuropsychiatric disorders* (pp. 288–311). New York: Oxford University Press.

Mesquita, B., & Fridja, N. H. (1992). Cultural variations in emotion. *Psychological Bulletin, 112,* 179–204.

Mishkin, M., & Appenzeller, T. (1987). The anatomy of memory. *Science, 256,* 80–89.

Morgan, M. A., & LeDoux, J. E. (1995). Differential contribution of dorsal and ventral medial prefrontal cortex to the acquisition and extinction of conditioned fear in rats. *Behavioral Neuroscience, 109,* 681–688.

Morris, J. S., Friston, K. J., Buechel, C., Frith, C. D., Young, A. W., Calder, A. J., & Dolan, R. J. (1998). A neuromodulatory role for the human amygdala in processing emotional facial expressions. *Brain, 12,* 47–57.

Morris, J. S., Frith, C. D., Perrett, D. I., Rowland, D., Young, A. W., Calder, A. J., & Dolan, R. J. (1996). A differential neural response in the human amygdala to fearful and happy facial expressions. *Nature, 383,* 812–815.

Morris, J. S., Ohman, A., & Dolan, R. J. (1999). A subcortical pathway to the right amygdala mediating "unseen" fear. *Proceedings of the National Academy of Sciences USA, 96,* 1680–1685.

Nobre, A. C., Coull, J. T., Frith, C. D., & Mesulam, M. M. (1999). Orbitofrontal cortex is activated during breaches of expectation in tasks of visual attention. *Nature Neuroscience, 2,* 11–12.

Ochsner, K. N., & Kosslyn, S. M. (1999). The cognitive neuroscience approach. In D. E. Rumelhart & B. O. Martin (Eds.), *Handbook of cognition and perception. Vol. X: Cognitive science* (pp. 319–365). San Diego, CA: Academic Press.

Ochsner, K. N., Kosslyn, S. M., Cosgrove, G. R., Price, B., Cassem, N., Nierenberg, A., & Rauch, S. (in press). Deficits in visual cognition and attention following bilateral anterior cingulotomy. *Neuropsychologia.*

Ochsner, K. N., & Lieberman, M. D. (2000). *The social cognitive neuroscience approach.* Harvard University, Cambridge, MA. Manuscript submitted for publication.

Ochsner, K. N., & Schacter, D. L. (2000). Constructing the emotional past: A social cognitive neuroscience approach to emotion and memory. In J. C. Borod (Ed.), *The neuropsychology of emotion* (pp. 163–193). New York: Oxford University Press.

Ohman, A. (1988). Preattention processes in the generation of emotions. In V. Hamilton, G. H. Bower, & N. H. Frijda (Eds.), *Cognitive perspectives on emotion and motivation* (Vol. 44, pp. 127–143). Dordrecht, Netherlands: Kluwer.

Panksepp, J. (1998). *Affective neuroscience: The foundations of human and animal emotions.* New York: Oxford University Press.

Paradiso, S., Facorro, B. C., Andreasen, N. C., O'Leary, D. S., Watkins, L. G., Ponto,

L. L. B., & Hichwa, R. D. (1997). Brain activity assessed with PET during recall of word lists and narratives. *Neuroreport, 8*, 3091–3096.

Pennebaker, J. W. (1997). Writing about emotional experiences as a therapeutic process. *Psychological Science, 8*, 162–166.

Petersen, S. E., Fox, P. T., Posner, M. I., Mintun, M., & Raichle, M. E. (1988). Positron emission tomomgraphic studies of the cortical anatomy of single-word processing. *Nature, 331*, 585–589.

Petersen, S. E., Fox, P. T., Posner, M. I., Mintun, M., & Raichle, M. E. (1990). Positron emission tomographic studies of the processing of single words. *Journal of Cognitive Neuroscience, 1*, 153–259.

Posner, M. I., & Rothbart, M. K. (1991). Attentional mechanisms and conscious experience. In A. D. Milner & M. Rugg (Eds.), *The neuropsychology of consciousness* (pp. 91–111). San Diego, CA: Academic Press.

Petit, L., Courtney, S. M., Ungerleider, L. G., & Haxby, J. V. (1998). Sustained activity in the medial wall during working memory delays. *Journal of Neuroscience, 18*, 9429–9437.

Phelps, E. A., Hyder, F., Blamire, A. M., & Shulman, R. G. (1997). fMRI of the prefrontal cortex during overt verbal fluency. *Neuroreport, 8*, 561–565.

Phillips, M. L., Bullmore, E. T., Howard, R., Woodruff, P. W. R., Wright, I. C., Williams, S. C. R., Simmons, A., Andrew, C., Brammer, M., & David, A. S. (1998). Investigation of facial recognition memory and happy and sad facial expression perception: An fMRI study. *Psychiatry Research: Neuroimaging, 83*, 127–138.

Pool, J. L., & Ransohoff, J. (1949). Autonomic effects on stimulating rostral portion of cingulate gyri in man. *Journal of Neurophysiology, 12*, 385–392.

Porro, C. A., Cettolo, V., Francescato, M. P., & Baraldi, P. (1998). Temporal and intensity coding of pain in human cortex. *Journal of Neurophysiology, 80*, 3312–3320.

Posner, M. I., & DiGirolamo, G. J. (1998). Executive attention: Conflict, target detection, and cognitive control. In R. Parasuraman (Ed.), *The attentive brain* (pp. 401–423). Cambridge, MA: MIT Press.

Quigley, K. S., & Feldman Barrett, L. (1999). Emotional learning and mechanisms of intentional psychological change. In J. Brandtstadter & R. M. Lerner (Eds.), *Action and development: Origins and functions of intentional self-development* (pp. 435–464). Thousand Oaks, CA: Sage.

Raichle, M. E. (1997). Automaticity: From reflective to reflexive information processing. In M. Ito & Y. Miyashita (Eds.), *Cognition, computation, and consciousness* (pp. 137–149). Oxford, UK: Oxford University Press.

Rainville, P., Duncan, G. H., Price, D. D., Carrier, B., & Bushnell, M. C. (1997). Pain affect encoded in human anterior cingulate but not somatosensory cortex. *Science, 277*, 968–971.

Rauch, S. L., Savage, C. R., Alpert, N. M., Fischman, A. J., & Jenike, M. A. (1997). The functional neuroanatomy of anxiety: A study of three disorders using positron emission tomography and symptom provocation. *Biological Psychiatry, 42*, 446–452.

Rauch, S. L., Savage, C. R., Alpert, N. M., Miguel, E. C., Baer, L., Fishman, A. J., Manzo, P. A., Moretti, C., & Jenike, M. A. (1995). A positron emission tomographic study of simple phobic symptom provocation. *Archives of General Psychiatry, 52,* 20–28.

Rauch, S. L., Savage, C. R., Brown, H. D., Curran, T., Alpert, N. M., Kendrick, A., Fischman, A. J., & Kosslyn, S. M. (1995). A PET investigation of implicit and explicit sequence learning. *Human Brain Mapping, 3,* 271–286.

Rauch, S. L., van der Kolk, B. A., Fisler, R. E., & Alpert, N. M. (1996). A symptom provocation study of posttraumatic stress disorder using positron emission tomography and script-driven imagery. *Archives of General Psychiatry, 53,* 380–387.

Reiman, E. M., Lane, R. D., Ahern, G. L., & Schwartz, G. E. (1997). Neuroanatomical correlates of externally and internally generated human emotion. *American Journal of Psychiatry, 154,* 918–925.

Robinson, M. D. (1998). Running from William James' bear: A review of preattentive mechanisms and their contributions to emotional experience. *Cognition and Emotion, 12,* 667–696.

Robinson, R. G., & Paradiso, S. (1996). Insights concerning the cerebral basis of emotions based on studies of mood disorders in patients with brain injury. In R. D. Kavanaugh & B. Zimmerberg (Eds.), *Emotion: Interdisciplinary perspectives* (pp. 297–314). Mahwah, NJ: Erlbaum.

Rolls, E. T. (1999). *The brain and emotion.* Oxford, UK: Oxford University Press

Rolls, E. T., Hornak, J., Wade, D., & McGrath, J. (1994). Emotion-related learning in patients with social and emotional changes associated with frontal lobe damage. *Journal of Neurology, Neurosurgery and Psychiatry, 57,* 1518–1524.

Rumelhart, D. E. (1989). The architecture of mind: A connectionist approach. In M. I. Posner (Ed.), *Foundations of cognitive science* (pp. 133–159). Cambridge, MA: MIT Press.

Russell, J. A., & Feldman Barrett, L. (1999). Core affect, prototypical emotional episodes, and other things called emotion: Dissecting the elephant. *Journal of Personality and Social Psychology, 76,* 805–819.

Saarni, C. (1993). Socialization of emotion. In M. Lewis & J. M. Haviland (Eds.), *Handbook of emotions* (pp. 435–446). New York: Guilford Press.

Saver, J. L., & Damasio, A. R. (1991). Preserved access and processing of social knowledge in a patient with acquired sociopathy due to ventromedial frontal damage. *Neuropsychologia, 29,* 1241–1249.

Saxena, S., Brody, A. L., Maidment, K. M., Dunkin, J. J., Colgan, M., Alborzian, S., Phelps, M. E., & Baxter, L. R. (1999). Localized orbitofrontal and subcortical metabolic changes and predictors of response to paroxetine treatment in obsessive–compulsive disorder. *Neuropsychopharmacology, 21,* 683–693.

Schneider, F., Grodd, W., Weiss, U., Klose, U., Mayer, K. R., Naegele, T., & Gur, R. C. (1997). Functional MRI reveals left amygdala activation during emotion. *Psychiatry Research: Neuroimaging, 76,* 75–82.

Schultz, W. (1998). Predictive reward signal of dopamine neurons. *Journal of Neurophysiology, 80,* 1–27.

Schultz, W., Apicella, P., Romo, R., & Scarnati, E. (1995). Context-dependent activity in primate striatum reflecting past and future behavioral events. In J. C. Houk, J. L. Davis, & D. G. Beiser (Eds.), *Models of information processing in the basal ganglia: Computational neuroscience* (pp. 11–27). Cambridge, MA: MIT Press.

Schwarz, N., & Clore, G. L. (1988). How do I feel about it? The informative function of affective states. In K. Fiedler & J. Forgas (Eds.), *Affect, cognition and social behavior* (pp. 44–62). Toronto, Ontario, Canada: Hogrefe.

Shallice, T. (1994). Multiple levels of control processes. In C. Umilta & M. Moscovitch (Eds.), *Attention and performance 15: Conscious and nonconscious information processing* (pp. 395–420). Cambridge, MA: MIT Press.

Shallice, T., & Burgess, P. (1993). Supervisory control of action and thought selection. In A. D. Baddeley & L. Weiskrantz (Eds.), *Attention: Selection, awareness, and control: A tribute to Donald Broadbent* (pp. 171–187). Oxford, UK: Clarendon Press/Oxford University Press.

Shaver, P., Schwartz, J., Kirson, D., & O'Connor, C. (1987). Emotion knowledge: Further exploration of a prototype approach. *Journal of Personality and Social Psychology, 52,* 1061–1086.

Shin, L. M., Kosslyn, S. M., McNally, R. J., Alpert, N. M., Metzger, L. J., Lasko, N. B., Orr, S. P. L., & Pitman, R. K. (1997). Visual imagery and perception in posttraumatic stress disorder: A positron emission tomographic investigation. *Archives of General Psychiatry, 54,* 233–241.

Shulz, W. (1998). Predictive reward signal of dopamine neurons. *Journal of Neurophysiology, 80,* 1–27.

Shweder, R. A. (1993). The cultural psychology of emotions. In M. Lewis & J. M. Haviland (Eds.), *Handbook of emotions* (pp. 417–431). New York: Guilford Press.

Speedie, L. J., Wertman, E., Ta'ir, J., & Heilman, K. M. (1993). Disruption of automatic speech following a right basal ganglia lesion. *Neurology, 43,* 1768–1774.

Stuss, D. T., Eskes, G. A., & Foster, J. K. (1994). Experimental neuropsychological studies of frontal lobe functions. In F. Boller & J. Grafman (Eds.), *Handbook of neuropsychology.* Amsterdam: Elsevier.

Talbot, J. D., Marrett, S., Evans, A. C., Meyer, E., Bushnell, M. C., & Duncan, G. H. (1991). Multiple representations of pain in human cerebral cortex. *Science, 251,* 1355–1358.

Taylor, S. T., Liberzon, I., Fig, L. M., Decker, L. R., Minoshima, S., & Koepe, R. A. (1998). The effect of emotional content on visual recognition memory: A PET activation study. *Neuroimage, 8,* 188–197.

Trabasso, T., Stein, N., & Johnson, L. R. (1981). Children's knowledge of events: A causal analysis of story structure. In G. Bower (Ed.), *Learning and motivation* (Vol. 15, pp. 237–282). New York: Academic Press.

Tulving, E., Kapur, S., Craik, F. I. M., Moscovitch, M., & Houle, S. (1994). Hemispheric encoding/retrieval asymmetry in episodic memory: Positron emission tomography findings. *Proceedings of the National Academy of Sciences USA, 91,* 2016–2020.

Van Lancker, D., & Pachana, N. (1995). Acquired dysprosodic speech production: Mood, motivational, cognitive or motor disorder. *Brain and Language, 51,* 193–196.

van Stegeren, A. H., Everaerd, W., Cahill, L., McGuagh, J. L., & Gooren, L. J. G. (1998). Memory for emotional events: Differential effects of centrally versus peripherally acting ß-blocking agents. *Psychopharmacology, 138,* 305–310.

Vogt, B. A. (1986). Cingulate cortex. In A. Peters & E. G. Jones (Eds.), *Cerebral cor-*

tex: Vol. 4. Association and auditory cortices (pp. 89–149). New York: Plenum Press.

Vogt, B. A., Sikes, R. W., & Vogt, L. J. (1993). Anterior cingulate cortex and the medial pain system. In B. A. Vogt & M. Gabriel (Eds.), *Neurobiology of cingulate cortex and limbic thalamus: A comprehensive handbook* (pp. 313–344). Boston: Birkhaeuser.

von Cramon, D., & Jurgens, U. (1983). The anterior cingulate cortex and the phonatory control in monkey and man. *Neuroscience and Biobehavioral Reviews, 7,* 423–425.

Wegner, D. M., & Bargh, J. A. (1998). Control and automaticity in social life. In D. T. Gilbert, S. T. Fiske, & D. Lindzey (Eds.), *The handbook of social psychology* (4th ed., Vol. 2, pp. 446–496). Boston: McGraw-Hill.

Whalen, P. J. (1998). Fear, vigilance, and ambiguity: Initial neuroimaging studies of the human amygdala. *Current Directions in Psychological Science, 7,* 177–188.

Whalen, P. J., Bush, G., McNally, R. J., Wilhelm, S., McInerney, S. C., Jenike, M. A., & Rauch, S. L. (1998). The emotional counting Stroop paradigm: A functional magnetic resonance imaging probe of the anterior cingulate affective division. *Biological Psychiatry, 44,* 1219–1228.

Whalen, P. J., Rauch, S. L., Etcoff, N. L., McInerney, S. C., Lee, M. B., & Jenike, M. A. (1998). Masked presentations of emotional facial expressions modulate amygdala activity without explicit knowledge. *Journal of Neuroscience, 18,* 411–418.

Williams, J. M. G., Watts, F. N., MacLeod, C., Mathews, A. (1990). *Cognitive psychology and emotional disorders.* Chichester, UK: Wiley. (Original work published 1988)

Young, A. W., Aggleton, J. P., Hellawell, D. J., & Johnson, M. (1995). Face processing impairments after amygdalotomy. *Brain, 118,* 15–24.

Zald, D. H., & Pardo, J. V. (1997). Emotion, olfaction, and the human amygdala: Amygdala activation during aversive olfactory stimulation. *Proceedings of the National Academy of Sciences USA, 94,* 4119–4124.

3

Emotion and Memory

PIERRE PHILIPPOT
ALEXANDRE SCHAEFER

> I raised to my lips a spoonful of the tea in which I had soaked
> a morsel of the cake. No sooner had the warm liquid, and the
> crumbs with it, touched my palate that a shudder ran through
> my all body. . . . An exquisite pleasure had invaded my senses,
> but individual, detached, with no suggestion of its origin. . . .
> Whence could it have come to me, this all-powerful joy? . . .
> And suddenly, the memory returns. The taste was that of the
> little crumb of madeleine which on Sunday morning at
> Combray . . . when I went to say good day to her in her
> bedroom, my aunt Léonie used to give me, dipping it first in
> her own cup of real or of lime-flower tea.
> —PROUST (1913/1922/1957, pp. 56–58)

We have all experienced that seemingly trivial events can trigger intense
emotional feelings because of their capacity to reactivate a memory of a
past emotional experience. In this famous excerpt from one of Marcel
Proust's novels, the simple taste of a biscuit evokes past memories in the
character who reexperiences the emotions he lived years ago. The same
phenomenon—an emotion being elicited by the activation of an autobiographical memory—is even more striking in the case of individuals suffering of posttraumatic stress: for them, any stimulus that can cue the memory
of the traumatic event induces intense feelings of distress (Saigh, 1991).

If there is a consensus on the fact that the activation of memories of
past emotional experiences can induce emotion (Cuthbert, Vrana, &
Bradley, 1991), the role of memory in the elicitation and regulation of emotion is not yet well established. Are emotional memories activated during

everyday emotional experiences? What role do such memories play in the appraisal of emotional situations? Is it possible to experience emotion without reactivating past memories? For instance, do individuals suffering from amnesia have emotional feelings similar to those of individuals without amnesia? How do we store our emotional experiences? The present chapter will address these questions by examining how memory and emotion processes interact.

We first examine the attention that these questions have received in the history of emotion theory. Next, we review models and empirical evidence from several domains, including models of emotional memory proposed by social and cognitive theorists as well as contributions of neuroscientists to emotional memory. Then we review research pertaining to eyewitness testimony, so-called flash-bulb memory, and autobiographical memory priming in emotion. Finally, these diverse theoretical and empirical evidences are integrated and an original model of emotional memory is proposed.

MEMORY: A TOPIC HISTORICALLY NEGLECTED BY EMOTION THEORISTS

We all have an intuitive sense that many events evoke emotion because we ascribe them a meaning based on past self-relevant experiences. However, memory has received very little emphasis in the history of emotion theories. The first author to explicitly mention memory in her model of emotion is Magda B. Arnold (1950, 1960, 1970a, 1970b). In contrast with previous theories (Cannon, 1927; James, 1884), her "excitatory theory of emotion" poses that the activation of emotion is not a mere mechanical linkage of conditioned and unconditioned stimuli on the one hand, and conditioned and unconditioned responses on the other. All new emotional experience requires memory as the basis of appraisal (Arnold, 1970b). More specifically, whatever is experienced, in any sensory modalities, arouses not only a memory of similar things experienced in the past, but also revives the corresponding affect. In other words, "The liking or dislike once felt toward a person or a thing is felt again as soon as we encounter something similar" (Arnold, 1970b, p. 264). In addition, the situation with the relevant memories induces the subject to anticipate possible future outcomes. Thus, memory and imagination are the two bases of the preliminary appraisal of emotion stimuli. As Arnold (1970a) puts it, in interpreting a situation, "we *remember* what has happened to us in the past, how this thing has affected us and what we did about it. Then, we *imagine* how it will affect us this time and estimate whether it will be harmful" (emphasis added, p. 174). This fusion of memories, expectancy, and information coming from our sensory organs represent what Arnold (1950) names a "psychological evaluation of the situation" or "preliminary appraisal."

This preliminary appraisal of "good or bad for me" produces an impulse toward or away from the thing so appraised (Arnold, 1970a, p. 174). Arnold (1950, p. 19) names this impulse an "emotional attitude," such as anger, fear, or disgust, which is consciously felt (Arnold, 1970a, p. 174). In turn, the felt emotional attitude initiates nerve impulses from the cortex to centers in the midbrain such as the thalamus and the hypothalamus, which touch off the appropriate patterns of emotional expression, as well as the corresponding peripheral changes.

Ideas similar to Arnold's were redeveloped much later by Mandler (1980, 1984). According to Mandler, emotion starts with the interruption of ongoing organized thought and behavior. Such an interruption automatically triggers autonomic nervous system (ANS) activity. In line with Lacey and Lacey (1970), Mandler considers the ANS as a structure that alerts the organism to important events in the environment. Among the most important events to which attention has to be drawn are the occasions when well-developed and well-organized adaptive actions fail or cannot be completed. Yet, ANS activity alone does not suffice to generate an emotion. As in Schachter's (1964) theory, parallel to arousal, emotion also requires cognitive evaluation about the situation and about the possible cause of the arousal. The source of this meaning analysis resides in the complex networks of past experiences, belief systems, and perceptual expectations of the individuals. Thus, meaning analyses are a function not only of the situation characteristics but also of the idiosyncrasies of individuals representations and emotional memories.

An important interaction between physiology and meaning is that physiological responding singles out the interrupted events by marking them in memory as being accompanied by ANS activity (Mandler, 1984). On subsequent retrieval, events marked as ANS triggers would call for special attention and for special memorial processing. Thus, not only the perception of ANS activity, but also the memory that a similar situation was accompanied by ANS arousal could trigger emotional processing.

Unfortunately, neither Arnold nor Mandler has specified the nature of the memory processes involved in emotional appraisal further than postulating that autobiographical memories of similar past experiences were activated and were ascribing meaning to the present situation. Are these "emotional memories" instances of unique experiences (i.e., specific episodic events) or more generic memories? What makes these memories "emotional"? In sum, at the beginning of the 1980s, our understanding of how memory processes could be instrumental in emotion phenomena was still very poor. There was at least the intuition that the memory of our past emotional experiences were serving as a "database" that enabled appraisal of ongoing emotional situations, but this intuition had never been subjected to empirical research. We now turn to more recent theoretical contributions accounting for emotional memories to examine how such memories might impact on emotional processes.

PSYCHOLOGICAL MODELS OF EMOTIONAL MEMORY

In the 1980s, an interest started to develop in the memory structure of emotion. In the following subsections, we present chronologically the major models of emotional memory. As we intend to show, the evolution of these models has followed the evolution of general models of memory.

Bower's Associative Semantic Network Model

Bower (1981) is the first author to have proposed a model of emotional memory. His model is conceived as an associative semantic network, rather like the network models of semantic memory (Collins & Loftus, 1975; Collins & Quillian, 1969). In this model, memory is constituted by a set of nodes connected by associative links. Nodes represent concepts or events; propositions consist of subsets of nodes connected by specific associative links. An event is retrieved in memory when the proposition or set of propositions that constitutes it is activated.

According to Bower's (1981) model, every basic emotion (such as joy, anger, or fear) is represented by a node in the memory network. Complex emotions would consist of the simultaneous activation of several nodes of basic emotions. Each basic emotion node is connected to several other nodes, such as expressive behaviors, autonomic patterns, evoking appraisal, or verbal labels. The architecture of Bower's model is represented in Figure 3.1.

According to the principle of spreading activation, when one emotion node is activated, the connected nodes are activated too. Thus, when the node of anger is activated, the corresponding nodes of elevated blood pressure, frowning, clenching fists, and so on, are activated. Each emotion node is also linked to propositional representation of the events during which that emotion has been experienced. Thus, the activation of an emotion also induces the activation of past experiences during which that emotion has been aroused.

Bower's (1981) model constitutes a theoretical basis on which empirical research has been developed. This research, however, has focused on how emotion can influence memory, not on testing the validity of the model concerning emotion representation or memory processes in emotion. It has provided data on two phenomena: *mood-congruent memory* and *mood-dependent memory* (Bower & Cohen, 1982).

The term "mood-congruent memory" refers to the phenomenon in

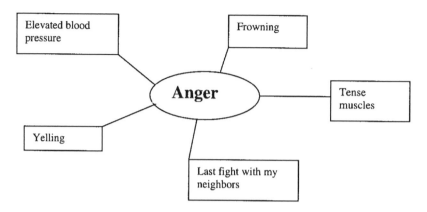

FIGURE 3.1. The architecture of Bower's (1981) associative network model of emotional memory.

which new information is more readily encoded in memory when its valence is congruent with the present mood state of the encoder. For instance, positive information would be better memorized if learned in a positive mood than if learned in a negative mood. The explanation of this phenomenon is that an emotional event activates its corresponding emotion node. If this node is already activated by a mood state, it will be much more strongly activated. This "double" activation strengthens the connection between the different nodes and propositions representing the emotion and the event.

The term "mood-dependent memory" refers to the phenomenon in which information encoded in a specific mood state is better retrieved when individuals are in the same mood state than when they are in a different mood state. The explanation is that when the information is encoded, a link is created with the nodes activated at that time, including emotion nodes if individuals are in a mood state as they are encoding the new information. During retrieval, the activation of the emotion node corresponding to the encoding mood constitutes an additional cue for information retrieval.

Bower's (1981) model and the phenomena of mood-dependent memory and mood-congruent memory have been used to account for emotional disorders such as depression: an individual in a depressive mood state would selectively retrieve depressogenic information that would in turn activate the depression node in memory. A positive feedback loop would thus be created.

Bower's (1981) memory model was the first attempting to explain how emotion is represented and how emotional events are stored in memory.

Like all first attempts, this model suffers from several shortcomings and has been the subject of thorough critiques (Teasdale, 1993). One critique is that it proposes a unique code of representation for elements as different as physiological responses, characteristics of eliciting event, or subjective feelings. It is unlikely that such different elements would be represented in the same code and structure in memory. A second critique is that this model cannot account for the distinction between the documented phenomena of "hot" and "cold" emotions. In Bower's model, once an emotion node is activated, spreading activation automatically arouses the whole structure. Thus, it would be impossible to think about emotion without being emotionally aroused. A third critique is that this model proposes a unique memory structure for semantic knowledge about emotion and episodic representations of emotional experience. Indeed, Bower's model is the direct application of a semantic memory model to the domain of emotion. However, it is now well established that semantic and episodic memories are quite distinct processes, organized in different structures (Wheeler, Stuss, & Tulving, 1997). Finally, at the empirical level, the effects of mood-dependent and -congruent memories do not seem to be reliable and are the subject of controversy (Kenealy, 1997; Ucros, 1989; Wetzler, 1985).

Lang's Bioinformational Model

Lang's (1979) bioinformational model is somewhat similar to Bower's model, as its general structure is also based on an associative semantic network. In Lang's conception, rather than a node, emotion representations are best understood as semantic networks tying together different types of proposition. Lang distinguishes between three proposition types: stimulus propositions, response propositions, and meaning propositions. Stimulus propositions define the characteristics of the emotion-eliciting stimulus: the event, context, and situation. Take, for instance, the case of the representation of snake fear. Stimulus propositions might define the perceptive characteristics of the snake (e.g., its shape, color, and movement pattern), the situation in which snakes can appear (e.g., in the woods or in the bushes), and the context in which the emotion takes place (e.g., the individual is alone). Response propositions comprise all the responses triggered by the emotion elicitors, such as "running away," acceleration of heart rate, opening the mouth, and frowning. Finally, meaning propositions ascribe the implications of the elements of the emotional representation for the individual. For instance, being alone in the woods and being confronted with a snake implies danger; the acceleration of heart rate, the desire to run away, and a fearful expression mean that the individual is afraid (see the schematic illustration in Figure 3.2). In Lang's conception, emotion is the mere activation of such memory structures.

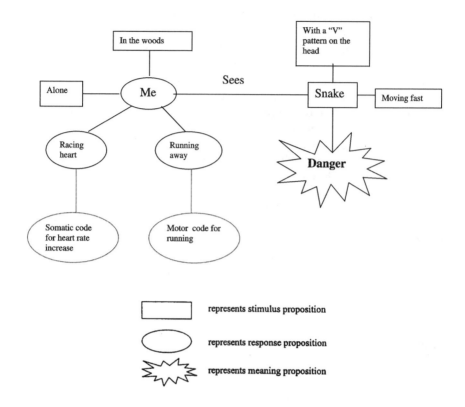

FIGURE 3.2. The architecture of Lang's (1979) model of emotional memory.

An important characteristic of Lang's model is that it postulates that response propositions are encoded in two different codes: a semantic code and a somatomotor code. The semantic code is conceptual and similar to the code of the stimulus and meaning propositions. They are accessible to consciousness and can readily be translated into language. The somatomotor code comprises the motor and visceral programs that trigger and organize body responses. These codes are not directly accessible to language or consciousness. However, Lang (1979) postulates that the two codes are connected in memory. Thus, activating the response proposition of heart rate acceleration at the semantic level—for instance, by thinking about it—will in turn activate the corresponding somatomotor program and should result in specific corresponding bodily changes.

In several respects, Lang's (1979) model is an improvement over Bower's. First, it postulates a double coding for somatic and motor responses. Second, emotion memory representation is conceived as a network and not as a node. Third, while Bower is postulating a specific node for each basic emotion, Lang's model is more idiosyncratic: emotion representations are developed as a function of the individual emotional history. As a consequence, emotion representation in Lang's conception is more specific than in Bower's: according to the former we would have different representations for different types of fear or anger, whereas according to the latter there would be only one representation for each basic emotion.

However, Lang's (1979) model suffers from at least two limitations. First, there is no strong empirical evidence for the postulated link between the semantic representation of body responses and the effector programs organizing them. It even goes against present empirical evidences. On the one hand, semantic representations of body response do not correspond to actual physiological changes (Philippot, 1993; Rimé, Philippot, & Cisamolo, 1991). On the other hand, the semantic activation of specific response propositions seems to elicit more a general state of arousal than the specific corresponding physiological changes (Acosta & Vila, 1990). Second, Lang's model accounts for the general representation of emotion in memory, but it does not account for specific memories of emotional episodes. In other words, like Bower, Lang proposes a semantic memory model of emotion but ignores specific episodic memories.

Leventhal's Hierarchical Processing Model

Leventhal (1984a) has proposed a model of emotional memory that does not account for the memory of specific episodes but that complements Lang's model in an important way. The central postulate of Leventhal's model is that adult emotions are complex behavioral reactions and processes organized hierarchically in three cognitive levels. The different levels covary with the degree of abstraction of the cognitive processes involved. These three levels are the sensorimotor, the schematic, and the conceptual (Leventhal, 1984a, 1984b).

The sensorimotor level of processing is the basic processor of emotional behavior and experience. It includes a set of innate and central expressive–motor programs for generating distinctive sets of expressive reactions, autonomic responses and feelings in response to specific releasing stimuli. These programs are activated automatically, that is, without volitional effort. In newborns, this is the only emotional system to be active (Leventhal & Mosbach, 1983).

The schematic level consists of concrete representations of the various components of emotions that were activated during specific emotional episodes. Schematic processes combine subjective feelings, expressive reactions, and visceral responses with stimulus inputs as they were encountered during emotional experiences. This system can be conceptualized as a record of conditioned emotional reactions (Leventhal & Mosbach, 1983). Generalized schemas (i.e., prototypes) emerge as similar emotional states are evoked and combined in memory with the perceptual features derived from multiple situations (Leventhal & Scherer, 1987). Once a schema is formed, the activation of anyone of its components will arouse the whole schema. Thus, not only the activation of the stimulus component, but also the activation of the expressive, or subjective, or visceral components has the ability to activate the other components.

Emotional schemas, which organize this second level, would develop from early childhood on. They would be highly dependent on individual experiences. According to Leventhal, individual specificity may be more pronounced in the autonomic responses component, which is less under social control than the expressive and subjective components. Leventhal and Scherer (1987) illustrate this by an example: If an infant is subjected regularly to vigorous stimulations, such as tickles, when he/she smiles at his/her parents, strong autonomic and motor reactions will be associated with the child's smiling responses and subjective pleasure. Hence, he/she will develop a schema of happiness that might be described as "euphoric" or "excited." By contrast, an infant whose smiles generate soft, parental coos and endearments will show mild visceral responses and will develop a schema of "calm" happiness. These authors conclude that "the intensity, and perhaps the patterns of autonomic responses associated with a specific emotion may depend upon prior conditioning" (Leventhal & Scherer, 1987, p. 11).

Finally, the third level, conceptual processing, is defined by two components: one stores information about past experiences, and one generates the voluntary performance of emotional acts. Both components are constituted by a propositional memory network in which specific elements are logically related. This level of processing is thus more abstract than the schematic level. The latter is the memory of the emotional responses themselves; the former reflects knowledge *about* emotional responses in a more general way. Such conceptual memories are formed when individuals are able to reflect on their emotional experience (Leventhal, 1984a). Conceptual processing is effortful and makes demands on conscious, attentional capacities. Importantly, it is conceptual processing that gives people the capacity to communicate about their emotions. As Leventhal and Mosbach (1983, p. 361) put it, conceptual processing allows reports such as "I seem to feel butterflies in my stomach and shaky all over whenever I have a close call with danger."

In adults, all three processing mechanisms are active in emotion-provoking situations. It would then not be possible to observe them separately. Leventhal and Mosbach (1983) also state that the entire system can be activated by processing at any level of the system. Hence, conscious and voluntary thoughts (conceptual system) can arouse the schematic and the perceptual motor systems, and visceral activity (perceptual motor system) can activate the conceptual system, for example, the identification of a sensation as "butterflies in the stomach" and its connection to certain types of experiences and feelings.

In sum, like Lang, Leventhal proposes a model of emotional memory that accounts for how emotional meaning is ascribed to a situation and for how the emotional responses are organized. They also share the same conception of how these memory structures are constructed in the course of development, even though Leventhal is more specific than Lang. Leventhal distinguishes different levels of processing that explain different emotional phenomena. One should not attempt to find similarities between Lang's three types of propositions and Leventhal's three levels; the two distinctions are best conceived as orthogonal to each other. For instance, Lang's stimulus propositions can be encoded at all three levels of Leventhal. The main weaknesses of Leventhal's model is that it has not been subjected to empirical testing and that it does not account for episodic memories of emotion.

We now turn to two recent cognitive models of emotion, based on memory processes.

Integrated Cognitive Subsystems

Teasdale developed the first of these models on the basis of a general model of cognitive architecture by Barnard (Barnard & Teasdale, 1991; Teasdale, 1993, 1996, 1999; Teasdale & Barnard, 1993). This integrated cognitive subsystems (ICS) model conceives cognition as a network of subsystems, each specialized in the processing of a certain type of information, and each having its own memory structure and code. Although the original model is more complex, one can distinguish between several subsystems. These include the following:

- The subsystems processing sensory information and body state
- The subsystem identifying the objects processed by the sensory subsystem
- The effector subsystem that organizes voluntary behavior
- The propositional subsystem
- The implicational subsystem

These last two systems are responsible for the attribution of meaning to sensory and object information and thus are central to this model. Another important specification of the model is that the information processed by a given subsystem can be translated and transferred to certain other subsystems, but not necessarily in both directions and not necessarily to any other subsystem. Figure 3.3 illustrates the general architecture of the model and the paths through which information can follow.

As can be seen in Figure 3.3, the sensory information processed by the sensory subsystem is passed to the object subsystem that identifies it, and according to the meaning ascribed to it by the propositional and implicational subsystems, a response is organized and operated by the effector subsystem. Central to Teasdale and Barnard's model is the distinction between the two meanings—ascribing subsystems—the propositional and implicational subsystems.

The former subsystem conveys specific meanings in terms of discrete concepts and the relationships among them. For example, the thought "my car is broken again" has a specific meaning that can be grasped easily given the direct relationship between language, concepts, and their correspondence to material reality. Meaning conveyed at this level has a "truth value" that follows the rules of logic and can be judged true or false. It can be verified by reference to evidence.

The latter type, the implicational subsystem, conveys a more generic, holistic level of meaning. It encodes recurring, high-order regularities across the sensory, propositional, and body state information codes. Meaning at this level is difficult to communicate, as it does not map directly onto language and is very abstract. It is better conveyed by metaphors or parables. Implicational meaning conveys the emotional significance for the individual of the information activated in other subsystems. In other words, it is what this information means or implies for his/her personal goals. Teasdale (1996, p. 29) notes that "subjectively, synthesis of generic meanings is marked by experience of particular holistic 'senses' or 'feelings' with

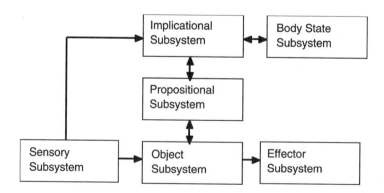

FIGURE 3.3. The architecture of Teasdale and Barnard's integrated cognitive subsystems (ICS) model of emotional memory.

implicit meaning content: 'something is wrong,' 'confidence,' ' hopeless-ness.' " From this perspective, the ICS model proposes that only the generic meaning conveyed by the implicational level is directly linked to emotion (Teasdale, 1996). The implicational subsystem generates the "hot" cog-nitions and conveys the deep emotional meaning. The knowledge encoded by the propositional subsystem represents the "cold" cognitions, including the ones about emotion.

As shown in Figure 3.3, the emotional meaning encoded by the implicational subsystem can be activated by three sources. First, the sensory subsystem can directly activate the implicational subsystem, without object recognition. For instance, a loud noise or the perception of something mov-ing very quickly toward us has the capacity to arouse the emotional mean-ing of danger. Second, the propositional subsystem can also feed into the implicational subsystem. For example, thoughts such as "my car is broken again" generated by the propositional subsystem can activate the implica-tional meaning of distress. Finally, the body state subsystem can also trigger a specific emotional meaning at the implicational level via body feedback. A well-documented example is the case of facial feedback (Matsumoto, 1987).

Once aroused in the implicational subsystem, an emotional meaning has two effects. First, it will directly impact on the body state subsystem and thus generate body changes. For instance, the distress induced by the thought "my car is broken again" might induce changes in the body subsys-tem resulting in elevated heart rate and hyperventilation. Second, the emo-tional meaning might also produce changes in the propositional system and generate thoughts like "My car is broken—what am I going to do?" Such conscious thinking might in turn determine voluntary behavior and coping strategies.

Although their architectures are very different, Leventhal's model and Teasdale and Barnard's model share some important features. The distinction between the implicational and propositional subsystems paral-lels that between the schematic and propositional levels. Likewise, the way knowledge would be built at these different levels of representation is somewhat similar, and so is their relationship to real-world evidence. Teasdale and Barnard's model has the advantage of a general structure compatible with several contemporary models of cognition and, because of its scope, the advantage of explaining a large range of phenomena. It has been used to explain depression and its maintenance through a locked feedback loop between the implicational and propositional subsys-tems, and it has generated valuable empirical evidences in this specific domain (Teasdale, 1996). Unfortunately, the central postulate of the model, the existence of two different systems for meaning ascription, has not yet been empirically tested.

Conclusions

Four models of the interrelationships between emotion and memory have just been presented. They all share a common cognitive account of emotion: emotion would be an emerging property of the activation of specific memory processes. The two older models, Bower's and Lang's, have a semantic network architecture. These models are still widely cited in the literature, especially to account for mood-congruent memory, mood-dependent memory, and imagery. Leventhal's model is intermediate and brings the distinctions between different levels of processing of emotional information. Finally, Teasdale and Barnard's ICS model proposes a new form of architecture in which emotion is the result of interactive modules, each specialized in a type of processing. This model integrates the concept of level of processing of emotional information introduced by Leventhal. It is to be noted that it is only in the older model, Bower's, that emotion is encoded as such in memory. In all the other models, emotion is an emerging property of a network or a set of modules but is not encoded per se.

An important limitation of the four models presented in this section is that they are very general and abstract and, consequently, difficult to test empirically. Indeed, with the exception of the research on mood-dependent or -congruent memory, there are very few studies that have directly tested the assumptions of these models regarding emotional processes. Later in this chapter, we review research from our laboratory that has addressed this issue. Another limitation of these models is that they do not consider the possible role of specific autobiographical memories in emotional processes.

The hierarchical processing model and the ICS model both suggest that emotional processes might be organized by schematic representations (Leventhal's schematic level and Teasdale and Barnard's implicational subsystem). These schematic representations would be constituted by the abstraction of the many similar emotional events experienced by individuals during their personal histories. Such representations would integrate multimodal aspects of experience, that is, perceptual, semantic, and sensorial information about a generic emotional event. For instance, the schematic representation of anger might encompass feelings of tension, the semantic concept of injustice, and the image of a threatening face.

NEUROPSYCHOLOGICAL APPROACHES OF EMOTIONAL MEMORY

Another approach to the study of the interactions between emotion and memory lies in the neurophysiological hypothesis of an emotional memory brain system. In this section, we consider two theoretical models describing the neural mechanisms that might underlie such an emotional memory system. Afterward, we discuss some empirical results that test predictions derived from these models and examine whether the conclusion of the former section fits with neuropsychological evidences.

Two Neuropsychological Models of Emotional Memory

A neuropsychological model of emotional memory must fulfill three requirements. First, it must conceive of emotion as a memory process, that is, as elicited through the activation of previously stored knowledge. Second, it must address the question of the specificity of the memory processes leading to emotion: is there a memory system specialized in emotional information, and can this system work independently of other memory systems? Third, it has to include assumptions about the brain mechanisms underlying emotional memory. In the neuroscience literature, LeDoux (1992, 1993, 1996) and Damasio (1994) have proposed models that meet these conditions.

LeDoux's Model of Emotional Memory

Joseph E. LeDoux studies the brain processes involved in fear conditioning. Most of his studies are designed on an animal model of emotion. LeDoux (1992, 1993, 1996) considers that emotion results from the activation of a special type of information stored in a particular memory system: the emotional memory system. This emotional memory system is independent of a conscious declarative memory system. It produces emotional reactions and operates outside consciousness. The conscious memory system processes factual knowledge about past events and generates conscious memories of these events. One of LeDoux's claims is that emotion does not need consciousness to occur. The existence of consciously experienced emotional feelings would only be an epiphenomenon, not essential to emotional processes. Emotional feelings would result from the simultaneous presence in working memory of the perception of an emotional situation and the perception of bodily responses provoked by connections between the emotional memory system and several effector systems like the ANS.

Following a large body of research on fear conditioning in rats, LeDoux suggests that the brain structure most likely to underlie the emotional memory system is the amygdala, a small structure situated in the internal part of the temporal lobe. The amygdala appraises the emotional meaning of a stimulus and encodes the association between this meaning and the situation characteristics. This is accomplished by two neural circuits: the first is the thalamic circuit, which includes sensory inputs coming from the thalamus to the amygdala, and the second is the thalamo-cortical circuit, including sensory inputs that pass through the thalamus and the sensory cortices before reaching the amygdala. These circuits make possible associations between perceptual elements of a situation and the emotional meaning of this situation. Hence, when a stimulus previously associated with an emotion reaches the amygdala, associated emotional information is activated. In addition, the amygdala has connections with several body response systems.

Despite the postulate of independence between the emotional memory system and the declarative memory system, LeDoux suggests that they can interact through several pathways between the amygdala and the hippocampus (Philips & LeDoux, 1992). The hippocampus is a temporal lobe structure that is central to declarative memory. Indeed, a very large body of research has showed that the hippocampus is involved in retrieving past memories of complex events (McClelland, McNaughton, & O'Reilly, 1995; Squire, 1992). Therefore, the pathways between the amygdala and the hippocampus make possible associations between emotional information and information about the complex context of a past event. This process explains how emotion can be elicited when one is thinking of a past emotional episode.

In sum, although mostly based on animal fear conditioning, the work of LeDoux offers interesting hypotheses for the role of memory in human emotions. Further, some links can be made between LeDoux's model and some of the psychological models of emotion discussed in the previous section. The implicit memory system, supported by the amygdala, can be related to the schematic level in Leventhal's model and the implicational subsystem in Teasdale and Barnard's ICS model. Indeed, both are information processing systems that operate through implicit processes and whose specific outputs are emotional responses. Another similarity between these processes and the amygdala rests in the integrative function combining sensory information with bodily responses that is attributed to these structures or processes. Further, the conscious declarative memory system, supported by a network including the hippocampus and some frontal areas, can easily be related to Teasdale and Barnard's propositional subsystem and Leventhal's conceptual level of processing.

Damasio's Theory of Primary and Secondary Emotion Systems

Based on the study of emotional behavior in brain-damaged humans, Damasio (1994) proposes a theory of emotion that distinguishes between a primary and a secondary emotion system. Primary emotions are biologically determined affective reactions to some basic perceptual features of a stimulus. For instance, some movements similar to reptilian movements would automatically generate a negative affective state. The activation of primary emotion would rely on genetically inherited neural representations situated in subcortical areas, more particularly in the amygdala and the anterior cingulate cortex (ACC).

Secondary emotions are learned emotional reactions. They depend mostly on neural representations situated in the medial prefrontal cortex. According to Damasio (1994), the contents of these neural representations are the linkages between categories of past events and their affective meanings. In other words, secondary emotions depend on the activation of neural structures that promote a link between a type of event and the emotional consequences of this event. These representations are shaped during the ontogenesis through the storage in memory of successive events and their emotional outcomes. The secondary emotion system does not work independently of the primary emotion system. The prefrontal structures are in constant interaction with the subcortical structures involved in primary emotions.

Like LeDoux, Damasio (1994) proposes that conscious emotional feelings are the result of the simultaneous conscious perception of (1) bodily changes generated by unconscious neural mechanisms and (2) the situation eliciting the emotion. But contrary to LeDoux, Damasio suggests that conscious emotional feelings play an important role in human emotion. Indeed, the awareness of a relation between a situation and emotional bodily changes increases the range of possible adaptive responses to the situation.

Several similarities can be noted between Damasio's (1994) model and some of the models reviewed earlier. Indeed, primary emotions, supported mostly by the amygdala and the ACC, seem to include, in Damasio's theory, the same mechanisms postulated by Leventhal in the sensory motor level of processing. Further, the secondary emotion processes of the medial prefrontal cortex are very similar to those accomplished by Teasdale and Barnard's implicational subsystem and Leventhal's schematic level. As a matter of fact, as in Damasio's neural representations of secondary emotions, both of these constructs are postulated to contain representations that are the result of linkages between summaries of emotional episodes and the emotional responses present during these episodes. Another similarity between Leventhal's model and Damasio's model lies in the relation between consciousness and emotion. Both postulate that consciousness is a necessary component of the emotional process since it makes possible to adopt a wide range of coping responses.

Conclusions

Both of these models conceive of emotion as a memory process: emotional responses are triggered by the activation of previously encoded information. In addition to that, these two models offer answers to the following questions: (1) Can emotional memory work independently of the conscious processes of declarative memory? (2) What are the brain structures underlying emotional memory? In response to the first question, LeDoux adopts a clear position: emotional memory is a specific process that can work independently of conscious declarative memory and, more generally, does not need consciousness to occur. Damasio is less explicit concerning the independence between a hypothetical emotional memory system and declarative memory, but he asserts that consciousness is useful and even necessary for many aspects of emotional life. As to the second question, LeDoux suggests that the amygdala is the crucial center of emotional memory, whereas Damasio thinks that the amygdala is only one piece in a more complex system in which the medial prefrontal cortex plays a more important role. These authors also diverge regarding the role of the amygdala and its relation to the different processes proposed by Leventhal and by Teasdale and Barnard. While LeDoux's theory suggests that the function of the amygdala is similar to the functions of the schematic processes, Damasio's model limits its role to primary emotions that are closer to processes at the sensorimotor level (i.e., body responses) than to the schematic processes.

In order to evaluate these points of view, we next review two bodies of research. First, studies evaluating emotions in amnesiac patients are examined in order to investigate the relations between emotional memory, declarative memory, and consciousness. Indeed, amnesiac patients are impaired in consciously remembering past episodes of their lives. If emotional memory is independent of conscious declarative memory processes, these patients should experience "normal" emotions. Second, we review studies on the role played by the amygdala in emotional learning in order to document the functions it serves in the emotional brain memory system.

Emotion in Amnesia

Studying emotion in amnesiac patients is a way of testing whether the emotional memory system is independent of a conscious declarative memory system. Indeed, amnesiac patients with lesions in the hippocampus and surrounding areas are impaired in retrieving conscious memories of past events. Hence, if the postulate of independence between emotional memory and declarative memory is true, an amnesiac patient without damage to the amygdala should experience normal emotions.

Some empirical evidences seem to confirm these predictions. First, amnesiac patients show a normal *mere exposure effect* (Johnson & Multhaup, 1992; Tobias, Khilstrom, & Schacter, 1992). The mere exposure effect consists of the preference for an item to which the subject has previously been exposed, without a conscious remembering of the first exposure. However, it is not clear if this effect depends on emotional processes. Indeed, the "preference" can be induced by a "feeling of knowing" elicited by the encounter of the previously perceived item rather than by an association with an affective meaning. Second, amnesiac patients can learn affective valence (Bechara et al., 1995; Johnson & Multhaup, 1992; Tranel & Damasio, 1993). They are able to encode an association between an unconditioned appetitive or aversive stimulus and a neutral one. They are also able to reinstate this association after the learning stage without consciously remembering the learning experience. Third, amnesiac patients are able to normally perceive the emotional meaning of a stimulus; that is, they have normal scores on self-report scales evaluating the arousal level of an emotional stimuli (Hamman, Cahill, & Squire, 1997). However, this third task does not depend necessarily on emotional memory. Indeed, for evaluating the emotionality level of a stimulus, accessing semantic knowledge about emotion is sufficient.

Although these results seem to confirm that emotional processing can work independently of a conscious declarative memory system, it remains that the tasks set in these experiments require only very simple emotional processes. Recently, in our laboratory, Chapelle (1998; see also Chapelle, Philippot, & Vanderlinden, 2000) tried to induce emotions in A.C., a severely amnesiac patient. Using different emotion-induction procedures, Chapelle found that A.C. was able to generate emotions when stimuli were external (emotional video clips or slides) but that he was severely impaired compared to controls when stimuli were internal (e.g., mental imagery). These results indicate that the autonomy between an emotional memory system and a conscious declarative memory system is task dependent. In other words, as suggested by Damasio, not all emotional behaviors can occur without an intact conscious memory system. In the case reported by Chapelle, internally generated emotions seem not to be possible without such a system. These data are congruent with the multiple entry memory (MEM) theory of Johnson and Multhaup (1992), which postulates two broad categories of emotions: emotions depending on perceptual, externally initiated processes, and emotions depending on reflexive, internally initiated processes. The latter would require more conscious and controlled processing than the former. According to Johnson and Multhaup, emotions depending on reflexive processes are impaired in amnesiac patients. In sum, the results of Chapelle challenge the postulate of independence between emotional memory and declarative memory.

Role of the Amygdala

A large body of research in animal studies has shown that ablation or pharmacological lesions of the amygdala in rats impair learning and expression of conditioned fear (see, e.g., Bailey, Kim, Sun, Thompson, & Helmstetter,

1999; Helmstetter, 1992; LeDoux, 1995; Maren, 1998; Rogan & LeDoux, 1996). An animal whose amygdala is damaged is unable to express a fear response (e.g., increase of heart rate or somatomotor immobility) when exposed to a conditioned stimulus, that is, a neutral stimulus (such as a light or a color) that has been previously paired to an unconditioned stimulus of fear (such as a loud noise or an electric shock).

In humans, some studies conducted with patients whose amygdala was damaged also suggest that the amygdala is involved in fear conditioning. LaBar, LeDoux, Spencer, and Phelps (1995) showed that patients with damage to the amygdala showed less autonomic conditioning associated to a loud noise than did patients with an intact amygdala. Other studies on patients with amygdalar lesions obtained similar results (Adolphs, Tranel, Damasio & Damasio, 1995; Bechara et al., 1995). Hamman and colleagues (1996) also showed that a patient with amygdalar damage was impaired in the recognition of faces expressing fear.

Some studies obtained evidence for the involvement of the amygdala in the effect of memory enhancement for emotional material. Amnesiac patients whose lesions did not include the amygdala showed a normal effect of memory enhancement for emotional information despite a general impairment of all memory tasks. Interestingly, amnesiac patients whose lesions included the amygdala did not show the same effect (Hamman, Cahill, & Squire, 1997). Patients whose lesions affected bilaterally only the amygdala did not show a general memory impairment, but rather an absence of the effect of enhancement for emotional material (Adolphs, Cahill, Schul, & Babinsky, 1997). Similarly, Mori and colleagues (1999) report that Alzheimer patients are able to remember a highly emotional episode (namely, the Kobe earthquake in Japan) and that the quality of this remembering was positively correlated with the amygdalar volume of these patients.

Although these data seem to provide strong arguments for LeDoux's ideas, other empirical evidence has challenged the hypothesized crucial role of the amygdala in an emotional memory system. First, Tranel and Damasio (1993) studied an amnesiac patient with a total lesion of the amygdala and hippocampus who was able to learn an affective valence. Second, some patients with a frontal lobe lesion that does not include the amygdala seem to be unable to learn emotional information. For instance, Bechara, Damasio, Damasio, and Anderson (1994) and Bechara, Tranel, Damasio, and Damasio (1993) devised an experiment that consisted of a poker-like card game. In this game, the player learns gradually which strategies are risky and which are safe. The investigators observed that patients with lesions in the medial prefrontal cortex adopted a much more risky strategy than did the controls, although they were aware that their strategy was risky and inefficient. Moreover, it has been shown that, when receiving a reward during the game (e.g., winning the money at stake), the patients with a frontal lobe lesion showed a normal electrodermal response. But, unlike the controls, these patients did not show an anticipatory electrodermal response, that is, just before engaging in a risky strategy. According to Damasio (1994), this result reflects the impairment of these prefrontal lobe patients in the activation of emotional representations. Indeed, to anticipate that a situation is risky or not, it would be necessary to activate in memory the associations between this kind of situation and its emotional consequences. Therefore, medial areas of the prefrontal cortex seem to play a role of emotional memory, as suggested by Damasio. Data from neuroimaging research is consistent with this assumption. Indeed, the medial prefrontal cortex seems to be significantly activated in all kinds of emotion-inducing tasks compared to nonemotional conditions (Drevets & Raichle, 1998; George et al., 1995; Lane, Reiman, Ahern, et al., 1997; Lane, Reiman, Bradley, et al., 1997; Reiman et al., 1997; Reiman, 1997). Third, animal studies have shown that many subcortical structures other than the amygdala also play an important role in the learning of emotional responses (Kiernan, Bailey, Sims, Lukes & Cranney, 1996; Maren, 1999; Maren & Fanselow, 1997; Riedel, Harrington, Hall, & Macphail, 1997; Westbrook, Good, & Kiernan, 1997).

In sum, these data suggest that the amygdala plays an important role in fear conditioning and in the processing of fear-inducing or -reducing information (e.g., facial expressions). It encodes the contingent associations between unconditioned and conditioned stimuli and emotional responses. However, there is as yet no strong evidence that it plays such an important role for other emotions. In addition, the evidence reviewed in the preceding paragraph shows that the amygdala is certainly not the only crucial structure involved in emotional memory in humans.

Conclusions

Even if empirical evidence is far from depicting a simple reality, tentative hypotheses can be formulated about the neural mechanisms of emotional memory. Regarding the independence between emotional memory and conscious declarative processes, neuropsychological data suggest an implicit emotional memory system that can produce emotional responses independently of conscious declarative processes. However, for some emotional processes (e.g., emotional induction by internal stimuli), conscious declarative processes are necessary.

The brain circuits associated with emotional memory seem to be rather complex. Looking at animal studies and at single-case human studies, we note that the amygdala appears to be a crucial structure for fear processing. However, some single-case studies by Damasio and neuroimaging experiments suggest that the medial prefrontal cortex plays a more important role. These results are not necessarily incompatible. The present literature even allows for some speculations regarding the brain structures implicated in the processes defined by Leventhal's and Teasdale and Barnard's models. Indeed, one can propose that the amygdala is responsible for (1) appraising the emotionality of stimuli on the basis of biologically driven dimensions and (2) making contingent associations between perceptual features of the stimuli and emotional responses. This suggests that, if we elaborate on the basis of the sensorimotor (Leventhal) or body response (Teasdale and Barnard) systems, the amygdala would be an important structure in the building of basic emotional schemas on the fringe of the schematic (Leventhal) or implicational (Teasdale and Barnard) system. The medial prefrontal cortex would be responsible for higher-order associations, that is, links between complex event summaries and emotional responses, paralleling more distinctly the functions of Leventhal's schematic system and Teasdale and Barnard's implicational subsystem. Finally, the third level of emotional processing, the propositional (Teasdale and Barnard) or conceptual (Leventhal) system, would operate in a network including the hippocampus for episodic declarative memory and probably the dorsolateral prefrontal cortex, usually associated with working memory tasks (Clark et al., 2000; Schumaker et al., 1996; Schwartz et al., 1996). Even though such proposals are tentative, this integration indicates that there are many parallels between the theories of Leventhal and of Teasdale and Barnard, and neuropsychological data, on the other.

AUTOBIOGRAPHICAL MEMORY AND EMOTION

The theories and research we have reviewed so far have addressed emotional memory in general, but little has been said about the memory of specific emotional events. Yet, judging from Proust's recounting of his madeleine experience (presented at the start of this chapter), investigation of the latter subject could be a promising approach for the study of memory processes underlying the elicitation of emotion. We now review the research integrating emotion and autobiographical memory as follows: first, we consider studies that investigated the effects of the emotions felt during an event on the quality of remembering of that event; second, we review studies, mainly from our laboratory, that investigated the role of autobiographical memory in the elicitation of emotion.

Memory for Emotional Events

We often have the impression that we remember better emotional events than neutral ones. Emotional autobiographical memories seem to be more accurate, closer to the original event. However, the opposite phenomenon can also occur: people who have experienced a highly negative emotional event like a rape or a road accident sometimes have difficulty remembering the event, a phenomenon often referred to as "repression." In fact, the emotion felt while one is experiencing an event seems to have an impact on how this event will be remembered later.

Eyewitness Studies

A large number of studies have investigated so-called eyewitness testimony. Such studies usually consist of asking people to remember real-life or laboratory-induced negative emotional events they witnessed or experienced, in order to measure recall accuracy. Some studies (Yuille & Cutshall, 1986; Yuille & Tollestrup, 1992) showed that witnesses of an emotional event (e.g., a crime) are able to retain accurately and consistently the circumstances of the event over several months, and that people who reported the highest levels of stress during the event are those who had the most accurate memories of it. Yet, contrary to these results, clinical observations have documented that an amnesiac syndrome might well be induced by a highly stressful, traumatic event (Christianson & Safer, 1996), suggesting that extreme levels of emotion can have a deleterious effect on memory. This notion has been confirmed by some experimental studies. For instance, Loftus and Burns (1982) showed that subjects who viewed a very violent film had a poor memory performance for details of the film. Some other studies found the "weapon focus" effect, namely, the fact that when one has suffered an armed aggression, memory performance for details other than the weapon is very poor (Steblay, 1992).

To account for these seemingly opposite results, Kassin, Ellsworth, and Smith (1989) suggested that the effect of negative emotion on memory follows the Yerkes–Dodson law, that is, an inverted-U curve. Low and high levels of emotion would impair memory performance, whereas moderate levels of emotion during the event would enhance it. However, some empirical evidence contradicts this assumption: several studies have shown that highly stressful events can lead to very accurate and detailed memories. For instance, Christianson and Hubinette (1993) found that eyewitnesses of bank robberies had detailed memories of what took place and that victims (i.e., the bank workers who were directly threatened) had more detailed memories than the bystanders. Thus, it seems that the effect of emotion on memory performance seems to follow a more complex function than the Yerkes–Dodson law.

An alternative approach is to distinguish different aspects of memory performance and to look for interactions between the emotionality of the event and the type of information to be remembered. Indeed, it was found that highly emotional events were well retained with respect to central aspects of the event compared to peripheral details, which were poorly remembered. For instance, the participants of the Christianson and Hubinette (1993) study remembered well detailed information concerning the action of the robbery and the weapons used, but they remembered poorly details like the time and date of the robbery, and information about other witnesses. Several experiments have shown that this is a strong and reliable effect (Burke, Heuer, & Reisberg, 1992; Christianson, 1992; Wessel & Merckelbach, 1998).

To account for this effect, Christianson (1992) formulated the following "attentional narrowing" hypothesis: More attentional resources would be allocated to emotion-provoking stimuli than to other stimuli present in the context but irrelevant for the emotional situation. This attentional focus would impact positively on emotional information encoding and later on recall performance. However, Christianson, Loftus, Hoffman, and Loftus (1991) showed that the interaction between emotion and the type of recalled information remains when the number of eye fixations on the central or peripheral details is controlled for. Christianson and colleagues conclude that attentional processes are not the unique factor accounting for these results. In addition to attentional narrowing at the encoding stage, there might be postevent elaborative processes that strengthen memory for central details. Compared to a neutral event, an emotional event would lead to more elaborative processing about the causes of the event and the emotional aspects of the situation. A neutral event would induce an elaborative processing concerning external, contextual details. Although this explanation is based on results that postulate a necessary link between eye fixation and attention allocation that is challenged by some authors (Posner, Walker, Friedrich, & Rafal, 1984), it introduces an interesting hypothesis: the specific characteristic of an emotional autobiographical memory would partially depend upon constructive processes occurring after the event.

The aforementioned studies have several limitations. Field studies often lack the control comparison with a neutral event. In addition, it is often difficult to reliably assess recall accuracy, that is, whether remembered details are not the results of equivocal recollections. In laboratory studies, the major limitations are (1) the artificiality of the emotional situations (e.g., slides depicting situations in which participants were not personally implicated) and (2) the absence of a measure of the emotional arousal elicited by the stimulus. Still, as whole, studies on eyewitness testimony suggest that the memory for emotional events is better than for neutral ones, especially if one considers memory for emotionally relevant details. This relationship might disappear in the case of extreme emotion, but experimental results have not as yet supported this clinical observation.

Flashbulb Memory

If, as a rule, the focal details of emotional memories are better memorized, there seems to be an exception. Indeed, a specific class of emotional events, namely, learning about important news, can generate vivid and abundant recall of contextual details irrelevant to the central emotional event. For instance, when we learn about a major emotional public event like the death of a head of state, we can often easily remember the details of the context in which we first heard this information. Do you remember where, when, and with whom you were when you first heard of the accidental death of Princess Diana? If this is the case, you have what is called a *flashbulb memory* (FBM) of this event, that is, a vivid and detailed recollection of the context in which you first learned of it. This memory can remain unchanged over a long period of time (Conway, 1990).

Brown and Kulik (1977) were the first to offer an explanation for FBM, the "now print" hypothesis: if an event is new and unexpected, then it produces surprise, a particularly effective emotion for encoding information for obvious adaptive reasons. FBM formation would also depend upon the personal importance of the event—its consequentiality, which is not differentiated from emotional arousal in their model. Finally, Brown and Kulik consider that rehearsal through conversation (overt rehearsal) or thinking (covert rehearsal) can enhance the phenomenon. Several studies have found evidences in favor of Brown and Kulik's model (Bohannon, 1988; Bohannon & Symons, 1992; Christianson, 1989; Pillemer, 1984; Rubin & Kozin, 1984).

Nearly 20 years later, Conway and colleagues (1994) extended Brown and Kulik's model by adding one explanatory factor: previous knowledge pertaining to the event. People who have such good prior knowledge about the persons and other elements involved in the public event would be more prone to develop a FBM. Conway and colleagues obtained results supporting this hypothesis. They studied people's memory of the resignation of British Prime Minister Margaret Thatcher and found that interest in politics and prior knowledge of Thatcher's government was associated with FBM formation.

In our laboratory, Finkenauer and colleagues (1998) proposed a model that differentiates the emotion components that impact on FBM formation. In this model, FBM is directly determined by surprise, by the emotional state felt during the original public event, and by the memory of it. Consequentiality, novelty and rehearsal would only have an indirect impact on FBM via the sense of shock, other emotional feelings, and memories generated by the event. Using structural equation modeling, our model was compared to the models of Brown and Kulik (1977) and of Conway and colleagues (1994). We investigated people's memory of the death of Belgian

King Baudouin, an event that generated high levels of emotion in Belgium. We found that (1) our model had the best fit compared to the two others; (2) when we applied the two other models to the data, it appeared that consequentiality had no direct effect on FBM; and (3) one hypothesized path of our model was nonsignificant—the direct effect of emotional feelings on FBM.

These findings have three implications: first, as predicted by the "now print" hypothesis, surprise is a strong predictor of FBM; second, FBM is directly predicted by the memory of the original public event; and, third, the emotional state felt during the event seem to have an indirect effect on FBM, through rehearsal, which in turn determines memory of the public event, which finally determines FBM. Bellelli and his collaborators (Bellelli, Curci, & Leone, 1999; Bellelli & Gallucci, 1999) reached similar conclusion in studying FBM related to the resignation in 1996 of Judge Antonio Di Pietro in Italy, a very popular magistrate who had incarnated the fight against corruption among Italian politicians. Hence, emotional feelings seem to have a long-term effect on FBM through postevent cognitive rehearsal.

Research on FBM suffers from several limitations. First, it is exclusively based on correlational studies. Second, the public events chosen by researchers often differ greatly in nature, and so the constructs assessed do not always have the same meaning across studies. Third, it is not well established whether memory for public events is different from memory for personal events, a finding that, if confirmed, might challenge the current status of the FBM concept. Finally, in FBM studies, the accuracy of the memory is not assessed. What is assessed is the subjective quality of the memory, that is, the quantity and quality of the details present in the memory, without controlling for their accuracy.

Implications of the Findings About Eyewitness Testimony and Flashbulb Memory

Despite the aforementioned limitations, research on eyewitness testimony and FBM provides interesting information about memory performance for emotional autobiographical events. Indeed, the studies reviewed in this section suggest that attentional processes can be enhanced during an emotional event, improving encoding processes, which increases subsequent memory performance about this event. Another important implication is that emotion can have a long-term enhancing effect on memory through rehearsal. This is mediated by the facts that (1) emotional events trigger more subsequent rehearsal than do neutral events and (2) rehearsal strengthens the event's memory traces. The first assumption is in accord with data showing that emotional events are generally followed by recurrent reinstatements of the event through social sharing and mental rumination

(Luminet, Bouts, Delie, Manstead, & Rimé, in press; Rimé, Finkenauer, Luminet, Zech, & Philippot, 1998). The second assumption is in accord with research that found that rehearsing a memory contributes to increasing the number of details present in the memory (Johnson & Chalfonte, 1994).

A contradiction remains to be solved: why is there impairment of memory of peripheral details in eyewitness research whereas there is an enhancement of memory of contextual irrelevant details in FBM research? This is probably because eyewitness research focuses on memory's accuracy, whereas in FBM research the main dependent variable is the memory's subjective quality. Therefore, the contradiction is only apparent, as these are two different factors that can vary independently. Further, as participants in eyewitness research are confronted with a situation in which the accuracy and reliability of their memories are evaluated, it is likely that they adopt more rigorous criteria of reality monitoring (Johnson, Hashtroudi, & Lindsay, 1993), rejecting more details. Consequently, memories assessed in eyewitness research should have fewer peripheral details than memories assessed in FBM studies.

The Activation of Autobiographical Memory and the Elicitation of Emotion

In the previous section, we have examined whether there is something specific to emotional event memory. In this section, we examine how memory from our past experience might influence ongoing emotional experiences. Reviewing a research program conducted in our laboratory, we now address the functions served by memory processes in the elicitation of emotion.

Building from the theories of Leventhal and of Teasdale and Barnard presented previously, we postulate that two memory systems are active in the elicitation of emotion. One is schematic and encodes the high-order recurrences of emotional events, that is, the associations between eliciting conditions and emotional responses. It constitutes a generic and implicit system of representation, similar to the "schematic level" of Leventhal and the "implicational subsystem" of Teasdale and Barnard. The other memory system is more specific and analytic; it corresponds to declarative knowledge about emotion, and it is responsible for the planning of voluntary action and coping strategies. It has been labeled "conceptual" and "propositional" by the aforementioned authors, respectively. In this theoretical perspective, "hot" cognitions, and hence emotional intensity, would be determined by the activation of the schematic memory system.

Our hypothesis was that one could draw a parallel between these emotional memory systems and the structure of emotional autobiographical memories. Indeed, autobiographical memory is organized hierarchically.

Generic or "overgeneral" memories are at the top of a pyramidal structure that encompasses specific memories (Conway, 1992, 1996; Conway & Rubin, 1993). An example of a "general" autobiographical memory (g-ABM) would be "the Sunday afternoon walks that the whole family was taking every weekend when I was a child." Such a memory condenses the information from many specific episodes, repeated over an extended period of time, and has a specific feeling state attached to it. An example of a "specific" autobiographical memory (s-ABM) would be "that very time when, during one of these family Sunday walks, I got bitten by a dog." This episode, fortunately for the individual, only happened once, and so can be located precisely in time and location. We propose that g-ABMs carry the emotional information processed by the schematic system. Indeed, g-ABMs and emotional schemas, both being generic summaries of specific emotional experiences, share the same level of emotional information processing. By contrast, s-ABMs are primarily concerned with information from the propositional system: both require more controlled processes, if only because of the strict criteria they use for source monitoring. In conclusion, the activation of "hot" cognitions, as well as emotional intensity, should be associated with the activation of g-ABMs rather than of s-ABMs.

Clinical research on depression by Williams (1996) suggests that this might be the case. Williams has shown that depressed individuals have a bias in accessing their autobiographical memory: they report preferentially g-ABMs and suffer from a limitation in accessing s-ABMs. According to Williams, this deficit in accessing s-ABMs handicaps depressed individuals in finding concrete instrumental coping strategies when confronted with emotional problems. Indeed, Williams found a negative relationship between the deficit in accessing s-ABMs and interpersonal problem solving. In our theoretical perspective, we suggest that the schematic system is overactivated in depressed individuals, who consequently fail to activate the propositional system sufficiently to process the emotional information in such a way as to decide on appropriate behavioral options and coping strategies.

To test whether emotional intensity was related to a greater accessibility of g-ABMs, we first conducted an exploratory correlational study (Philippot & Dozier, 1996). Students were exposed to a movie excerpt inducing anger. Immediately after the movie, participants reported the ABMs that had spontaneously occurred and the emotion intensity felt while viewing the movie. Afterward, they rated each ABM for its emotional intensity. ABMs were subsequently classified as g-ABMs and s-ABMs by independent judges. The emotional intensity felt during the movie was positively correlated with the number and the emotional intensity of the reported g-ABM ($r = .51$ and $.53$, respectively), but no relationship was observed with the s-ABM.

In a subsequent study, the emotional intensity was manipulated. Participants were exposed to either a rather neutral film excerpt or to an anger-inducing excerpt (Philippot, Schaefer, & Herbette, 2000). They had to push a button each time a personal memory came to mind as they were watching the movie. After the movie, the videotape was shown again, but this time the experimenter stopped the tape each time the participant had pressed the button. The participant was then invited to report the evoked memory. Subsequent analyses revealed that g-ABMs were proportionally larger in the emotional condition than in the neutral condition.

These studies show that emotional intensity facilitates the access to g-ABM as compared to s-ABM. According to our theoretical perspective, this should be the case because both emotional intensity and g-ABM accessibility depend upon the schematic system. If this is correct, priming an individual with a g-ABM should result in the activation of the schematic system and, consequently, in increased emotional intensity. This should not be the case if the individual is primed with a s-ABM. This hypothesis was tested in the following two studies:

In the first study (Philippot, 1997), participants reported in a diary for 12 consecutive days any negative emotional events they were experiencing. After having turned in their diary, they came to the laboratory for the first of two sessions. Participants were asked to freely associate the personal memories evoked by three events from their diary chosen by the experimenter. These memories were subsequently classified as s-ABMs or g-ABMs. During the second laboratory session, participants were invited to reexperience in mental imagery the three emotional events selected in their diary and to report the emotionality intensity felt during that imagery task. However, an experimental manipulation took place just before the imagery task: participants were primed either with two g-ABMs they had associated with the event or with two s-ABMs. In a control condition, participants performed a semantic task: they had to find the antonyms of a list of words that were read to them. The analysis of the results fully supported our hypothesis: participants reported more intense emotional experience during the imagery task when primed with g-ABMs than with s-ABMs, the latter condition not differing from the control condition.

This finding was replicated in a subsequent study (Philippot et al., 2000) in which emotion was induced by showing five movie excerpts to the participants, one of a neutral nature, the others inducing either anger, fear, sadness, or happiness. In a preliminary session, participants had read the script of each excerpt and they had reported the personal memories aroused by each script. These memories were subsequently classified as s-ABMs or g-ABMs. Before each movie excerpt, participants were primed with the same procedure as described in the preceding paragraph. Again, the results supported the hypothesis, participants in the g-ABM condition reporting more emotion than participants in the two other conditions did.

The results of these four studies are congruent with our hypothesis: overgeneral memories are linked to cognitive structures that generate "hot" cognition and emotional arousal. Following previous theoreticians such as Leventhal or Teasdale and Barnard, we conceive of these structures as a schematic system. Specific memories, however, seem to be less potent in activating this system. Our hypothesis is that specific memories activate the propositional system and hence should lead to enhanced capacities in coping with the emotional situation. We intend in future studies to test this assumption.

It should be noted that there is something counterintuitive in the observation that priming with g-ABMs results in greater emotional arousal. For instance, Lang (1979) insists on giving detailed instructions during emotion induction via mental imagery producing emotional arousal. The present empirical evidence contradicts this notion and the theoretical conception of emotional memory that underlies it. This important point is further elaborated in the next and last section of this chapter.

INTEGRATION

We began this chapter by asking some key questions pertaining to the role of memory in emotional processes: What is the function served by memory from our past experiences in the elicitation and regulation of emotion? How are emotional experiences stored in our memory? Is it possible to experience emotion without accessing memories from our past emotional experiences? To answer these questions, we have reviewed different domains of the psychological literature.

We have seen that historically very little attention was given to the role of memory in the emotional processes. A notable exception was the work of Magda Arnold, who ascribed to emotional memory a central role in the automatic and implicit attribution of emotional meaning to a situation. Unfortunately, this pioneering proposal was not followed by further theoretical or empirical developments. Since the 1980s, however, interest has developed in the memory of emotions. The first models to be proposed, those of Bower and of Lang, were network models. They tend to conceptualize emotional memory as a unitary, one-level process. In Bower's model, emotional memory is not distinguished from memory in general: it obeys the same rules and uses the same structure and codes that any other memory would. Lang improved this model by proposing that body responses would be doubly coded in memory: at one level, there would be a declarative propositional code; at another level, there would be effector or motor codes that would directly command and organize the body responses. Yet, in this model, with the exception of the link to effector codes for body responses, emotional memory would not be different from memory in general.

More recent models clearly agree on the fact that emotional memory is best conceived of as a multilevel or multisystem structure. In fact, there is a remarkable convergence in the two models we presented in the second section of this chapter: those of Leventhal and of Teasdale and Barnard. According to these models, an emotional memory can be encoded at different levels. Moreover, emotional meaning can be ascribed to a situation and emotional responses can be elicited and organized by any of these levels. A large consensus can be found for at least two levels. One level is declarative and has been labeled propositional. Its information is directly accessible to consciousness and maps easily onto language. It follows the rules and structure of propositional logic. It organizes voluntary action and coping strategies. The other level is implicit and schematic. It encodes recurring, high-order regularities in emotional experiences and is primarily based on spatial and temporal contingencies in perceptual inputs. It obeys the rules of conditioning, and its content is not easily translated into language. Processing at this level is automatic and much faster than at the propositional level.

Some authors (Leventhal & Scherer, 1987; Teasdale & Barnard, 1993) have proposed that the schematic level is directly connected to the cognitive system organizing body responses. This is congruent with neuropsychological evidences and the model of LeDoux (1996). This basic body system could be conceived of as the set of innate neural structures that organize basic behavioral and emotional tendencies such as fighting, fleeing, or appetitive drives (Frijda, 1986; Panksepp, 1989). Teasdale and Barnard (1993) have proposed that this system might be activated only by inputs from the schematic (or "implicational," as they label it) system.

The notion that emotional memory, and hence the cognitive organization of emotion, is best conceived as a multilevel process is also supported by neuropsychological evidences. For instance, LeDoux (1996) has shown that emotional processes organized by emotional memory in the amygdala can occur automatically, outside of awareness, and that this level is independent of declarative processes. This distinction shares a lot of similarities with the distinction between the schematic and propositional systems just described. Likewise, what we called the body system is similar to the concept of "primary emotions" in the model of Damasio (1994). In both cases, these structures consist of innate, biologically determined reactions. In Damasio's model, "secondary emotions" correspond to what we labeled the schematic system. Damasio also proposes that conscious emotional feelings, arising from the perception of bodily changes and of the eliciting situation, play an important role in human emotion by increasing the range of adaptive responses. This latter consideration corresponds to the function ascribed to the propositional system.

Finally, the results of our research on the role of autobiographical memory in the elicitation of emotion are perfectly congruent with the notion that emotional memory is a multilevel process. The priming of generic emotional memories, supposed to activate schematic processes, induces a greater intensity in emotional feelings than the priming of specific emotional memories, which are supposed to activate primarily propositional processes.

A Model of Emotional Memory

Based on the preceding integration of theories and research findings, we propose a model for memory processes in emotion illustrated in Figure 3.4. This model distinguishes between two cognitive systems, each based on a different type of memory. One system, labeled "schematic processes," is based on schemas; it is automatic and implicit. The other system, labeled "propositional and reflexive processes," is more complex and is based on episodic and semantic knowledge. It can be consciously accessed. The further definition of these systems, as well as of the model, is easier to achieve from a developmental perspective.

At birth, neither of the two systems exists. Emotional reactions are coordinated by a set of innate neural circuits organizing behavior in key domains for survival and social binding. In Figure 3.4, these circuits are labeled the "body response system." These responses are what Damasio (1994) called "primary emotions." They are similar to the concept of sensorimotor processes developed by Leventhal (1984). They are also the basis of emotional action tendencies (Frijda, 1986). These innate responses can be triggered by extremely simple perceptual indices, like the perception of a movement pattern, or somesthesic sensations. For instance, the sensation of losing support automatically triggers panic in a newborn.

The system of schematic processes develops on the basis of the activation of "primary emotions." The first schemas to constitute it are abstract representations that are the mere records of the links between sensory indices and body responses, as they occurred during emotional events actually experienced by the individuals. Thus, it encodes emotional conditioning according to the rule of temporal contingency: two elements are connected only because they have been repetitively activated simultaneously. Schemas are automatically activated, and they are processing information very rapidly but with no flexibility. Schemas are based on concrete and actual experiences, but their content is abstract and general, as they encode the high-order recurrences among these concrete experiences and not the experiences themselves. As they are based on associations, the links are

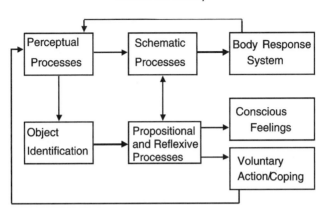

FIGURE 3.4. An integrative model of emotional memory.

bidirectional: schemas can activate body response systems, and vice versa. Damasio (1994) reports evidence for such a bidirectional link, which is also documented by the facial feedback effect (Matsumoto, 1987) or by the maintenance of a depressogenic schema via a body response loop (see, e.g., Teasdale, 1996). Being based on actual experiences, schema are idiosyncratic to the individual. Thus, according to previous experiences, different individuals might develop different schemas for, say, anger: some could develop preferentially a schema for inward anger, whereas others would develop a schema for outward anger. The schematic system concept bears a resemblance to the concepts of "secondary emotion" (Damasio, 1994), of "implicational processes" (Teasdale & Barnard, 1993), and of a "schematic level" (Leventhal, 1984). One could say that the schematic system constitutes the "cognitive heart" of emotion, that is, the seat of "hot" cognition.

With cognitive maturation and the development of perceptual systems, more elaborate processes rapidly develop during ontogeny. Objects are extracted from perceptual indices and identified as such. They are the basis of concept formation. From concepts, a new type of knowledge develops—the system of propositional and reflexive processes. It consists of specific meanings: discrete concepts are related through specified semantic links. Thus, the "logic" of connection markedly differs from that of the schematic system: links between elements do not follow the rules of temporal contingency but those of semantic logic. This knowledge system can be consciously and voluntarily accessed. It corresponds to "cold" cognition. It allows analytic processing of information in a much more flexible way than the schematic system. Indeed, the propositional and reflexive system is more diversified than the schematic system; it contains many more units of representation (concepts vs. schemas), and the links between these representations are more diverse (semantic links vs. contingency connections). However, it necessitates more cognitive resources and more processing time. While information in the schematic system is very slow to change because it encodes recurrences, information in the propositional and reflexive system can be changed very rapidly. For instance, a single new fact can change the information in the propositional and reflexive system.

Because of its reflexive nature, this system can initiate its own processes, allowing self-reflexive processes. Mental ruminations—induction of emotion through mental imagery—initiate emotional processes via the self-reflexive capacity of the propositional and reflexive system. This capacity is also necessary for choosing between behavioral responses to a situation and to voluntarily initiate coping strategies (Wheeler et al., 1997). Finally, the propositional and reflexive system is also necessary for the conscious identification of a feeling state. Even if schematic processes give an experiential quality to emotional states, propositional and reflexive processes are necessary for the conscious acknowledgment by individuals that they are experiencing an emotion. The propositional and reflexive system bears a resemblance to the "propositional subsystem" of Teasdale and Barnard (1993) and the "conceptual level" of Leventhal (1984).

Given that in everyday life the two systems are often activated together, associations between elements of both are frequently established. Thus, information from one system might acquire the capacity to arouse the other. This is represented by the reciprocal arrow between the two systems at the center of Figure 3.4. Hence, consciously thinking about an emotional experience might arouse the schematic system. Similarly, the automatic activation of the schematic system by perceptual input might generate specific thoughts at the propositional and reflextive system level. In fact, such links are integrated to the schemas that can be redefined as encoding high-level recurrences between sensory indices, thoughts from the propositional and reflexive system, and body responses.

In conclusion, this model attempts to integrate the different recent models of emotional memory and to account for the empirical evidences reviewed earlier. Although quite general, this model is sufficiently specified to be empirically tested, as exemplified by the different research programs from our laboratory reviewed earlier. For instance, it offers an explanation for the emotion-enhancing effect of g-ABMs. It also accounts for the dissociation observed in the emotional life of individuals suffering from amnesia. Clearly, much more empirical work is needed to further test and refine this model. Still, we believe that such a theoretical framework might well be heuristic for empirical research in the many domains related to emotional memory.

Future Research Directions

The current state of the literature on memory processes in emotion is two-fold. On the one hand, this domain suffers from a remarkable paucity of empirical studies: compared to other domains of emotion research, such as facial expression or appraisal, very little experimental work has been done on memory processes in emotion. On the other hand, as we noted in the foregoing sections, there is currently a remarkable convergence of the psychological and neuropsychological models of memory processes in emotion. In other words, it appears that this domain is reaching a sufficient degree of theoretical integration to allow for programmatic research.

In our opinion, several avenues of research seem particularly promising. One would be to distinguish the effect of "cold" versus "hot" cognition about emotion on information processing. Indeed, a frequent criticism of experiments on the effects of emotion on cognitive and social processes is that they do not disentangled effects of emotional feeling from those of mere emotion knowledge activation (Clore et al., in press; Wyer & Carlston, 1979). In other words, it is not possible to say whether the activation of "cold" cognition about emotion is sufficient to obtain the observed effects or whether the activation of "hot" cognition—and thus of emotional body responses—is necessary. A multilevel approach of emotional processing would answer this question. Memory process can be primed at two distinct levels of emotional processing—one that yields actual emotional feeling, and another that only activates "cold" emotional knowledge. Innes-Ker and Niedenthal (2000) have already pioneered this approach and found different effects of emotional priming on social categorization.

Another avenue would be to investigate the relationships between episodic memory for specific events and generic schematic memory structures for emotion. Indeed, as demonstrated in this chapter, the literature on the memory of specific emotional experience has developed independently from the research on the cognitive structures of emotion. The recent development of episodic memory theory (see, e.g., Wheeler et al., 1997) provides a theoretical basis on which to design studies linking memories for specific emotional events and the schematic structure of emotional memory.

A third avenue consists of pursuing brain imagery research on memory processes in emotion by a multilevel approach. Activating different levels of processing in emotional memory tasks while recording brain images would enable further exploration of the observed convergence between psychological and neuropsychological models of memory processes in emotion. The observation of neural paths differentiated according to the level of emotional information processing would bring further evidence in support of the multilevel approach.

ACKNOWLEDGMENT

The writing of this chapter has been facilitated by Grant Nos. 8.4508.95 and 8.4512.98 from the Fonds National de la Recherche Scientifique de Belgique.

REFERENCES

Acosta, A. & Vila, J. (1990). Emotional imagery: Effect of autonomic response information on physiological arousal. *Cognition and Emotion, 4*, 145–160.

Adolphs, R., Cahill, L., Schul, R., & Babinsky, R. (1997). Impaired declarative memory for emotional material following bilateral amygdala damage in humans. *Learning and Memory, 4*, 291–300.

Adolphs, R., Tranel, D., Damasio, H., & Damasio, A. (1995). Fear and the human amygdala. *Journal of Neuroscience, 15*, 5879–5892.

Arnold, M. B. (1950). An exitatory theory of emotion. In M. L. Reymert (Ed.), *Feelings and emotions* (pp. 11–33). New York: McGraw-Hill.

Arnold, M. B. (1960). *Emotion and personality.* New York: Columbia University Press.

Arnold, M. B. (1970a). Perennial problems in the field of emotion. In M. B. Arnold (Ed.), *Feelings and emotions* (pp. 149–185). New York: Academic Press.

Arnold, M. B. (1970b). Brain function in emotion: A phenomenological analysis. In P. Black (Ed.), *Physiological correlates of emotion* (pp. 261–285). New York: Academic Press.

Bailey, D. J., Kim, J. J., Sun, W., Thompson, R. F., & Helmstetter, F. J. (1999). Acquisition of fear conditioning in rats requires the synthesis of mRNA in the amygdala. *Behavioral Neuroscience, 113*, 276–282.

Barnard, P. J., & Teasdale, J. D. (1991). Interactive cognitive subsystems: A systemic approach to cognitive–affective interaction and change. *Cognition and Emotion, 5*, 1–39.

Bechara, A., Damasio, A. R., Damasio, H., & Anderson, S. (1994). Insensitivity to future consequences following damage to human prefrontal cortex. *Cognition, 50*, 7–12.

Bechara, A., Tranel, D., Damasio, H., Adolphs, R., Rockland, C., & Damasio, A. (1995). Double dissociation of conditioning and declarative knowledge relative to the amygdala and hippocampus in humans. *Science, 289*, 1115–1118.

Bechara, A., Tranel, D., Damasio, A. R., & Damasio, H. (1993). Failure to respond autonomically in anticipation of future outcomes following damage to human prefrontal cortex. *Society for Neuroscience Abstracts, 19*, 791.

Bellelli, G., Curci, A., & Leone, G. (1999). La ricerca. In G. Bellelli (Ed.), *Ricordo di un giudice: Uno studio sulle Flashbulb memories* (pp. 189–222). Naples: Liguori.

Bellelli, G., & Gallucci, M. (1999). Il modello strutturale. In G. Bellelli (Ed.), *Ricordo di un giudice: Uno studio sulle Flashbulb memories* (pp. 223–240). Naples: Liguori.

Bohannon, J. N. (1988). Flashbulb memories for the space shuttle disaster: A tale of two stories. *Cognition, 29*, 179–196.

Bohannon, J. N., & Symons, V. L. (1992). Flashbulb memories: Confidence, consistency, and quantity. In E. Winograd & U. Neisser (Eds.), *Affect and accuracy in recall: Studies of flashbulb memories* (pp. 65–91). New York: Cambridge University Press.

Bower, G. H. (1981). Mood and memory. *American Psychologist, 36,* 129–148.

Bower, G. H., & Cohen, P. R. (1982). Emotional influence in memory and thinking: Data and theory. In M. S. Clark & S. T. Fiske (Eds.), *Affect and cognition* (pp. 291–332). Hillsdale, NJ: Erlbaum.

Brown, R., & Kulik, J. (1977). Flashbulb memories. *Cognition, 5,* 73–99.

Burke, A., Heuer, F., & Reisberg, D. (1992). Remembering emotional events. *Memory and Cognition, 20,* 277–290.

Chapelle, G. (1998). *Processus de mémoire et processus émotionnel: Étude de cas d'un patient amnésique.* Unpublished doctoral thesis, Université Catholique de Louvain, Louvain-la-Neuve, Belgium.

Chapelle, G., Philippot, P., & Vanderlinden, M. (2000). *Dissociation between perceptual and reflexive emotional processing in an amnesiac patient.* Manuscript submitted for publication.

Christianson, S. A. (1989). Flashbulb memories: Special, but not so special. *Memory and Cognition, 17,* 433–443.

Christianson, S. A. (1992). Emotional stress and eyewitness memory: A critical review. *Psychological Bulletin, 112,* 284–309.

Christianson, S. A., & Hubinette, B. (1993). Hands up! A study of witnesses' emotional reactions and memories associated with bank robberies. *Applied Cognitive Psychology, 7,* 365–379.

Christianson, S. A., Loftus, E. F., Hoffman, H., & Loftus, G. R. (1991). Eye fixations and memory for emotional events. *Journal of Experimental Psychology: Learning, Memory and Cognition, 17,* 693–701.

Christianson, S. A., & Safer, M. A. (1996). Emotional events and emotions in autobiographical memories. In D. C. Rubin (Ed.) *Remembering our past: Studies in autobiographical memory* (pp. 218–243). Cambridge, UK: Cambridge University Press.

Clark, C. R., Egan, C. F., McFarlane, A. C., Morris, P., Weber, D., Sonkkilla, C., Marcina, J., & Tochon-Danguy, H. J. (2000). Updating working memory for words: A PET activation study. *Human Brain Mapping, 9,* 42–54.

Clore, G. L., Wyer, R. S., Dienes, B., Gasper, K., Gohm, C., & Isbell, L. (in press). Affective feelings as feedback: Some cognitive consequences. In L. L. Martin & G. L. Clore (Eds.), *Mood and cognition: Contrasting theories.* Mahwah, NJ: Erlbaum.

Collins, A. M., & Loftus, E. F. (1975). A spreading activation theory of semantic processing. *Psychological Review, 82,* 407–428.

Collins, A. M., & Quillian, M. R. (1969) Retrieval time from semantic memory. *Journal of Verbal Learning and Verbal Behavior, 8,* 240–247.

Conway, M. A. (1990). *Autobiographical memory: An introduction.* Philadelphia: Open University Press.

Conway, M. A. (1992). A structural model of autobiographical memory. In M. A. Conway, D. C. Rubin, H. Spinnler & W. A. Wagenaar (Eds.), *Theoretical perspectives on autobiographical memory* (pp. 167–193). Dordrecht, Netherlands: Kluwer.

Conway, M. A. (1996). Autobiographical knowledge and autobiographical memories. In D. C. Rubin (Ed.), *Remembering our past: Studies in autobiographical memory* (pp. 67–93). Cambridge, UK: Cambridge University Press.

Conway, M. A., Anderson, S. J., Larse, S. F., Donnely, C. M., McDaniel, M. A., McClelland, A. G. R., Rawles, R. E., & Logie, R. H. (1994). The formation of flashbulb memories. *Memory and Cognition, 22*, 326–343.

Conway, M. A., & Rubin, D. C. (1993). The structure of autobiographical memory. In A. F. Collins, S. E. Gathercole, M. A. Conway, & P. E. Morris (Eds.), *Theories of memory* (pp. 103–137). Hove, East Sussex, UK: Erlbaum.

Cuthbert, B. N., Vrana, S. R., & Bradley, M. M. (1991). Imagery: Function and physiology. *Advances in Psychophysiology, 4*, 1–42.

Damasio, A. R. (1994). *Descartes' error: Emotion, reason and the human brain.* New York: Grosset/Putnam.

Drevets, W. C., & Raichle, M. E. (1998). Reciprocal suppression of regional cerebral blood flow during emotional versus higher cognitive processes: Implications for interactions between emotion and cognition. *Cognition and Emotion, 12*, 353–385.

Finkenauer, C., Luminet, O., Gisle, L., El-Ahmadi, A., Van der Linden, M., & Philippot, P. (1998). Flashbulb memories and the underlying mechanisms of their formation: Toward an emotional–integrative model. *Memory and Cognition, 26*, 516–531.

Frijda, N. H. (1986). *The emotions.* Cambridge, UK: Cambridge University Press.

George, M. S., Ketter, T. E., Parekh, P. I., Horwitz, B., Herscovitch, P., & Post, R. M. (1995). Brain activity during transient sadness and happiness in healthy women. *American Journal of Psychiatry, 152*, 341–351.

Hamman, S. B., Cahill, L., & Squire, L. R. (1997). Emotional perception and memory in amnesia. *Neuropsychology, 11*, 104–113.

Hamman, S. B., Stefanecci, L., Squire, L. R., Adolphs, R., Tranel, D., Damasio, H., & Damasio, A. (1996). Recognizing facial emotion. *Nature, 379*, 497.

Helmstetter, F. J. (1992). Contribution of the amygdala to learning and performance of conditional fear. *Physiology and Behavior, 51*, 1271–1276.

Innes-Ker, A., & Niedenthal, P. M. (2000). *Emotion concepts and emotional states in social judgment and categorization.* Manuscript submitted for publication.

Johnson, M. K., & Chalfonte, B. L. (1994). Binding complex memories: The role of reactivation and the hippocampus. In D. L. Schacter & E. Tulving (Eds.), *Memory systems 1994* (pp. 311–350). Cambridge, MA: MIT Press.

Johnson, M. K., Hashtroudi, S., & Lindsay, D. S. (1993). Source monitoring. *Psychological Bulletin, 114*, 3–28.

Johnson, M. K., & Multhaup, K. S. (1992). Emotion and MEM. In S. A. Christianson (Ed.), *The handbook of emotion and memory* (pp. 33–66). Hillsdale, NJ: Erlbaum.

Kassin, S. M., Ellsworth, P. C., & Smith, V. L. (1989). The "general acceptance" of psychological research on eyewitness testimony: A survey of the experts. *American Psychologist, 44*, 1089–1098.

Kenealy, P. M. (1997). Mood-state-dependent retrieval: The effects of induced mood on memory reconsidered. *Quarterly Journal of Experimental Psychology, 50*, 290–317.

Kiernan, M. J., Bailey, G., Sims, J., Lukes, D., & Cranney, J. (1996). Accumbal lesions attenuate contextual fear conditioning in the rat. *Society for Neuroscience Abstracts, 22,* 1381.

LaBar, K. S., LeDoux, J. E., Spencer, D. D., & Phelps, E. A. (1995). Impaired fear conditioning following unilateral temporal lobectomy in humans. *Journal of Neuroscience, 15,* 6846–6855.

Lacey, J. I., & Lacey, B. C. (1970). Some autonomic-central nervous system interrelationships. In P. Black (Ed.), *Physiological correlates of emotion* (pp. 205–228). New York: Academic Press.

Lane, R. D., Reiman, E. M., Ahern, G. L., Schwartz, G. E., & Davidson, R. J. (1997). Neuroanatomical correlates of happiness, sadness and disgust. *American Journal of Psychiatry, 154,* 926–933.

Lane, R. D., Reiman, E. M., Bradley, M. M., Lang, P. J., Ahern, G. L., Davidson, R. J., & Schwartz, G. E. (1997). Neuroanatomical correlates of pleasant and unpleasant emotion. *Neuropsychologia, 35,* 1437–1444.

Lang, P. J. (1979). A bio-informational theory of emotional imagery. *Psychophysiology, 16,* 495–512.

LeDoux, J. E. (1992). Emotion as memory: Anatomical systems underlying indelible neural traces. In S. A. Christianson (Ed.), *The handbook of emotion and memory* (pp. 269–288). Hillsdale, NJ: Erlbaum.

LeDoux, J. E. (1993). Emotional memory systems in the brain. *Behavioural Brain Research, 58,* 69–79.

LeDoux, J. E. (1995). Emotion: Clues from the brain. *Annual Review of Psychology, 46,* 209–235.

LeDoux, J. E. (1996). *The emotional brain: The mysterious underpinnings of emotional life.* New York: Simon & Schuster.

Leventhal, H. (1984a). A perceptual-motor theory of emotion. In L. Berkowitz (Ed.), *Advances in experimental social psychology* (Vol. 17, pp. 117–182). New York: Academic Press.

Leventhal, H. (1984b). A perceptual motor theory of emotion. In K. Scherer & P. Ekman (Eds.), *Approaches to emotion* (pp. 271–291). Hillsdale, NJ: Erlbaum.

Leventhal, H., & Mosbach, P. A. (1983). The perceptual–motor theory of emotion. In J. T. Cacioppo & R. E. Petty (Eds.), *Social psychophysiology* (pp. 353–388). New York: Guilford Press.

Leventhal, H., & Scherer, K. (1987). The relationship of emotion to cognition: A functional approach to a semantic controversy. *Cognition and Emotion, 1,* 3–28.

Loftus, E. F., & Burns, T. E. (1982). Mental shock can produce retrograde amnesia. *Memory and Cognition, 10,* 318–323.

Luminet, O., Bouts, P., Delie, F., Manstead, A. S. R., & Rimé, B. (in press). Social sharing of emotion following exposure to a negatively valenced situation. *Cognition and Emotion.*

Mandler, G. (1980). The generation of emotion: A psychological theory. In R. Plutchik & H. Kellerman (Eds.), *Emotion: Theory, research, and experience* (Vol. 1, pp. 219–243). New York: Academic Press.

Mandler, G. (1984). *Mind and body.* New York: Norton.

Maren, S. (1998). Overtraining does not mitigate contextual fear conditioning deficits produced by neurotoxic lesions of the basolateral amygdala. *Journal of Neuro-science, 18,* 3088–3097.

Maren, S. (1999). Neurotoxic or electrolytic lesions of the ventral subiculum produce deficits in the acquisition and expression of Pavlovian fear conditioning in rats. *Behavioral Neuroscience, 113,* 283–290.

Maren, S., & Fanselow, M. S. (1997). Electrolytic lesions of the dorsal hippocampus, fimbria/fornix, or entorhinal cortex produce anterograde deficits in contextual fear conditioning in rats. *Neurobiology of Learning and Memory, 67,* 142–149.

Matsumoto, D. (1987). The role of facial responses in the experience of emotion: More methodological problems and a meta-analysis. *Journal of Personality and Social Psychology, 52,* 769–774.

McClelland, J. L., McNaughton, B. L., & O'Reilly, R. C. (1995). Why there are complementary learning systems in the hippocampus and neocortex: Insights from the successes and failures of connectionist models of learning and memory. *Psychological Review, 102,* 419–457.

Mori, E., Ikeda, M., Hirono, N., Kitagaki, H., Imamura, T., & Shimomura, T. (1999). Amygdalar volume and emotional memory in Alzheimer's disease. *American Journal of Psychiatry, 156,* 216–222.

Panksepp, J. (1989). The neurobiology of emotions: Of animals brains and human feelings. In H. Wagner & A. S. R. Manstead (Eds.), *Handbook of social psychophysiology* (pp. 5–26). Chichester, UK: Wiley.

Philippot, P. (1993). Actual physiological changes and perceived bodily sensations in emotion. *Psychophysiology, 30,* S51.

Philippot, P. (1997, May 21). *Autobiographical memory priming in the emotion.* Paper presented at the annual meeting of the Belgian Psychological Society, Brussels.

Philippot, P., & Dozier, S. (1996, August 12–17). Subjective and physiological consequences of associating emotional memories. *Proceedings of the 9th Conference of the International Society for Research on Emotion,* 155–159.

Philippot, P., Schaefer, A., & Herbette, G. (2000). *Autobiographical memory in emotion: Impact of number, intensity and level of memory priming on emotional intensity.* Manuscript in preparation.

Philips, R. G., & LeDoux, J. E. (1992). Differential contribution of amygdala and hippocampus to cued and contextual fear conditioning. *Behavioral Neuroscience, 106,* 274–285.

Pillemer, D. B. (1984). Flashbulb memories of the assassination attempt on President Reagan. *Cognition, 16,* 63–80.

Posner, M. I., Walker, J. A., Friedrich, F. J., & Rafal, R. D. (1984). Effects of parietal injury on covert orienting of attention. *Journal of Neuroscience, 4,* 1863–1874.

Proust, M. (1957). *Swann's way* (C. K. Scott Moncrieff, Trans.). London: Penguin Books. (Original work published in English 1922; original work published in French 1913)

Reiman, E. M. (1997). The application of positron emission tomography to the study of normal and pathological emotions. *Journal of Clinical Psychiatry, 58*(Suppl. 16), 4–12.

Reiman, E. M., Lane, R. D., Ahern, G. L., Schwartz, G. E., Davidson, R. J., Friston, K. J., Yun, L.-S., & Chen, K. (1997). Neuroanatomical correlates of externally and internally generated human emotion. *American Journal of Psychiatry, 154*, 918–925.

Riedel, G., Harrington, N. R., Hall, G., & Macphail, E. M. (1997). Nucleus accumbens lesions impair context but not cue conditioning in rats. *Neuroreport, 8*, 2477–2481.

Rimé, B., Finkenauer, C., Luminet, O., Zech, E., & Philippot, P. (1998). Social sharing of emotion: new evidence and new questions. In W. Stroebe & M. Hewstone (Eds.), *European review of social psychology* (Vol. 7., pp. 145–189). Chichester, UK: Wiley.

Rimé, B., Philippot, P., & Cisamolo, D. (1990). Social schemata of peripheral changes in emotion. *Journal of Personality and Social Psychology, 59*, 38–49.

Rogan, M., & LeDoux, J. E. (1996). Emotion: Systems, cells, synaptic plasticity. *Cell, 85*, 469–475.

Rubin, D. C., & Kozin, M. (1984). Vivid memories. *Cognition, 16*, 81–95.

Saigh, P. A. (1991). The development of PTSD following 4 different types of traumatization. *Behaviour Research and Therapy, 29*, 249–252.

Schacter, S. (1964). The interaction of cognitive and physiological determinants of emotional state. In L. Berkowitz (Ed.), *Advances in experimental social psychology* (Vol. 1, pp. 49–79). New York: Academic Press.

Schumacher, E. H., Lauber, E., Awh, E., Jonides, J., Smith, E. E., & Koeppe, R. A. (1996). PET evidence for an amodal verbal working memory system. *Neuroimage, 3*, 79–88.

Schwartz, B. E., Halgren, E., Simpkins, F., Fuster, J., Mandelkern, M., Krisdakmutorn, T., Gee, M., Brown, C., Ropchan, J. R., & Blahd, W. H. (1996). Primary or working memory in frontal lobe epilepsy: An (18)FDG-PET study of dysfunctional zones. *Neurology, 46*, 737–747.

Squire, L. R. (1992). Memory and the hippocampus: A synthesis from findings with rats, monkeys, and humans. *Psychological Review, 99*, 195–231.

Steblay, N. M. (1992). A meta-analytic review of the weapon focus effect. *Law and Human Behavior, 16*, 413–424.

Teasdale, J. D. (1993). Emotion and two kinds of meaning: Cognitive therapy and applied cognitive science. *Behaviour Research and Therapy, 31*, 339–354.

Teasdale, J. D. (1996). Clinically relevant theory: Integrating clinical insight with cognitive science. In P. Salkovskis (Ed.), *Frontiers of cognitive therapy* (pp. 26–47). New York: Guilford Press.

Teasdale, J. D. (1999). Multi-level theories of cognition-emotion relations. In T. Dalgleish & M. Power (Eds.), *Handbook of cognition and emotion* (pp. 665–681). Chichester, UK: Wiley.

Teasdale, J. D., & Barnard, P. J. (1993). *Affect, cognition and change*. Hove, East Sussex, UK: Erlbaum.

Tobias, B. A., Khilstrom, J. F., & Schacter, D. L. (1992). Emotion and implicit memory. In S. A. Christianson (Ed.), *The handbook of emotion and memory* (pp. 67–92). Hillsdale, NJ: Erlbaum.

Tranel, D., & Damasio, A. (1993). The covert learning of affective valence does not require structures in hippocampal system or amygdala. *Journal of Cognitive Neuroscience, 5*, 79–88.

Ucros, C. G. (1989). Mood state-dependent memory: A meta-analysis. *Cognition and Emotion, 3*, 139–167.

Wessel, I., & Merckelbach, H. (1998). Memory for threat-relevant and threat-irrelevant cues in spider phobics. *Cognition and Emotion, 12*, 93–104.

Westbrook, R. F., Good, A. J., & Kiernan, M. J. (1997). Microinjections of morphine into the nucleus accumbens impairs contextual learning in rats. *Behavioral Neuroscience, 111*, 996–1013.

Wetzler, S. (1985). Mood-state-dependent retrieval: A failure to replicate. *Psychological Reports, 56*, 759–765.

Wheeler, M. A., Stuss, D. A. T., & Tulving, E. (1997). Toward a theory of episodic memory: The frontal lobes and autonoetic consciousness. *Psychological Bulletin, 121*, 331–354.

Williams, J. M. G. (1996) Depression and the specificty of autobiographical memory. In D. C. Rubin (Ed.), *Remembering our past: Studies in autobiographical memories* (pp. 244–270). Cambridge, UK: Cambridge University Press.

Wyer, R. S., & Carltson, D. E. (1979). *Social cognition, inference and attribution.* Hillsdale, NJ: Erlbaum.

Yuille, J. C., & Cutshall, J. L. (1986). A case study of eyewitness memory of a crime. *Journal of Applied Psychology, 71*, 291–301.

Yuille, J. C., & Tollestrup, P. A. (1992). A model of the diverse effects of emotion on eyewitness memory. In S. A. Christianson (Ed.), *The handbook of emotion and memory* (pp. 201–215). Hillsdale, NJ: Erlbaum.

4

Positive Emotions

BARBARA L. FREDRICKSON
CHRISTINE BRANIGAN

Readers may wonder why positive emotions merit their own chapter in this book whereas negative emotions do not. It's analogous to why you might find courses at your university on women's history but not men's history. The scientific literature on emotions has been, by and large, a literature on negative emotions. Emotions like fear, anger, sadness, and disgust have taken center stage in both theory and research, whereas emotions like joy, contentment, interest, and love have played only minor roles. Fortunately, this imbalance is beginning to change. In recent years, special issues of journals (Aspinwall, 1998) and symposia at national and international conferences (Fredrickson, 1998a, 1999) have featured work relevant to the study of positive emotions. This recent emergence of work calls for a consolidation of what's known and what's new about positive emotions. This chapter aims to provide that consolidation, while underscoring how positive emotions may differ from negative emotions. We hope this review will generate curiosity about positive emotions and spur readers to join the scientific exploration of this relatively new frontier.

WHY HAVE POSITIVE EMOTIONS BEEN NEGLECTED?

There are multiple, intertwined reasons why research on negative emotions has far outpaced that on positive emotions. One reason, which has plagued psychology more generally (see Seligman & Csikszentmihalyi, 2000), is the traditional focus on psychological problems alongside remedies for those problems. Negative emotions—when extreme, prolonged, or contextually inappropriate—produce many grave problems for individuals and society, including phobias and anxiety disorders, aggression and violence, depression and suicide, eating disorders and sexual dysfunction, and a host of stress-related physical disorders. Although positive emotions do at times pose problems (e.g., mania, drug addiction), these problems have often assumed lower priority among psychologists and emotion researchers. So, due in part to their association with problems and dangers, negative emotions have captured the majority of research attention. Not surprisingly, given the human suffering they can cause, the push to understand negative emotions has been immense. Arguably, efforts to understand positive emotions should take a backseat to solving these problems. The misfortune of this triage strategy is that even though positive emotions may not spark problems of the same magnitude as negative emotions do, they may in fact provide some important solutions to the problems negative emotions generate (Fredrickson, 1998b, 2000a). We return to this point in a later section.

A second reason why positive emotions may have garnered so little empirical attention is that, relative to negative emotions, positive emotions appear to be fewer in number and rather diffuse (de Rivera, Possell, Verette, & Weiner, 1989; Ellsworth & Smith, 1988b). For instance, scientific taxonomies of discrete or basic emotions (Ekman, 1992; Izard, 1977; Tomkins, 1982) typically identify only one positive emotion for every three or four negative emotions (Ellsworth & Smith, 1988b), an imbalance also reflected in English-language emotion words (Averill, 1980). Interestingly, the relative lack of differentiation among the positive emotions is apparent across the various components of the emotion process. For instance, although specific negative emotions have specific facial configurations that imbue them with unique and universally recognized signal value (Ekman et al., 1987), specific positive emotions appear to have no unique signal value, but instead all share the Duchenne smile (i.e., raised lip corners accompanied by muscle contraction around the eyes; Ekman, 1992). Further diluting the signal value of positive emotions, non-Duchenne smiles (i.e., those absent muscle contraction around the eyes) are often indistinguishable from Duchenne smiles to untrained observers and appear in social circumstances replete with negative emotions or devoid of all emotion (but see Frank, Ekman, & Friesen, 1993; Keltner & Bonanno, 1997). Similarly, although autonomic specificity has been demonstrated between negative and positive emotions and, to some degree, among the negative emotions (Cacioppo, Klein, Berntson, & Hatfield, 1993; Levenson, 1992; Levenson, Ekman, & Friesen, 1990), the positive emotions have not yielded distinguishable autonomic responses (Fredrickson, Mancuso, Branigan, & Tugade, 2000; Levenson et al., 1990). Likewise, whereas self-reports of subjective experience yield differentiation among various negative emotion terms (Ellsworth & Smith, 1988a), positive emotion terms yield greater intercorrelations, reflecting a greater degree of blending (Ellsworth & Smith, 1988b). In speculating on the origins of these asymmetries, Nesse (1990) suggested that "natural selection shapes emotions only for situations that contain threats or opportunities. There are more negative than positive emotions because there are more different kinds of threats than opportunities" (p. 280). Others have noted that positive emotions do not require differentiation comparable to the negative emotions because the cost of failure to respond appropriately to a life threat could be death, whereas the cost of failure to respond appropriately to a life opportunity is unlikely to be so dire (Pratto & John, 1991; Rozin & Fallon, 1987).

Perhaps in part because of their lesser differentiation, research on positive emotions may have been slowed because distinctions among positive emotions and other, closely related affective states like sensory pleasure and positive mood have often been blurred, not sharpened. Although working definitions of emotions vary somewhat across researchers, consensus is emerging that emotions (both positive and negative) are best conceptualized as multicomponent response tendencies that unfold over relatively short time spans. Typically, emotions begin with an individual's assessment, or appraisal, of the personal meaning of some antecedent event—what Lazarus (1991) called the person–environment relationship, or the adaptational encounter. Either conscious or unconscious, this appraisal process triggers a cascade of response tendencies, which may be manifest across loosely coupled component systems, such as subjective experience, facial expressions, and physiological changes.

Sometimes various forms of sensory pleasure (e.g., sexual gratification, satiation of hunger or thirst) are taken to be positive emotions because they share with positive emotions a pleasant subjective feel and include physiological changes, and because sensory pleasure and positive emotions often co-occur (e.g., sexual gratification within a loving or exciting context). Yet emotions differ from physical sensations in that emotions require appraisals or meaning assessments to be initiated. In contrast to positive emotions, pleasure can be caused simply by changing the immediate physical environment (e.g., eating, or otherwise stimulating the body). Moreover, whereas pleasure depends heavily on real or imagined bodily stimulation, positive emotions more often occur in the absence of such physical sensation (e.g., joy at receiving good news, or interest in a new idea). Pleasurable sensations, then, are best considered automatic responses to fulfilling bodily needs. In fact, Cabanac (1971) suggested that people experience sensory pleasure with any external stimulus that "corrects an internal trouble." A cool bath, for instance, is only pleasant to someone who is overheated (who thus needs to be cooled). Likewise, food is pleasant to the hungry person, but becomes less pleasant—even unpleasant—as this person becomes satiated.

Emotions also differ from moods in that they are *about* some personally meaningful circumstance (i.e., they have an object) and are typically short lived and occupy the foreground of consciousness. In contrast, moods are typically free floating or objectless, more long lasting, and occupy the background of consciousness (Oatley & Jenkins, 1996; Rosenberg, 1998). This distinction between moods and emotions, however, is guarded more at theoretical levels than at empirical levels. In research practice, virtually identical techniques are used for inducing positive moods and positive emotions (e.g., giving gifts, viewing comedies). By consequence, much of the sizable literature on the effects of positive mood on cognition and behavior (Aspinwall, 1998; Isen, 1987, 2000) is directly relevant to positive emotions. When dependent measures (of cognition or behavior) are placed in close temporal sequence with induction procedures, the effects are likely attributable to positive emotions (see Rosenberg, 1998). Studies from this tradition suggest that positive emotions such as joy and amusement produce patterns of thought that are notably unusual (Isen, Johnson, Mertz, & Robinson, 1985), flexible (Isen & Daubman, 1984), creative (Isen, Daubman, & Nowicki, 1987), and receptive (Estrada, Isen, & Young, 1997). In general terms, positive emotions and moods "enlarge the cognitive context" (Isen, 1987, p. 222), an effect recently linked to increases in brain dopamine levels (Ashby, Isen, & Turken, 1999).

Another reason why positive emotions have been understudied is the habit among emotion theorists of creating models of emotions *in general.* Such models are typically built to the specifications of those attention-grabbing negative emotions (e.g., fear and anger), with positive emotions squeezed in later, often seemingly as an afterthought. For instance, key to many theorists' models of emotions is the idea that emotions are, by definition, associated with *specific action tendencies* (Frijda, 1986; Frijda, Kuipers, & Schure, 1989; Lazarus, 1991; Levenson, 1994; Tooby & Cosmides, 1990). Anger, for instance, creates the urge to attack, fear the urge to escape, disgust the urge to expel, guilt the urge to make amends, and so on. No theorist argues that people invariably act out these urges when feeling particular emotions. But rather, people's ideas about possible courses of action narrow in on these specific behavioral urges. A key element in these models is that having specific action tendencies come to mind is what made emotions evolutionarily adaptive: these were among the actions that worked best in getting our ancestors out of life-or-death situations. Another key idea is that specific action tendencies and organized physiological change go hand in hand. So, for example, when you have the urge to escape when feeling fear, your body reacts by mobilizing appropriate autonomic support for the possibility of running

Although specific action tendencies have been invoked to describe the form and function of positive emotions as well, the action tendencies identified for positive emotions are notably vague and underspecified (Fredrickson & Levenson, 1998). Joy, for instance, is linked with aimless activation, interest with attending, and contentment with inactivity (Frijda, 1986). These tendencies are far too general to be called specific (Fredrickson, 1998b). Although a few theorists had earlier noted that fitting positive emotions into emotion-general models posed problems (Ekman, 1992; Lazarus, 1991), this acknowledgment was not accompanied by any new or revised models to better accommodate the positive emotions. Instead, the difficulties inherent in "shoehorning" the positive emotions into emotion-general models merely tended to marginalize them further. Many theorists, for instance, minimize challenges to their models by maintaining their focus on negative emotions, paying little or no attention to positive emotions.

To date, then, numerous theorists have argued that emotions (in general) evolved because they promoted specific actions in life-threatening circumstances and thereby increased the odds of our ancestors' survival. To be sure, models based on specific action tendencies provide sound and compelling descriptions of the form and function of many negative emotions. Yet these same models fail to fit the positive emotions well (Fredrickson, 1998b). First of all, positive emotions do not typically arise in life-threatening circumstances and, perhaps by consequence, do not seem to create well-defined urges to pursue specific courses of action. What good are positive emotions then? From a functional perspective, do positive emotions have any adaptive value? It appears that the traditional approach of building models to explain all emotions has hindered psychology's ability to answer these questions adequately.

TAKING POSITIVE EMOTIONS SERIOUSLY

If many positive emotions do not share the hallmark feature with the negative emotions of promoting and supporting specific actions, then what is their form and possible function? To answer this question, Fredrickson (1998b) proposed that models based on specific action tendencies be retained for negative emotions and that new models be developed for positive emotions.

Working toward this end, Fredrickson (1998b) questioned two common presumptions within contemporary emotion theory. The first was that emotions must necessarily yield *specific* action tendencies. Although positive emotions do often produce urges to act, they appear to be less prescriptive than negative emotions about which particular actions should be taken. The second was that emotions must necessarily spark tendencies for *physical* action. Some of the positive emotions, Fredrickson argued, seem instead to spark changes primarily in cognitive activity. So, in place of action tendencies, Fredrickson introduced the term *thought–action tendencies*. Additionally, instead of presuming that thought–action tendencies are specific, Fredrickson explored the *relative breadth* of the momentary thought–action repertoire.

Using this new terminology, traditional action-oriented models for negative emotions can be paraphrased as follows: Negative emotions *narrow* a person's momentary thought–action repertoire. They do so by calling to mind and body the time-tested, ancestrally adaptive actions represented by specific action tendencies. This effect is clearly adaptive in life-threatening situations that require quick action to survive. Yet, because positive emotions are not linked to threats requiring quick action, Fredrickson (1998b) proposed that positive emotions *broaden* a person's momentary thought–action repertoire. Indeed, in a recent laboratory experiment, we demonstrated that, compared to neutral states, two phenomenologically distinct positive emotions—joy and contentment—each widen the array of thoughts and actions that come to people's minds. By contrast, two distinct negative emotions—fear and anger—shrink this same thought–action repertoire (Fredrickson & Branigan, 2000). In the next section, we review further evidence for the broadening hypothesis as we describe several distinct positive emotions in turn.

DESCRIPTIONS OF FOUR POSITIVE EMOTIONS

We next consider in detail four phenomenologically distinct positive emotions: joy, interest, contentment, and love. In using these specific emotion terms, we rely on Ekman's (1992) notion of emotion families. For instance, the term "joy" does not necessarily represent a single affective state but rather a family of related states characterized by a common theme plus variations on that theme. To reflect this concept of emotion families, as we describe each emotion, we also note closely related emotion terms. Additionally, for each emotion we describe the circumstances that tend to elicit that emotion, apparent changes in the momentary thought–action repertoire, and the consequences or outcomes of these changes.

Joy

Joy is often used interchangeably with happiness (Lazarus, 1991) and shares conceptual space with other relatively high-arousal positive emotions such as amusement (sometimes called exhilaration or mirth; Ruch, 1993), elation, and gladness (de Rivera et al., 1989). Feelings of joy arise in contexts appraised as safe and familiar (Izard, 1977) and as requiring low effort (Ellsworth & Smith, 1988b); in some cases, such feelings are triggered by events construed as accomplishments or signs of progress toward a person's goals (Izard, 1977; Lazarus, 1991). Frijda (1986) offered the clearest statement on the action tendency associated with joy, which he termed free activation: "[it] is in part aimless, unasked-for readiness to engage in whatever interaction presents itself and in part readiness to engage in enjoyments" (p. 89). The paradigmatic case of joy, in Frijda's view, is a "young child jumping out of bed on a sunny morning, running around and seeking things to play with and to enjoy" (personal communication, September 6, 1996). In other words, joy creates the urge to play and be playful in the broadest sense of the word, encompassing not only physical and social play but also intellectual and artistic play. Play, especially imaginative play, is to a large degree unscripted. It involves exploration, invention, and just plain fooling around. Pointing to no single set of actions, play takes many forms. To our minds, then, the urge to play represents a quite generic, nonspecific thought–action tendency. Joy and related positive emotions can thus be described as broadening an individual's thought–action repertoire.

Even though the playfulness inspired by joy is often aimless, it does appear to have reliable outcomes. Certainly, social play builds and strengthens friendships and attachments (Lee, 1983; Martineau, 1972). In addition, play promotes skill acquisition: physical skills are developed and practiced in rough-and-tumble play, manipulative–cognitive skills are developed and practiced in object play, and social-affective skills are developed and practiced in social play (Boulton & Smith, 1992; Caro, 1988; Dolhinow & Bishop, 1970; Pellegrini, 1992; Sylva, Bruner, & Genova, 1976). Play also fosters creativity: it involves experimentation with a wide range of possible behaviors, ways of viewing the world, and ways of being in the world (Schaefer, 1993), thereby establishing an inventory of ideas and objects that can later be combined in new and innovative ways (Dansky, 1980; Sutton-Smith, 1992; Vytgotsky, 1967). The effects of play also appear to be long lasting: Playfulness in childhood is associated with increased creativity in adulthood (Sherrod & Singer, 1989; Singer, 1973). Childhood play may also fuel brain development, especially in the frontal lobes responsible for executive functions and implicated in attention-deficit/hyperactivity disorder (ADHD; Panksepp, 1998). Joy, then, not only broadens an individual's momentary thought–action repertoire through the urge to play but also, over time, and as a product of recurrent play, can have the incidental effect of building an individual's physical, intellectual, and social resources. Importantly, these new resources are durable and can be drawn on later, long after the instigating experience of joy has subsided.

Interest

Interest is sometimes used interchangeably with curiosity, intrigue, excitement, or wonder, and shares conceptual space with challenge and intrinsic motivation (Deci & Ryan, 1985). Also, what Csikszentmihalyi (1990) calls flow, or the enjoyment experienced when a person's perceived skills match the perceived challenges of a particular activity, represents a form of interest. While not all emotion theorists consider interest a basic emotion (see, e.g., Ekman, 1992; Lazarus, 1991), building on the work of Tomkins (1962), Izard (1977) made a compelling case for its inclusion. Interest, according to Izard, is the emotion experienced most frequently. Interest arises in contexts appraised as safe and as offering novelty, change, and a sense of possibility (Izard, 1977) or mystery (Kaplan, 1992). These contexts also tend to be appraised as important and as requiring effort and attention (Ellsworth & Smith, 1988b). Some theorists have posited that the momentary thought–action tendency of interest is simply to attend to something or orient oneself (see, e.g., Frijda, 1986). But this stops short of fully describing the impact of interest. Instead, we favor Izard's treatment of interest. The momentary thought–action tendency sparked by interest, according to Izard, is exploration, explicitly and actively aimed at increasing knowledge of and experience with the target of interest. Interest generates "a feeling of wanting to investigate, become involved, or extend or expand the self by incorporating new information and having new experiences with the person or object that has stimulated the interest" (Izard, 1977, p. 216). Although interest may or may not be accompanied by overt physical action, it is nonetheless associated with feeling animated and enlivened (Izard, 1977); Tomkins (1962) characterized interest as thinking with excitement. Importantly, the openness to new ideas, experiences, and actions is what characterizes the mindset of interest as broadened rather than narrowed.

Although interested individuals explore for intrinsic reasons, to satisfy their own inner curiosity, such exploration has reliable outcomes. Most obviously, interest-inspired exploration increases knowledge (Deci, Vallerand, Pelletier, & Ryan, 1991; Hazen & Durrett, 1982; Renninger, Hidi, & Krapp, 1992). One example comes from evolutionary analyses of environmental aesthetics (Kaplan, 1992; Orians & Heerwagen, 1992). Studies have demonstrated that pictures of landscapes that are at once mysterious and easy to read reliably arouse people's interest (for a review, see Kaplan, 1992). Being intrigued by such landscapes, Kaplan (1992) argued, encouraged our ancestors to explore and seek new information, which in turn served to update and extend their cognitive maps. This expanded knowledge base could then be drawn on in later instances that threatened survival (e.g., finding water, food, escape routes, or hiding places). Beyond simply incrementing knowledge, interest and related states also appear to foster psychological complexity, defined by Csikszentmihalyi and Rathunde (1998) as the ability to integrate and differentiate complex relationships with people and among concepts and strivings. Similarly, Izard (1977), again building on Tomkins (1962), wrote that interest is the primary instigator of personal growth, creative endeavor, and the development of intelligence. Interest, then, not only broadens an individual's momentary thought–action repertoire as the individual is enticed to explore, but over time and as a product of sustained exploration, interest also builds the individual's store of knowledge and cognitive abilities. Again, these become durable resources that can be accessed in later moments and in other emotional states.

Contentment

Contentment is the positive emotion most often inappropriately confused with sensory pleasure, the affective response to meeting bodily needs (see above, p. 125). The term is also often used interchangeably with other low-arousal positive emotion terms such as tranquility or serenity (Ellsworth & Smith, 1988b), and it shares conceptual space with mild or receptive joy (Izard, 1977) and, to some degree, relief (Lazarus, 1991). Contentment may also be the positive emotion least appreciated in Western cultures. In part, contentment is captured by the Japanese emotion term *amae*, which refers to the sense of being accepted and cared for by others in a passive relationship of reciprocal dependence (Markus & Kitayama, 1991). Contentment arises in situations appraised as safe and as having a high degree of certainty and a low degree of effort (Ellsworth & Smith, 1988b). At first blush, contentment appears to have no real action tendency, inasmuch as Frijda (1986) links contentment with inactivity, Ellsworth and Smith (1988b) link tranquility with "doing nothing," and Lazarus (1991) links relief with ceasing vigilance. It may be, however, that the changes sparked by contentment are more cognitive than physical. A closer look at theoretical writings on contentment and related positive emotions suggests that this emotion prompts individuals to savor their current life circumstances and recent successes, experience "oneness" with others and the world around them, and integrate recent events and achievements into their overall self-concept and worldview (de Rivera et al., 1989; Izard, 1977). Notably, this integrative mindset appears to facilitate creativity and insight. Anecdotally, key elements of Charles Darwin's theory of evolution occurred to him while he was traveling peacefully in his carriage, and for mathematicians solutions often present themselves during vacations or other times of serene relaxation (Beveridge, 1950). Contentment, then, is not simply behavioral passivity, but rather a reflective broadening of a person's self-views and worldviews. It is a mindful emotion that involves full awareness of and openness to momentary experiences; it carries the urge to savor and integrate those experiences, which in turn creates a new sense of self and new worldviews. These links to mindfulness, receptivity, integration, and increasing self-complexity and insight characterize contentment as an emotion that broadens individuals' momentary thought–action repertoires and builds their personal resources.

Love

Love is conceptually different than the positive emotions already considered. First, most theorists acknowledge that love is not a single emotion and that people experience varieties of love (e.g., romantic or passionate love, companionate love, caregiver love, and attachment to caregivers; see Hatfield & Rapson, 1993; Oatley & Jenkins, 1996). Second, experiences of love are felt toward specific individuals (e.g., one's mother, confidant, lover, or child) and therefore are necessarily contextualized by these relationships (Oatley & Jenkins, 1996). Following Izard (1977), we hold that love experiences are made up of many positive emotions, including interest, joy, and contentment, among others. As Izard put it, "acquaintances or friends renew your interest by revealing new aspects of themselves and the resulting increase in familiarity (deeper knowledge of the person) brings joy [and contentment]. In lasting friendships or love relationships this cycle is repeated endlessly" (p. 243). Supporting the idea that love represents a fusion of other specific positive emotions, Ellsworth and Smith (1988b) found that love, interest, and playfulness (what we have been calling joy) were the least differentiated positive emotions they examined. So, to the extent that love triggers the more specific positive emotions of interest, contentment, and joy, it also broadens the momentary thought–action repertoire as people explore, savor, and play with the people they love.

   In the moment, exploring, savoring, and being playful with loved ones seems to have no obvious aim other than intrinsic enjoyment. Over time, however, the interactions inspired by love help to build and strengthen social bonds and attachment. Humor, amusement, and smiling, for instance, facilitate social interaction and intimacy at every stage of relationship formation (Swartz, 1990). For infants, smiling and other expressions of positive emotion serve as a means of communication between the child and caretaker (Simons, McClusky-Fawcett, & Papini, 1986) and enable the child to shape the caretaker's behavior in response to his/her needs (Foss, 1969). Beyond infancy, humor strengthens social and family bonds (Martineau, 1972). These social bonds are not only satisfying in and of themselves but are also likely to be the locus of subsequent social support. In this sense, love and the various positive emotions experienced in love relationships (e.g., joy, interest, and contentment) build and solidify an individual's social resources. Like intellectual and physical resources, social resources can accumulate and be drawn on later.

THEORETICAL PERSPECTIVES ON FUNCTION

Classic Views: Approach/Continue

Most commonly, the function of positive emotions has been identified as facilitating approach behavior (Cacioppo, Priester, & Berntson, 1993; Davidson, 1993; Frijda, 1994) or continued action (Carver & Scheier, 1990; Clore, 1994). Experiences of positive emotions, according to this classic perspective, prompt individuals to engage with their environments and partake in activities, many of which are evolutionarily adaptive for the individual, its species, or both. This link between positive emotions and activity engagement provides an explanation for the often-documented positivity offset, or the tendency for individuals to experience mild positive affect frequently, even in neutral contexts (Diener & Diener, 1996; Ito & Cacioppo, 1999). Without such an offset, individuals would most often be unmotivated to engage with their environments. Yet, with such an offset, individuals exhibit the adaptive bias to approach and explore novel objects, people, or situations.

Although positive emotions do often appear to function as internal signals to *approach* or *continue,* we argue that they share this function with other positive affective states. Sensory pleasure, for instance, motivates people to approach and continue consuming whatever stimulus is biologically useful for them at the moment (Cabanac, 1971). Likewise, free-floating positive moods motivate people to continue along any line of thinking or action that they have initiated (Clore, 1994). As such, functional accounts of positive emotions that primarily emphasize tendencies to approach or continue may only capture the lowest common denominator across all affective states that share a pleasant subjective feel. We contend that this classic approach leaves functions that are unique to positive emotions uncharted and argue that positive emotions have additional functions beyond those shared with sensory pleasure and positive moods. As we have seen, joy carries the urge to play, interest the urge to explore, contentment the urge to savor and integrate, and love a combination of many of these urges. These broader thought–action tendencies, we argue, have functions beyond simply instigating approach or continued action.

A New View: The Broaden-and-Build Model

The broaden-and-build model of positive emotions (Fredrickson, 1998b) offers a new view of their functional significance, beyond those functions shared with other positive affective states. This model posits that distinct positive emotions like joy, interest, contentment, and love not only share the feature of broadening individuals' momentary thought–action repertoires but also share the feature of building individuals' personal resources, including physical, intellectual, social, and psychological resources. Importantly, these resources are more durable than the transient emotional states that led to their acquisition. By consequence, then, the often incidental effect of experiencing a positive emotion is an increment in lasting personal resources that can be drawn on later, in other contexts and in other emotional states (Fredrickson, 1998b).

The functional account of positive emotions that the broaden-and-build model offers also draws on evolutionary psychology. One route to arguing that a particular psychological phenomenon is an evolved adaptation is to take a form-to-function approach: First one notes the form of some existing psychological phenomenon, then thinks back to the lives of our hunter–gatherer ancestors and tries to locate the sort of adaptive problem that might have been solved by this form (Tooby & Cosmides, 1992). The form that characterizes positive emotions, Fredrickson (1998b) argued, is a momentarily broadened thought–action repertoire. The common denominator across the contexts that elicit positive emotions is perceived safety and satiation. The ability to recognize and take advantage of the opportunities inherent in safe and satiated moments is, at face value, of obvious importance. Of all the things a hunter–gatherer could do in a such a moment—sleep, sit around, continue to run, attack, or be vigilant—why might being playful or exploratory have led to a reproductive advantage?

The key is in the "build" part of the broaden-and-build model. Through the experiences of positive emotions, our ancestors built their personal resources, including *physical resources* (e.g., the ability to outmaneuver a predator), *intellectual resources* (e.g., a detailed cognitive map for navigation), *social resources* (e.g., someone to turn to for help), and *psychological resources* (e.g., an optimistic worldview). These links between positive emotions and resource building also suggest that positive emotions may be essential to early child development. Indeed, Panksepp argued that "youth may have evolved to give complex organisms time to play" (1998, p. 96). Importantly, the personal resources accrued during positive states were durable. When these same ancestors later faced threats to life and limb, these resources could translate into increased odds of survival and, in turn, increased odds of living long enough to reproduce. Thus, the adaptive problem that appears to be solved by positive emotions is this: When and how should individuals build resources for survival? The answer is to build resources during safe and satiated moments by playing, exploring, and/or savoring and integrating (Fredrickson, 1998b, 2000a). The evolutionary functional analysis within the broaden-and-build model offers a new perspective on what positive emotions have been good for—their ancestral function—and explains why they are now part of our universal human nature. (Readers interested in a review of empirical support for the broaden-and-build model are directed to Fredrickson, 1998b, in press.)

It is critical to note that the evolutionary functional analysis provided within the broaden-and-build model does *not* mean that experiences of positive emotions necessarily have adaptive advantages in present-day circumstances, nor that present-day humans pursue positive emotions to maximize their odds of survival, reproduction, or inclusive fitness. Indeed, positive emotions may now serve multiple purposes in people's lives. At times, the "pursuit of happiness" may solely reflect the fact that positive emotions are hedonically pleasant and therefore inherently rewarding. Present-day motivations aside, the adaptationist account within the broaden-and-build model makes the more modest claim that the structure and effects of positive emotions evident in present-day humans have been shaped by the recurrent conditions faced by our ancestors over the course of their evolution.

Although we cannot assume that positive emotions inevitably "do good," the insights that the broaden-and-build model offers into the psychological form and ancestral function of positive emotions can illuminate ways that present-day humans might deploy positive emotions to optimize their own health and well-being (Fredrickson, 2000a). Moreover, the broaden-and-build model claims that positive emotions can have effects beyond making people "feel good" or improving their subjective experiences of life. They also have the potential to broaden people's habitual modes of thinking and build their physical, intellectual, and social resources. These processes, we will argue, can help people overcome current stresses faster and make them more resilient to future adversities. Cataloging these beneficial effects is a primary focus of current research on positive emotions. We use the rest of this chapter to highlight and discuss important advances in this area.

RESEARCH FOCUS: BENEFICIAL EFFECTS OF POSITIVE EMOTIONS

Positive Emotions Regulate Negative Emotions

As we have discussed, the broaden-and-build model states that positive emotions broaden individuals' momentary thought–action repertoires (Fredrickson, 1998b, 2000a). If true, then positive emotions should also serve as particularly effective antidotes for the lingering effects of negative emotions, which narrow individuals' thought–action repertoires. In other words, positive emotions should have an *undoing effect* on negative emotions. The basic observation that positive emotions (or their key components) are somehow incompatible with negative emotions is not new; it has been demonstrated over several decades by a range of researchers working on affect-related processes (Baron, 1976; Cabanac, 1971; Nezu, Nezu, & Blissett, 1988; Solomon, 1980; Wolpe, 1958). Even so, the precise mechanism(s) ultimately responsible for this long-noted incompatibility have not been adequately identified.

Broadening may turn out to be the operative mechanism. By broadening the momentary thought–action repertoire, positive emotions may loosen the hold that (no longer relevant) negative emotions gain on an individual's mind and body by dismantling or *undoing* the narrowed psychological and physiological preparation for specific action. In other words, the broadened thought–action repertoire of positive emotions may be psychologically incompatible with the narrowed thought–action repertoire of negative emotions (Fredrickson, 2000a). In addition, to the extent that a negative emotion's narrowed thought–action repertoire (i.e., specific action tendency) evokes physiological changes to support the indicated action (Levenson, 1994), a counteracting positive emotion—with its broadened thought–action repertoire—should quell or undo this physiological preparation for specific action. By returning the body to baseline levels of physiological activation, positive emotions create physiological support for pursuing the wider array of thoughts and actions called forth.

Building on this reasoning, Fredrickson and colleagues hypothesized that positive emotions should have a unique ability to down-regulate the lingering cardiovascular aftereffects of negative emotions. Our laboratory has tested this aspect of the undoing hypothesis in a series of experiments (Fredrickson & Levenson, 1998; Fredrickson et al., 2000). Our empirical strategy was first to induce negative emotional arousal in all participants, using either a fear-eliciting film clip (Fredrickson & Levenson, 1998) or an anxiety-eliciting speech task (Fredrickson et al., 2000). Next, into this context of negative emotional arousal (and using a between-groups design), we induced mild joy, contentment, neutrality, or sadness, again using film clips. We tested our hypothesis by measuring how long it took for the initial negative emotional arousal to return to baseline levels once the randomly assigned film was introduced. Across three independent samples, we found that two positive emotions—mild joy and contentment—each significantly accelerated cardiovascular recovery relative to neutrality and sadness (Fredrickson & Levenson, 1998; Fredrickson et al., 2000, Study 1). Importantly, in another study (Fredrickson et al., 2000, Study 2), we found that the positive and neutral films used in this research, when viewed following a resting baseline, elicited virtually no cardiovascular reactivity whatsoever. So, although the positive and neutral films do not differ in what they *do* to the cardiovascular system, they do differ in what they can *undo* within this system. We obtained further evidence for the undoing effect from a correlational study that linked spontaneous smiles during negative emotional arousal to faster cardiovascular recovery from that arousal (Fredrickson & Levenson, 1998). Experiments have thus documented that positive emotions can undo the cardiovascular reactivity that lingers following a negative emotion and that this undoing effect is both reliable and generalizable (Fredrickson & Levenson, 1998; Fredrickson et al., 2000). Importantly, the evidence suggests that smiles and two phenomenologically distinct positive emotions—mild joy and contentment—all share the ability to undo negative emotional arousal.

Beyond speeding physiological recovery, the undoing effect implies that positive emotions should counteract any aspect of negative emotions that stems from a narrowed thought–action repertoire. For instance, negative emotions can entrain people toward narrowed lines of thinking consistent with the specific action tendencies they trigger: when angry, individuals may dwell on getting revenge or getting even; when anxious or afraid, they may dwell on escaping or avoiding harm; when sad or depressed, they may dwell on the repercussions of what has been lost. The undoing hypothesis predicts that positive emotions should restore flexible thinking in these circumstances. To the best of our knowledge, no experiments have yet tested this prediction. Even so, indirect supportive evidence can be drawn from a collection of correlational studies. Individuals who express or report higher levels of positive emotion show more constructive and flexible coping, more abstract and long-term thinking, and greater emotional distance following stressful negative events (Keltner & Bonanno, 1997; Lyubomirsky & Tucker, 1998; Martin, Kuiper, Olinger, & Dance, 1993; Stein, Folkman, Trabasso, & Richards, 1997). More generally, positive emotions may undo the psychological or cognitive narrowing engendered by negative emotions. Although additional studies are needed, we suspect that the undoing effect occurs because positive emotions broaden people's momentary thought–action repertoires in a manner that is incompatible with the continuance of negative emotion.

Closely related to Fredrickson and colleagues' research on the undoing effect of positive emotions, there is a long tradition of studies suggesting that humor is an effective means of coping with negative emotions and stress (Martin & Lefcourt, 1983; Nezu et al., 1988). For instance, individuals who participated in a humorous intervention activity reported significantly lower levels of anxiety and depression relative to controls (Houston, McKee, Carroll, & Marsch, 1998). In addition to its effects on anxiety and depression, humor has been found to help alleviate the effects of anger (Baron, 1976; Berkowitz, 1970; Dworkin & Efran, 1967; Singer, 1968) and sadness (Labott & Martin, 1987; Moran & Massam, 1999). Thus, humor may serve a protective function, guarding individuals from negative stimuli as well as mitigating the effects of exposure to such stimuli. Humor, then, harnesses the coping benefits of positive emotions to regulate negative emotions. For compatible discussions of how positive emotions can facilitate the regulation of negative emotions, see Folkman (1997) and J. T. Moskowitz (Chapter 10, this volume).

Positive Emotions Trigger Upward Spirals toward Emotional Well-Being

Research and theory on depression often describes a "downward spiral" in which initial experiences of depressed moods and the narrowed, pessimistic thinking they engender influence each other reciprocally, leading to ever-worsening moods and at times resulting in clinical levels of depression (Peterson & Seligman, 1984; Teasdale, 1983). The broaden-and-build model predicts a comparable "upward spiral" in which experiences of positive emotions and the broadened thinking they engender also influence one another reciprocally, leading to appreciable increases in subjective well-being. In other words, experiences of positive emotions are hypothesized to accumulate and compound: the psychological broadening sparked by one positive emotion can increase an individual's receptiveness to subsequent pleasant or meaningful events, increasing the odds that the individual will find positive meaning within these subsequent events and experience additional positive emotions (Fredrickson, 2000a). Moreover, the broaden-and-build model posits that an important side effect of experiencing positive emotions is an increment in personal resources. Thus, through incremental processes attributable to psychological broadening, experiences of positive emotions might, over time, not only facilitate coping and alleviate negative affective states but also, with time and repeated experience, positive emotions might also increment people's enduring personal resources. These resources could include both intraindividual resources, like increased psychological and physical resilience, and interpersonal resources, like enhanced social relationships, which can be the locus of both pleasant activities and positive meaning. Taken together, these new resources—gained through positive emotion experiences—should enhance people's emotional well-being.

In part, positive emotions may trigger this upward spiral toward enhanced emotional well-being by building psychological resilience and influencing the ways people cope with adversity. Consistent with this view, research has shown that people who experienced positive emotions during bereavement were more likely to develop long-term plans and goals. Together with positive emotions, plans and goals predicted greater psychological well-being 12 months post-bereavement (Stein et al., 1997; for related work, see Bonanno & Keltner, 1997, and Moskowitz, Chapter 10, this volume).

More directly, Fredrickson and Joiner (2000) tested the hypothesis that, through cognitive broadening, positive emotions build psychological resilience, producing an upward spiral toward enhanced emotional well-being. They did this by assessing positive and negative emotions, as well as a concept called broad-minded coping, at two time points, 5 weeks apart. The measure of broad-minded coping drew items from Moos's (1988) Coping Responses Inventory that tap broadened thinking, such as "think of different ways to deal with the problem" and "try to step back from the situation and be more objective." The aim was to predict changes in positive emotions and broad-minded coping over time. Through a series of regression analyses and tests of mediation, the data revealed evidence for an upward spiral effect. First, controlling for initial levels of broad-minded coping, initial levels of positive emotion predicted improvements in broad-minded coping from Time 1 to Time 2. These improvements in broad-minded coping in turn predicted subsequent increases in positive emotions. Next, the data revealed evidence for the reciprocal relations: Controlling for initial levels of positive emotion, initial levels of broad-minded coping predicted improvements in positive emotions from Time 1 to Time 2. These improvements in positive emotions in turn predicted subsequent increases in broad-minded coping. Importantly, these effects were unique to positive emotions; substituting negative emotions into the same regression equations yielded no significant relations whatsoever (Fredrickson & Joiner, 2000).

These findings suggest that, over time, positive emotions and broad-minded coping mutually build on one another. Because broad-minded coping can be viewed as a form of psychological resilience, these data support the hypothesis, drawn from the broaden-and-build model, that momentary experiences of positive emotion can build enduring psychological resources and trigger upward spirals toward emotional well-being. So, positive emotions not only make people feel good in the present moment but also—through their effects on broadened thinking—positive emotions increase the likelihood that people will feel good in the future. (For related work on the relations between positive emotions and physical well-being, see T. J. Mayne, Chapter 12, this volume.)

As an aside, the propensity for positive emotions to instigate an "upward spiral" toward emotional well-being may be another feature that distinguishes positive emotions from sensory pleasure and positive moods. Positive states that lead only to approach—but not to broadening—would not by consequence create greater openness to subsequent positive experiences and would not therefore initiate the upward spiral described above. Perhaps that is why people appear to value positive emotions more than they value mere pleasure or good moods. For instance, although love and sensory pleasure are both positive states, experiences of love seem to matter more to most people than do experiences of sensory pleasure (Fredrickson, 2000b). This may be, in part, because love and other positive emotions carry relatively more personal meaning than do other pleasant states and—

because they trigger upward spirals—love and other positive emotions are more likely to influence people's future life outcomes.

THE FUTURE OF RESEARCH ON POSITIVE EMOTIONS

One goal of the broaden-and-build model of positive emotions has been to describe the psychological form and ancestral function of positive emotions. Even so, a more critical, overarching goal has been to inject positive emotions into the minds of researchers and theorists invested in emotions research, in an effort to begin a substantive and empirical dialogue on the often neglected and trivialized topic of positive emotions. The model itself provides one road map for future research on positive emotions. In this section, we describe some critical directions that such future research should take.

A first critical direction for future research will be to further test the *broaden* component of the broaden-and-build model. Although the twin hypotheses that, relative to neutral states, positive emotions broaden individuals' momentary thought–action repertoires whereas negative emotions narrow these same repertoires have received direct support in an initial experiment (Fredrickson & Branigan, 2000), many questions remain. For instance, are these effects replicable, and do they extend to other measures of the breadth of thought–action repertoires? If so, what changes in basic cognitive processes possibly underlie changes in the scope of thoughts and actions called forth? Is the scope of attention enlarged during experiences of positive emotions, as suggested by a handful of inconclusive studies? (Basso, Schefft, Ris, & Dember, 1996; J. L. Brandt, D. Derryberry, & M. A. Reed, 1992, cited in Derryberry & Tucker, 1994). Alternatively (or additionally), is the scope of working memory expanded during experiences of positive emotions? Finally, do emotion-related changes in the scopes of attention and cognition generate emotion-related differences in openness to information? In set switching and creativity? In coping and interpersonal problem solving? Relatedly, what are the neurological underpinnings of the broadening effects of positive emotions? Are these effects mediated by changing levels of circulating brain dopamine, as Ashby and colleagues (1999) have suggested? What brain structures, circuits, and processes are involved?

A second critical direction for future research will be to test the *build* component of the broaden-and-build model. Although the evidence that positive emotions trigger an upward spiral toward enhanced emotional well-being (Fredrickson & Joiner, 2000) provides initial support for the hypothesis that positive emotions build psychological resilience, the building hypothesis merits much additional testing. Is this upward spiral effect replicable, and can it be demonstrated over more and more distal time points? Can experiences of positive emotions, over time, build other enduring personal resources (beyond broad-minded coping), such as optimism, hopefulness, wisdom, and creativity? Can experiences of positive emotions, over time, build enduring social resources, such as empathy, altruism, intimacy motive, and relationship satisfaction? If so, are increments in these personal and social resources mediated by psychological broadening and followed by increases in emotional and physical well-being? These hypotheses should be tested with both clinical and nonclinical samples, in both longitudinal studies and field experiments. The field experiments should test the psychological, social, and physical outcomes of interventions aimed at cultivating positive emotions in daily life (see Fredrickson, 2000a, in press). Additional support for the twin hypotheses that positive emotions build enduring personal resources and trigger upward spirals would provide evidence that, over time, positive emotions not only help to alleviate disorders and illnesses rooted in negative emotions but also go beyond to build individual character, solidify social bonds, and optimize people's health and well-being.

A third important direction for future research will be to assess the hypothesized link between the psychological and physiological effects of positive emotions. Specifically, does the psychological broadening effect track or mediate the physiological undoing effect? To test this hypothesis, repeated measures of cognitive broadening might be introduced into the aforementioned cardiovascular aftereffects down-regulation, or undoing, paradigm (Fredrickson et al., 2000), assessing the breadth of cognition at baseline, then immediately following negative emotion induction, and a third time following the experimental manipulation of positive, neutral, or negative states. The prediction from the broaden-and-build model would be that negative emotions simultaneously increase cardiovascular activation and narrow the scope of cognition, whereas positive emotions simultaneously undo cardiovascular activation and broaden the scope of cognition, and that changes in broadening mediate cardiovascular recovery. Research in this direction would illuminate the mechanisms through which positive emotions regulate experiences of negative emotions.

A fourth direction for future research will be to explore the specific physiological mechanisms that link positive emotions to improved physical health. A number of studies provide indirect evidence for the health-promoting role of positive emotions (see Mayne, Chapter 12, this volume). For instance, over several decades, research on social support has indicated that those individuals who have more of it exhibit healthier physiological profiles, including lower heart rates and systolic blood pressures, as well as lower serum cholesterol, uric acid, and urinary norepinephrine levels (for reviews, see Ryff & Singer, 1998; Uchino, Cacioppo, & Kiecolt-Glaser,

1996). Although emotional support appears to be a key dimension through which social support impacts physiology, the possible roles of specific positive emotions remain unknown. Commenting on this state of knowledge, Ryff and Singer (1998) wrote:

> We see a troubling paucity of knowledge regarding the physiology of deeply felt life purposes or richly experienced emotional ties to others. Biochemical processes are inevitably set in motion by these higher forms of human experience, although the exact nature of the physiological cascade is unknown. We hypothesize that . . . enduring experiences with personally meaningful life goals and love relationships facilitate . . . optimal operating ranges for multiple biological systems as well as enduring patterns of high left prefrontal [brain] activation, which modulates immune factors and neuroendocrine response to challenge. (p. 17)

Like Ryff and Singer, we note that much indirect evidence points to a role for positive emotions in maintaining and promoting physical health. Even so, the details regarding the specific physiological substrates associated with specific positive emotions potentially responsible for these various health benefits will emerge only when health researchers begin to take positive emotions seriously.

A fifth direction for future research will be to examine whether positive emotions in addition to joy, interest, contentment, and love also fit the broaden-and-build model. For instance, Haidt (2000) has recently proposed that the positive emotion of elevation fits the broaden-and-build model. Conceptualized as the opposite of disgust, which is triggered by witnessing others exhibiting their lower, baser, less God-like nature (Haidt, Rozin, McCauley, & Imada, 1997), elevation occurs when people see others exhibit their higher, better, more saintly nature, for instance, when witnessing another perform an unexpected altruistic act (Haidt, 2000). The momentary thought–action tendency sparked by elevation, according to Haidt, is a generalized desire to become a better person and perform altruistic acts oneself. This thought–action tendency is broadened, rather than narrowed, because it does not steer elevated individuals simply to mimic the prosocial act they witnessed, but rather to creatively consider a wide range of prosocial acts as paths toward becoming better people. Experiences of elevation, then, carry the potential to change people. To the extent that people act on the urges sparked by elevation, they may reach higher ground themselves, becoming better, more moral persons. In doing so, they create a new sense of self and more compassionate and optimistic worldviews. In this way, as with other positive emotions, the broadened mindset that accompanies elevation can build personal resources that can be drawn on in the future. A recent conceptual analysis of gratitude suggests that this positive emotion may function similarly (McCullough, Kilpatrick, Emmons, & Larson, in press).

We suggest that the positive emotion of pride may also fit the broaden-and-build model. Previous theorists have suggested that the momentary thought–action tendency for pride is a combination of physical expansiveness (e.g., erect posture, cheers, "bursting with pride") and the urge to share the news or event widely with others (Lazarus, 1991; Mascolo & Fischer, 1995). Yet, that analysis may place too much emphasis on the overt action tendencies linked with pride, and not enough on the covert thought tendencies that may also arise. Drawing from Lewis (1993), we propose that the momentary thought–action tendency sparked by pride also includes the urge to envision even greater achievements. So, while a proud individual may publicly share his/her accomplishments in a modest way (as most cultures have strong sanctions against excessive displays of pride), he/she may privately dream big about further accomplishments in the given domain. For instance, a student who feels proud about meriting a prestigious academic honor at his/her university may fantasize about one day being awarded the Nobel prize. We conceptualize this urge to "dream big" associated with pride as a broadened mindset. And although the bold visions generated during proud moments may be largely unbidden, they may have the incidental effect of helping individuals set and prioritize their goals for the future. To reproduce the pleasing experience of pride, individuals seek out opportunities to behave in ways that conform to social standards of worth or merit (Mascolo & Fischer, 1995). In other words, experiences of pride may fuel achievement motivation (Lewis, 1993). Pride, then, not only broadens a person's momentary thought–action repertoire with the urge to dream big, but it can also have the incidental effect of building a person's lasting personal resources of achievement motivation, not to mention self-esteem.

Beyond such theorizing, however, the degree to which each distinct positive emotion—joy, interest, contentment, love, elevation, gratitude, and pride—functions to broaden the scope of people's momentary thought–action repertoires and build their personal and social resources remains an empirical question in need of testing. Perhaps multiple positive emotions fit the broaden-and-build model, but each to varying degrees.

A sixth direction for future research concerns the relation between positive emotions and spirituality. Religion and spirituality have been linked to a wide range of psychological and physical health benefits (for reviews, see Levin, 1996; Levin & Chatters, 1998; McCullough, 1995). Notably, religious and spiritual beliefs often help people find positive meaning in ordinary daily events as well as in major life adversities. Finding positive meaning, in turn, predicts experiences of positive emotions (Folkman, 1997). Might then the effects of spirituality on psychological and physical health be carried by positive emotions? We suspect that they are, and postulate that the broadening and building effects of positive emotions play critical roles. For instance, spirituality itself may involve psychological broadening, as it often requires people to open themselves up to something larger than the self. This broadened mindset may be what allows spiritual individuals to find positive meaning in both major and minor life events, and accrue the personal and social resources that enable them to cope and thrive. As spirituality becomes a larger focus of empirical inquiry, these questions will be worth pursuing.

We suspect that empirical ventures down these six paths will yield intriguing and useful results. Even so, these are just a few of the directions that future research on positive emotions could take. Many other paths are also possible and will likely be uncovered as future emotion researchers begin to take positive emotions as seriously as past emotion researchers have taken negative emotions. We hope that this chapter can inspire both curiosity and seriousness about this long-neglected domain of emotional experience.

SUMMARY OF KEY POINTS

1. To date, positive emotions have received less empirical attention than negative emotions. This imbalance reflects multiple probable causes, including the following:
- Excessive negative emotions cause more problems than do positive emotions.
- Positive emotions are less differentiated than negative emotions.
- Positive emotions are often confused with other pleasant affective states, like sensory pleasure and positive moods.
- Models of emotions are typically built to the specifications of negative emotions, such as anger and fear, and suggest that all emotions produce specific action tendencies.

2. Positive emotions do not fit well within emotion models centered on specific action tendencies. A new view is that whereas negative emotions narrow people's momentary thought–action repertoires toward specific action tendencies, positive emotions broaden people's momentary thought–action repertoires.

3. This broadening hypothesis is supported by existing theoretical accounts of four distinct positive emotions: joy produces the urge to play; interest, the urge to explore; contentment, the urge to savor and integrate; and love, a combination of many of these urges.

4. Classic theoretical perspectives on the function of positive emotions

emphasize their role in motivating approach behavior and continued action. A new theoretical perspective on the function of positive emotions is offered within the broaden-and-build model. By broadening people's momentary thought–action repertoires, positive emotions have the incidental effect of building people's personal and social resources for survival.

5. Contemporary research has demonstrated many beneficial effects of positive emotions, including the following:

- Positive emotions facilitate the regulation of negative emotions.
- Positive emotions trigger upward spirals toward enhanced emotional well-being.

6. The future of research on positive emotions should include empirical tests of the following:

- The broadening component of the broaden-and-build model.
- The building component of the broaden-and-build model.
- Whether psychological broadening accounts for physiological undoing.
- The physiological mechanisms that connect positive emotions to improved physical health.
- The extent to which a wide range of positive emotions fit the parameters of the broaden-and-build model.
- The links between the benefits of spirituality and the benefits of positive emotions.

REFERENCES

Ashby, F. G., Isen, A. M., & Turken, A. U. (1999). A neuropsychological theory of positive affect and its influence on cognition. *Psychological Review, 106*, 529–550.

Aspinwall, L. G. (1998). Rethinking the role of positive affect in self-regulation. *Motivation and Emotion, 22*, 1–32.

Averill, J. R. (1980). On the paucity of positive emotions. In K. R. Blankstein, P. Pliner, & J. Polivy (Eds.), *Advances in the study of communication and affect: Vol. 6. Assessment and modification of emotional behavior* (pp. 7–45). New York: Plenum Press.

Baron, R. A. (1976). The reduction of human aggression: A field study of the influence of incompatible reactions. *Journal of Applied Social Psychology, 6*, 260–274.

Basso, M. R., Schefft, B. K., Ris, M. D., & Dember, W. N. (1996). Mood and global–local visual processing. *Journal of the International Neuropsychological Society, 2*, 249–255.

Berkowitz, L. (1970). Aggressive humor as a stimulus to aggressive responses. *Journal of Personality and Social Psychology, 16*, 710–717.

Beveridge, W. D. (1950). *The art of scientific investigation.* New York: Vantage Books.

Bonanno, G. A., & Keltner, D. (1997). Facial expressions of emotion and the course of conjugal bereavement. *Journal of Abnormal Psychology, 106*, 126–137.

Boulton, M. J., & Smith, P. K. (1992). The social nature of play fighting and play chasing: Mechanisms and strategies underlying cooperation and compromise. In J. H. Barkow, L. Cosmides, & J. Tooby (Eds.), *The adapted mind: Evolutionary psychology and the generation of culture* (pp. 429–444). New York: Oxford University Press.

Cabanac, M. (1971). Physiological role of pleasure. *Science, 173*, 1103–1107.

Cacioppo, J. T., Klein, D. J., Berntson, G. G., & Hatfield, E. (1993). The psychophysiology of emotion. In M. Lewis & J. M. Haviland (Eds.), *Handbook of emotions* (pp. 119–142). New York: Guilford Press.

Cacioppo, J. T., Priester, J. R., & Berntson, G. G. (1993). Rudimentary determinants of attitudes: II. Arm flexion and extension have differential effects on attitudes. *Journal of Personality and Social Psychology, 65*, 5–17.

Caro, T. M. (1988). Adaptive significance of play: Are we getting closer? *Tree, 3*, 50–54.

Carver, C. S., & Scheier, M. F. (1990). Origins and functions of positive and negative affect: A control-process view. *Psychological Review, 97*, 19–35.

Clore, G. L. (1994). Why emotions are felt. In P. Ekman & R. Davidson (Eds.), *The nature of emotion: Fundamental questions* (pp. 103–111). New York: Oxford University Press.

Csikszentmihalyi, M. (1990). *Flow: The psychology of optimal experience.* New York: HarperPerennial.

Csikszentmihalyi, M., & Rathunde, K. (1998). The development of the person: An experiential perspective on the ontogenesis of psychological complexity. In W. Damon (Series Ed.) & R. M. Lerner (Vol. Ed.), *Handbook of child psychology: Vol. 1. Theoretical models of human development* (5th ed., pp. 635–684). New York: Wiley.

Dansky, J. L. (1980). Make-believe: A mediator of the relationship between play and associative fluency. *Child Development, 51*, 576–579.

Davidson, R. J. (1993). The neuropsychology of emotion and affective style. In M. Lewis & J. M. Haviland (Eds.), *Handbook of emotions* (pp. 143–154). New York: Guilford Press.

Deci, E. L., & Ryan, R. M. (1985). *Intrinsic motivation and self-determination in human behavior.* New York: Plenum Press.

Deci, E. L., Vallerand, R. J., Pelletier, L. G., & Ryan, R. M. (1991). Motivation and education: The self-determination perspective. *Educational Psychologist, 26*, 325–346.

de Rivera, J., Possel, L., Verette, J. A., & Weiner, B. (1989). Distinguishing elation, gladness, and joy. *Journal of Personality and Social Psychology, 57*, 1015–1023.

Derryberry, D., & Tucker, D. M. (1994). Motivating the focus of attention. In P. M. Neidenthal & S. Kitayama (Eds.), *The heart's eye: Emotional influences in perception and attention* (pp. 167–196). San Diego, CA: Academic Press.

Diener, E., & Diener, C. (1996). Most people are happy. *Psychological Science, 7*, 181–185.

Dolhinow, P. J., & Bishop, N. (1970). The development of motor skills and social relationships among primates through play. In J. P. Hill (Ed.), *Minnesota Symposia on Child Psychology* (Vol. 4, pp. 141–198). Minneapolis: University of Minnesota Press.

Dworkin, E. S., & Efran, J. S. (1967). The angered: Their susceptibility to varieties of humor. *Journal of Personality and Social Psychology, 6,* 233–236.

Ekman, P. (1992). An argument for basic emotions. *Cognition and Emotion, 6,* 169–200.

Ekman, P., Friesen, W. V., O'Sullivan, M., Chan, A., Diacoyanni-Tarlatzis, I., Heider, K., Krause, R., LeCompre, W. A., Ritcairn, T., Ricci-Bitti, P. E., Scherer, K., Tomita, M., & Tzavras, A. (1987). Universals and cultural differences in the judgments of facial expressions of emotions. *Journal of Personality and Social Psychology, 53,* 712–717.

Ellsworth, P. C., & Smith, C. A. (1988a). From appraisal to emotion: Differences among unpleasant feelings. *Motivation and Emotion, 2,* 271–302.

Ellsworth, P. C., & Smith, C. A. (1988b). Shades of joy: Patterns of appraisal differentiating pleasant emotions. *Cognition and Emotion, 2,* 301–331.

Estrada, C. A., Isen, A. M., & Young, M. J. (1997). Positive affect facilitates integration of information and decreases anchoring in reasoning among physicians. *Organizational Behavior and Human Decision Processes, 72,* 117–135.

Folkman, S. (1997). Positive psychological states and coping with severe stress. *Social Science Medicine, 45,* 1207–1221.

Foss, B. M. (1969). *Determinants of infant behavior* (Vol. 4). New York: Barnes & Noble.

Frank, M., Ekman, P., & Friesen, W. (1993). Behavioral markers and recognizability of the smile of enjoyment. *Journal of Personality and Social Psychology, 64,* 83–93.

Fredrickson, B. L. (Chair). (1998a, August 5–9). *Perspectives on positive emotions.* Symposium conducted at the biannual meeting of the International Society for Research on Emotions, Wuerzburg, Germany.

Fredrickson, B. L. (1998b). What good are positive emotions? *Review of General Psychology, 2,* 300–319.

Fredrickson, B. L. (Chair). (1999, June 3–6). *Beneficial repercussions of positive affect.* Symposium conducted at the annual meeting of the American Psychological Society, Denver, CO.

Fredrickson, B. L. (2000a). Cultivating positive emotions to optimize health and well-being. *Prevention and Treatment* [Online serial], *3.* Available: http://journals.apa.org/prevention

Fredrickson, B. L. (2000b). Extracting meaning from past affective experiences: The importance of peaks, ends, and specific emotions. *Cognition and Emotion, 14,* 577–606.

Fredrickson, B. L. (in press). Positive emotions. In C. R. Snyder & S. J. Lopez (Eds.), *Handbook of positive psychology.* New York: Oxford University Press.

Fredrickson, B. L., & Branigan, C. (2000). *Positive emotions broaden thought–action repertoires: Evidence for the broaden-and-build model.* Manuscript in preparation.

Fredrickson, B. L., & Joiner, T. (2000). *Positive emotions trigger upward spirals toward emotional well-being.* Manuscript submitted for publication.

Fredrickson, B. L., & Levenson, R. W. (1998). Positive emotions speed recovery from the cardiovascular sequelae of negative emotions. *Cognition and Emotion, 12,* 191–220.

Fredrickson, B. L., Mancuso, R. A., Branigan, C., & Tugade, M. (2000). *The undoing effect of positive emotions*. Manuscript submitted for publication.

Frijda, N. H. (1986). *The emotions*. Cambridge, UK: Cambridge University Press.

Frijda, N. H. (1994). Emotions are functional, most of the time. In P. Ekman & R. Davidson (Eds.), *The nature of emotion: Fundamental questions* (pp. 112–122). New York: Oxford University Press.

Frijda, N. H., Kuipers, P., & Schure, E. (1989). Relations among emotion, appraisal, and emotional action readiness. *Journal of Personality and Social Psychology, 57*, 212–228.

Haidt, J. (2000). The positive emotion of elevation. *Prevention and Treatment* [Online serial], 3. Available: http://journals.apa.org/prevention

Haidt, J., Rozin, P., McCauley, C. R., & Imada, S. (1997). Body, psyche, and culture: The relationship between disgust and morality. *Psychology and Developing Societies, 9*, 107–131.

Hatfield, E., & Rapson, R. (1993). Love and attachment processes. In M. Lewis & J. M. Haviland (Eds.), *Handbook of emotions* (pp. 595–604). New York: Guilford Press.

Hazen, N. L., & Durrett, M. E. (1982). Relationship of security of attachment and cognitive mapping abilities in 2-year-olds. *Developmental Psychology, 18*, 751–759.

Houston, D. M., McKee, K. J., Caroll, L., & Marsch, H. (1998). Using humour to promote psychological wellbeing in residential homes for older people. *Aging and Mental Health, 2*, 328–332.

Isen, A. M. (1987). Positive affect, cognitive processes, and social behavior. *Advances in Experimental Social Psychology, 20*, 203–253.

Isen, A. M. (2000). Positive affect and decision making. In M. Lewis & J. M. Haviland-Jones (Eds.), *Handbook of emotions* (2nd ed., pp. 417–435). New York: Guilford Press.

Isen, A. M., & Daubman, K. A. (1984). The influence of affect on categorization. *Journal of Personality and Social Psychology, 47*, 1206–1217.

Isen, A. M., Daubman, K. A., & Nowicki, G. P. (1987). Positive affect facilitates creative problem solving. *Journal of Personality and Social Psychology, 52*, 1122–1131.

Isen, A. M., Johnson, M. M. S., Mertz, E., & Robinson, G. F. (1985). The influence of positive affect on the unusualness of word associations. *Journal of Personality and Social Psychology, 48*, 1413–1426.

Ito, T. A., & Cacioppo, J. T. (1999). The psychophysiology of utility appraisals. In D. Kahneman, E. Diener, & N. Schwartz (Eds.), *Well-being: Foundations of hedonic psychology* (pp. 470–488). New York: Russell Sage Foundation.

Izard, C. E. (1977). *Human emotions*. New York: Plenum Press.

Kaplan, S. (1992). Environmental preference in a knowledge-seeking, knowledge-using organism. In J. H. Barkow, L. Cosmides, & J. Tooby (Eds.), *The adapted mind: Evolutionary psychology and the generation of culture* (pp. 581–598). New York: Oxford University Press.

Keltner, D., & Bonanno, G. A. (1997). A study of laughter and dissociation: Distinct correlates of laughter and smiling during bereavement. *Journal of Personality and Social Psychology, 73*, 687–702.

Labott, S. M., & Martin, R. B. (1987). The stress-moderating effects of weeping and humor. *Journal of Human Stress, 13,* 159–164.

Lazarus, R. S. (1991). *Emotion and adaptation.* New York: Oxford University Press.

Lee, P. C. (1983). Play as a means for developing relationships. In R. A. Hinde (Ed.), *Primate social relationships* (pp. 82–89). Oxford, UK: Blackwell.

Levenson, R. W. (1992). Autonomic nervous system differences among emotions. *Psychological Science, 3,* 23–27.

Levenson, R. W. (1994). Human emotions: A functional view. In P. Ekman & R. Davidson (Eds.), *The nature of emotion: Fundamental questions* (pp. 123–126). New York: Oxford University Press.

Levenson, R. W., Ekman, P., & Friesen, W. V. (1990). Voluntary facial action generates emotion-specific autonomic nervous system activity. *Psychophysiology, 27,* 363–384.

Levin, J. S. (1996). How religion influences morbidity and health: Reflections on natural history, salutongenesis, and host resistance. *Social Science and Medicine, 43,* 849–864.

Levin, J. S., & Chatters, L. M. (1998). Research on religion and mental health: An overview of empirical findings and theoretical issues. In H. G. Koenig (Ed.), *Handbook of religion and mental health* (pp. 33–50). San Diego, CA: Academic Press.

Lewis, M. (1993). Self-conscious emotions: Embarrassment, pride, shame, and guilt. In M. Lewis & J. M. Haviland (Eds.), *Handbook of emotions* (pp. 563–573). New York: Guilford Press.

Lyubomirsky, S., & Tucker, K. L. (1998). Implications of individual differences in subjective happiness for perceiving, interpreting, and thinking about life events. *Motivation and Emotion, 22,* 155–186.

Markus, H. R., & Kitayama, S. (1991). Culture and the self: Implications for cognition, emotion, and motivation. *Psychological Review, 98,* 224–253.

Martin, R. A., Kuiper, N. A., Olinger, J., & Dance, K. A. (1993). Humor, coping with stress, self-concept, and psychological well-being. *Humor, 6,* 89–104.

Martin, R. A., & Lefcourt, H. M. (1983). Sense of humor as a moderator of the relation between stressors and moods. *Journal of Personality and Social Psychology, 45,* 1313–1324.

Martineau, W. H. (1972). A model of the social functions of humor. In J. H. Goldstein & P. E. McGee (Eds.), *The psychology of humor: Theoretical perspectives and empirical issues* (pp. 101–128). New York: Academic Press.

Mascolo, M. F., & Fischer, K. W. (1995). Developmental transformations in appraisals for pride, shame, and guilt. In J. P. Tangney & K. W. Fischer (Eds.), *Self-conscious emotions: The psychology of shame, guilt, embarrassment, and pride* (pp. 64–113). New York: Guilford Press.

McCullough, M. E. (1995). Prayer and health: Conceptual issues, research review, and research agenda. *Journal of Psychology and Theology, 23,* 15–29.

McCullough, M. E., Kilpatrick, S. D., Emmons, R. A., & Larson, D. B. (in press). Is gratitude a moral affect? *Psychological Bulletin.*

Moos, R. H. (1988). *Coping Responses Inventory manual.* Palo Alto, CA: Stanford University and U.S. Department of Veterans Affairs Medical Centers.

Moran, C. C., & Massam, M. M. (1999). Differential influences of coping humor and humor bias on mood. *Behavioral Medicine, 25,* 36–42.

Nesse, R. M. (1990). Evolutionary explanations of emotions. *Human Nature, 1*, 261–289.

Nezu, A. M., Nezu, C. M., & Blissett, S. E. (1988). Sense of humor as a moderator of the relation between stressful events and psychological distress: A prospective analysis. *Journal of Personality and Social Psychology, 54*, 520–525.

Oatley, K., & Jenkins, J. M. (1996). *Understanding emotions.* Cambridge, MA: Blackwell.

Orians, G. H., & Heerwagen, J. H. (1992). Evolved responses to landscapes. In J. H. Barkow, L. Cosmides, & J. Tooby (Eds.), *The adapted mind: Evolutionary psychology and the generation of culture* (pp. 555–579). New York: Oxford University Press.

Panksepp, J. (1998). Attention deficit hyperactivity disorders, psychostimulants, and intolerance of childhood playfulness: A tragedy in the making? *Current Directions in Psychological Science, 7*, 91–98.

Pellegrini, A. D. (1992). Rough-and-tumble play and social problem solving flexibility. *Creativity Research Journal, 5*, 13–26.

Peterson, C., & Seligman, M. E. P. (1984). Causal explanations as a risk factor for depression: Theory and evidence. *Psychological Review, 91*, 347–374.

Pratto, F., & John, O. P. (1991). Automatic vigilance: The attention-grabbing power of negative social information. *Journal of Personality and Social Psychology, 61*, 380–391.

Renninger, K. A., Hidi, S., & Krapp, A. (Eds.). (1992). *The role of interest in learning and development.* Hillsdale, NJ: Erlbaum.

Rosenberg, E. L. (1998). Levels of analysis and the organization of affect. *Review of General Psychology, 2*, 247–270.

Rozin, P., & Fallon, A. E. (1987). A perspective on disgust. *Psychological Review, 94*, 23–41.

Ruch, W. (1993). Exhilaration and humor. In M. Lewis & J. M. Haviland (Eds.), *Handbook of emotions* (pp. 605–616). New York: Guilford Press.

Ryff, C. D., & Singer, B. (1998). Contours of positive human health. *Psychological Inquiry, 9*, 1–28.

Schaefer, C. E. (1993). What is play and why is it therapeutic? In C. E. Schaefer (Ed.), *The therapeutic powers of play* (pp. 1–15). Northvale, NJ: Jason Aronson.

Seligman, M. E. P., & Csikszentmihalyi, M. (2000). Positive psychology: An introduction. *American Psychologist, 55*, 5–14.

Sherrod, L. R., & Singer, J. L. (1989). The development of make-believe play. In J. Goldstein (Ed.), *Sports, games and play* (pp. 1–38). Hillsdale, NJ: Erlbaum.

Simons, C. J. R., McCluskey-Fawcett, K. A., & Papini, D. R. (1986). Theoretical and functional perspective on the development of humor during infancy, childhood, and adolescence. In L. Nahemow, K. A. McCluskey-Fawcett, & P. E. McGhee (Eds.), *Humor and aging* (pp. 53–77). San Diego, CA: Academic Press.

Singer, J. L. (1968). The importance of daydreaming. *Psychology Today, 1*, 18–27.

Singer, J. L. (1973). *The child's world of make-believe: Experimental studies of imaginative play.* New York: Academic Press.

Solomon, R. L. (1980). The opponent-process theory of acquired motivation: The costs of pleasure and benefits of pain. *American Psychologist, 35*, 691–712.

Stein, N. L., Folkman, S., Trabasso, T., & Richards, T. A. (1997). Appraisal and goal processes as predictors of psychological well-being in bereaved caregivers. *Journal of Personality and Social Psychology, 72,* 872–884.

Sutton-Smith, B. (1992). The role of toys in the instigation of playful creativity. *Creativity Research Journal, 5,* 3–11.

Swartz, L. (1996). Building relationships through humor. *Dissertation Abstracts International, 56*(10-B), 5840. (University Microfilms No. AAM96–04628)

Sylva, K., Bruner, J. S., & Genova, P. (1976). The role of play in the problem-solving of children 3–5 years old. In J. Bruner, A. Jolly, & K. Sylva (Eds.), *Play* (pp. 244–257). New York: Basic Books.

Teasdale, J. D. (1983). Negative thinking in depression: Cause, effect or reciprocal relationship? *Advances in Behavior Research and Therapy, 5,* 3–26.

Tomkins, S. S. (1962). *Affect, imagery, consciousness: Vol 1. The positive affects.* New York: Springer.

Tomkins, S. S. (1982). Affect theory. In P. Ekman (Ed.), *Emotions in the human face* (2nd ed., pp. 353–395). New York: Cambridge University Press.

Tooby, J., & Cosmides, L. (1990). The past explains the present: Emotional adaptations and the structure of ancestral environments. *Ethology and Sociobiology, 11,* 375–424.

Tooby, J., & Cosmides, L. (1992). The psychological foundations of culture. In J. H. Barkow, L. Cosmides, & J. Tooby (Eds.), *The adapted mind: Evolutionary psychology and the generation of culture* (pp. 19–136). New York: Oxford University Press.

Uchino, B. N., Cacioppo, J. T., & Kiecolt-Glaser, J. K. (1996). The relationship between social support and physiological processes: A review with emphasis on underlying mechanisms and implications for health. *Psychological Bulletin, 119,* 488–531.

Vytgotsky, L. S. (1967). Play and its role in the mental development of the child. *Soviet Psychology, 5,* 6–18.

Wolpe, J. (1958). *Psychotherapy by reciprocal inhibition.* Stanford, CA: Stanford University Press.

5

The Evolution of Emotional Expression

A "Selfish-Gene" Account of Smiling and Laughter in Early Hominids and Humans

MICHAEL J. OWREN
JO-ANNE BACHOROWSKI

Perhaps because they are the only aspect that can be directly perceived by an observer, the external expressions of internal emotional states have long been of great interest to researchers in affective science. This particular area of inquiry is also arguably unique in the science of human behavior in that Darwin's (1872/1998) early and formative examination of the biological underpinnings of these expressions put evolution in a central role in the discussion from the very beginning. However, while biological conceptions of evolution have undergone important changes since Darwin's time, the original principles he proposed have tended to persist relatively unchanged in applications to human emotional expression. An update is therefore in order, specifically one that brings a more contemporary version of critical precepts in biological evolution to bear, takes account of concomitant progress that has been made in applicable areas of animal communication, and grounds itself in the larger context of primate evolutionary history.

Doing so puts some human expressions in a rather new light, especially with respect to the facial and nonlinguistic vocal signals associated with positive emotional states. These expressions stand out in particular because they are much more uniquely human than are signals of negative affect. Thus, smiling and laughter appear to have arisen specifically over the course of early hominid and human evolution, and one must therefore infer that their emergence was critically linked to other unique aspects of this

152

phylogeny. In this chapter, we examine human smiles and laughs from a "selfish-gene" perspective, an approach to natural selection that emphasizes the role of individual organisms or genes in evolutionary change, rather than the role of social groups or entire species. While the selfish-gene framework has dominated evolutionary biology for several decades, it has to date played little if any role in affective science. Self-conscious incorporation of this new perspective is therefore long overdue, particularly as it has striking implications for the evolution of communication. Examining these implications in detail means considering a number of diverse topics, but seems well worth the trouble in light of the new questions and hypotheses that can result. The particular scenario described here was generated in exactly that fashion, and our presentation of it therefore includes a variety of background information we deem to be important but that has largely been omitted from previous work. As the chapter is rather lengthy as a result, the remainder of this introduction briefly reviews each of the most important themes that are later discussed in detail, including our account of both the origins and chronology of the evolution of expressions of positive affect in hominids and humans.

EMOTIONAL EXPRESSIONS IN HUMANS AND NONHUMAN PRIMATES

While prosimians, monkeys, and apes produce a range of negatively toned expressions that are recognizably related to states like fear or aggressive anger, these species do not have comparably clear-cut analogues to the positively toned human expressions of smiling and laughter (reviewed by Chevalier-Skolnikoff, 1973; van Hooff, 1967; and Redican, 1975). In fact, nonhuman primates appear to use only one facial expression that is unequivocally positive in nature, namely, the "play-face" associated with friendly rough-and-tumble play among youngsters. While this gesture is very widespread, only two species are known to use a clearly positively toned sound. These animals, common chimpanzees and pygmy chimpanzees, both use a pant-like vocalization that is particularly likely to be heard in circumstances involving tickling or roughhousing among younger animals (de Waal, 1988; Marler & Tenaza, 1977). While reminiscent of human laughter and therefore often given the same label, this vocalization is unmistakably different (Provine, 1996).

In other words, while the same terms may be used, smiles and laughs in humans are different from the expressions of any nonhuman primate. However, one comparison that can still be made is to attempt to identify homologous relationships between human expressions and those of monkeys and apes (Preuschoft, 1992; Preuschoft & van Hooff, 1995). Here, a homology is said to exist if features being compared in two or more different species occur in each through descent from a common ancestor (discussed by Preuschoft & van Hooff, 1995). The features in question need not even be exactly the same, as species-specific variations may have arisen subsequent to evolutionary divergence. In addition, similarities among species can also occur as analogies—similar-looking solutions to common adaptive problems that are not specifically influenced by common descent. These comparisons have been fruitful in pointing out some likely relationships between human facial and vocal expressions and those of nonhuman primates, while also underscoring that there are many more questions than answers for the positively toned variants.

Overall, we are particularly struck by the general lack of unabashedly positive facial or vocal expressions among other members of the primate order. While the play-face display is widespread, for instance, it is predominantly seen in infants and juveniles, and then virtually disappears from the expressive repertoire of adults. In contrast, humans routinely produce smiles at high rates throughout life, using them in every sort of social situation. The comparison between laughter and the arguably laugh-like pants of chimpanzees parallels that of smiling and play-faces. Laughter is ubiquitous and distinct among humans, while positively toned panting is not prominent in either of the other two species' vocal repertoires. Nonetheless, it is important to note that similarities do exist between human laughter and this clearly pleasure-related but relatively undeveloped vocalization found in the two nonhuman species that are by far our closest primate relatives (Fleagle, 1999).

APPLYING THE SELFISH-GENE FRAMEWORK

While many theorists have commented on the evolutionary origins and functions of human smiling and laughter, no complete satisfying explanations are currently available. Most accounts have in fact focused on tracing the human expressions by examining physical similarities to nonhuman signaling, with less detailed attention being paid to the question of why these signals emerged in the first place. This "why" aspect seems especially interesting, however, particularly given the prominent and evidently unique role these expressions play in human interactions. We therefore offer a hypothesis on this aspect in particular, one which differs from previous work in self-consciously sticking as closely as possible throughout to the selfish-gene logic of contemporary evolutionary biology.

It becomes particularly important to hew to those principles when examining communicative phenomena, as it is very difficult to think of signaling behavior as other than a cooperative sort of event. Adopting a selfish-gene approach, however, we note that it is not enough to assume that a signal will evolve due to having adaptive value to the participants. The approach instead demands that selection pressures operating on senders of signals be explicitly separated from those affecting receivers in the communication event. The critical insight is that while the two parties may in some cases both benefit, their inherent interests are never exactly the same. Selection pressure on senders favors those who benefit themselves by effectively influencing receiver behavior, whereas success for the latter means showing responses that act to maximize their own fitness. While many scenarios concerning the evolution of signals emphasize mutual benefit to both parties, even in these situations each side will be under constant selection pressure to gain some advantage over the other—in inverse proportion to their genetic relatedness. Signals and responses must therefore be considered to coevolve over time, a process more fundamentally grounded in competition than in cooperation. Even if a communication system specifically allows unrelated individuals to coordinate their behavior in useful ways at a global level, signaling will not become prevalent or persist in stable form if either of the parties involved are sacrificing any fraction of their own long-term reproductive interests relative to those who do not produce or respond to the signal.

We begin with the following assumption: While the panoply of human emotions and emotional expressions is necessarily derived from features that were present in the common ancestor of modern chimpanzees and humans, key changes in smiling and laughter evidently occurred after these two lines had diverged. In other words, these expressive behaviors emerged in response to selection pressures operating specifically on our hominid ancestors—species whose increasingly terrestrial lifestyles became more and more separated from the conservative arboreal ecologies of chimpanzees. We infer that smiling and laughter arose as mechanisms that allowed these early hominids to adapt to new ecological niches as ape species were increasingly facing extinction due to their general inadaptability in the face of rapid and widespread habitat loss. Modern humans are descended from the particular species that were successful under these challenging circumstances, and we propose that increases in the ability of genetically unrelated individuals to form and maintain cooperative relationships was a significant factor. Finally, we hypothesize that smiling and laughter were instrumental as mechanisms of the affective bonding involved.

While only modestly novel at this point, the proposal becomes more substantive when the selfish-gene perspective is applied. Taking this approach, one must assume that truly cooperative behavior among unrelated individuals will be the exception rather than the rule, since natural selection inherently favors those who are able to extract more benefit from relationships with others than they give up to the other parties themselves. In order to be successful, then, a strategy of cooperating with others for mutual benefit must evolve in a form that makes it resistant to the countervailing selection pressure favoring behavior that brings short-term selfish gain to one party but not the other. In fact, as the nascent signaling system emerges and spreads, any facilitation of truly cooperative behavior that results will in and of itself create the selection pressure for dishonesty. To whatever extent true cooperation provides benefits, individuals who can exploit the willingness of others who cooperate while failing to reciprocate themselves will be favored. We therefore further infer that if the tendencies of apes and early hominids to form cooperative relationships did indeed become adaptively magnified to the level routinely observed in modern humans, the mechanisms involved in forming the underlying affective bonds must have included some means by which cooperative individuals could also predict the likely behavior of prospective behavioral partners. We argue both that smiling and laughter evolved as reliable indicators of positive emotional states for precisely this reason and that these signals initially emerged in a safeguarded form that at least for a time guaranteed their reliability in the face of selection pressure favoring dishonest versions.

The reasoning is that if a sender's expressive behavior in smiling or laughing is inherently dependent on a positive internal state, the receiver of such signals knows that the other individual is experiencing positive emotions while in the receiver's presence. This point is important because such feelings, whether positive or negative, can be assumed to be an important influence on how the sender actually does behave toward the other individual. Specifically, if the sender consistently experiences positive rather than negative or neutral emotions when in the presence of a particular companion, the latter becomes requisitely more likely to experience favorable cooperative treatment. When the sender also provides reliable cues to this affect through concomitant smiling and laughter, the receiver can use these signals as a means of predicting this potentially advantageous outcome. The greater the quantity and consistency of these positive signals over time, the more the receiver can afford to show positive, cooperative behavior toward the other party.

If the mechanism in question also responds to smiles and laughs from others, this single adaptation can create a feedback loop between two individuals that begins with even just a mildly positive emotional stance toward the other. In other words, if one person's positive emotional expressions evoke corresponding affect in another, the positive expressions thereby elicited in this second party will then amplify positive affect in the original signaler. This feedback loop fosters growth of mutual and positive affect between the two, which constitutes an important causal component of reciprocal cooperative behavior. Naturally, senders of such signals also put themselves at risk of exploitation by providing these reliable indicators of their otherwise unobservable emotional states. If some individuals show such cues but others do not, receivers will do better by soliciting cooperative behavior specifically from those who do in fact exhibit positive emotions toward them. However, the senders have no inherent assurance that their favorable treatment will subsequently be repaid by the receivers unless those individuals also provide reliable cues to positive affective states. Conversely, if a sender is able to sway a receiver's emotional stance through smiling and laughter, the latter becomes vulnerable. In this case, a sender that is able to produce these signals in the absence of a corresponding positive stance can exploit their impact on the other's behavior without being emotionally committed to showing that individual favorable treatment. Thus, natural selection should work against individuals that "fall for" smiles and laughs that are not associated with positive emotional states and are not predictive of subsequent sender behavior.

OUR HYPOTHESIS IN OVERVIEW

Putting these pieces together, we propose that selection pressure from dramatic habitat changes produced an elevated payoff for cooperative behavior in an early hominid. However, the emotional and communication mechanisms that subsequently appeared could only arise in an inherently safeguarded form, meaning that the associated signaling system was not susceptible to dishonesty by either senders or receivers. A system in which such cheating could readily occur would not have been stable and would therefore not develop into a species-wide adaptation. Therefore, thinking that smiling and laughter first evolved as reliable indicators of positive affect, we will refer to these honest versions as "emotion-dependent" signaling. We also propose that the emerging brain mechanisms underlying smiling and laughing were themselves subject to influence by smiles and laughs experienced from others, thereby inherently creating the possibility of more explosive growth of mutually positive affective regard in a relationship.

Both aspects are crucial as part of the hypothesized unitary adaptation, because either one occurring in isolation would be subject to exploitation and thus be unstable. In contrast, a mechanism that included both components would both resist exploitation and guide the individuals having it to form positive affective bonds specifically with others showing the same adaptation. This last point follows from noticing that signal-induced feedback fostering mutual growth of positive affect would only occur when both parties produce smiles and laughs and respond positively to such signals. The feedback effect disappears if either component is missing, with corresponding dampening of positive affect growth.

Again, however, the very existence of this honest communication would have increased the benefit to be derived from using dishonest signals. Inauthentic smiles and laughs would be effective if a sender could use them to elicit favorable treatment from another without actually feeling as positively toward that individual as would necessarily be the case if the signals were genuine. If smiling and laughter originally arose in a form that ensured authenticity, then these facsimile versions must have arisen at some later time and have a different neural foundation. Thus, we also propose that the success of spontaneous and honest smiles and laughs created selection pressure that eventually allowed senders to produce dishonest versions of these same expressions by gaining voluntary control of the facial and vocal musculature involved. In each case, the emotion-dependent system would necessarily have appeared first, thereby setting the stage for a volitional system. This chronology makes sense of well-established neuropsychological evidence that "involuntary" and "voluntary" emotional expressions are in fact controlled by separable motor systems in the brain (see an additional discussion of this topic in K. N. Ochsner & L. Feldman Barrett, Chapter 2, this volume). Finally, the same general logic also suggests that as the simpler of the two signals, spontaneous, authentic smiling must have evolved first. While dishonest smiling was therefore sooner or later sure to follow, decreasing the predictiveness of the honest version inherently created selection pressure for a new, more reliable way of signaling positive affect. The last piece of our argument is therefore that honest, spontaneous laughter emerged third in this sequence of events, with this vocal version helping to restore the predictive value of the by-then compromised smiling strategy. Because it represented a counterpunch in this cyclical arms race, the new emotion-dependent signal would necessarily have to be more complex and more difficult than the previous one to mimic on a volitional basis. Laughter appears to be exactly this sort of signal, which arguably completes the explanation of the current state of human positive-affect signaling.

THE CHAPTER IN OVERVIEW

As indicated by the length of these introductory remarks, there are many disparate threads to weave in fleshing out our arguments. The scenario we describe is also admittedly speculative and as yet untested. However, the selfish-gene logic that we adhere to throughout increases our deductive power by greatly narrowing the range of possible outcomes in the evolution of this communication system. Furthermore, we believe that simply being able to present a credible hypothesis in this form is in and of itself a constructive step toward more defensible evolutionary theorizing about communication. In order to make this case, we begin the body of the chapter with a brisk overview of critical concepts of selfish-gene evolution, thereafter examining why the occurrence of honest signaling poses a special problem for this framework. The next section then briefly reviews the evolutionary history of primates and describes some of the circumstances that were particularly important in shaping hominid evolution. That background creates the foundation for presenting our hypothesis in more detailed form, including two critical corollaries and some relevant empirical evidence. We then compare our proposal to some other hypotheses concerning smiling, laughter, and emotional expressions in general, and conclude with some thoughts about evolutionary theorizing in emotions research.

THE SELFISH-GENE PERSPECTIVE IN EVOLUTIONARY THEORY

Some History

Although no definitive date can be set for such changes, the publication of Williams's (1966) book refuting the "group-selection" approach to evolution provides a convenient marker of the emergence of the now dominant "selfish-gene" perspective in evolutionary biology. In previous decades, biologists had tended to focus on evolutionary effects at the species level, for example, examining processes of species divergence and population genetics. Much less attention was paid to lower levels of organization. Classical ethologists—biologists who had pioneered the scientific study of naturally occurring animal behavior—also emphasized species-level analysis. Their work contributed to the position that natural selection must favor species (or social groups within species) whose individual members routinely sacrifice themselves for the greater good of group-mates or other members of their species (hereafter "conspecifics"). Williams's powerful counterargument was that any individual with a gene whose effect was to promote such behavior would necessarily be at a disadvantage compared to others that did not—no matter how slight or profound. Any individual with this sort of "altruism" gene would necessarily be their own worst enemy in within-species competition, behaving in ways that decreased reproductive success for themselves while increasing the number of offspring that the beneficiaries of their altruism could produce. As the gene promoting this behavior would also be requisitely less represented in each successive generation, it would eventually be entirely replaced in the gene pool by one that could play the same role in every way except not encouraging altruism.

"Kin Selection" and "Reciprocal Altruism"

Arguments like these led evolutionary biologists to focus on natural selection occurring at the level of individual organisms and their individual genes, and this selfish-gene view quickly displaced previous approaches (see Dawkins, 1989, for a lucid and accessible overview). According to selfish-gene theory, natural selection favors genes whose effects on an organism ultimately increase the number of viable offspring the individual can produce that them-selves go on to successful reproduction. Therefore, genes that tend to benefit an individual's own reproductive success more than that of any other being become more prevalent, while other genes disappear. In other words, evolu-tion selects for selfish behavior, and the observable behaviors of individual members of all species should be explicable in this fashion. However, this harsh equation is notably softened for behaviors involving genetic relatives. Because biological kin share genes, favorable behavior directed toward rela-tives can indirectly help create additional copies of some of the altruist's own genetic material (Hamilton, 1964). This kin-selection effect can account for the strongly kin-biased behavior shown by individual members of virtually all sexually reproducing species, particularly in the case of their own offspring, with whom they share 50% of their genes.

Another rider to the selfish-gene contract is the phenomenon of recip-rocal altruism (Axelrod & Hamilton, 1981; Trivers, 1971). Here again, genes promoting apparently self-sacrificing behavior can be successful. In this case, individuals whose behavior benefits nonkin can nonetheless be successful if the favorable acts in question are repaid by the beneficiary of this altruism at some later time. There are constraints involved, of course, including that species members must encounter one another more than once during their lives if reciprocation is to be possible and that individuals must be able to recognize past benefactors and beneficiaries. Finally, they must also remember the past behavior of those individuals, particularly so as to withhold any further altruism from "cheaters" who do not recipro-cate. The occurrence of reciprocal altruism has been convincingly demon-strated in a number of species (Zahavi & Zahavi, 1997), but it is nonethe-less much less in evidence than kin-selection effects, which are ubiquitous in the animal kingdom.

One compelling reason that reciprocal altruism is much less important than kin selection in most species is that it requires inherent safeguards against cheating. In other words, any nascent tendency toward genetically based reciprocal altruism must gain its foothold in a world populated by in-herently selfish individuals. In fact, if the genes that favor such behavior do become more prevalent, the potential payoff to others for exploiting such tendencies grows in requisite fashion. Selection will thus favor individuals whose genes promote a tendency to "accept" altruism from genetically un-related individuals while withholding reciprocation whenever possible. Suc-cessful reciprocal altruism thereby creates selection pressure that under-mines itself, and it can become a stable species-wide behavior only if some sort of safeguard inherently limits the opportunity to cheat. An example al-luded to earlier is that when species members encounter one another multi-ple times, altruistic behavior can be selectively withheld from those who fail to reciprocate, thereby limiting the overall payoff for cheating. In addi-tion, altruists are likely to be very cautious with unfamiliar individuals, reserving their riskiest favorable behavior for those with whom they have established a long-term relationship already marked by repeated instances of reciprocated altruism.

Some Implications of the Selfish-Gene Perspective

Overall, the basic stance of a selfish-gene approach is that no two individuals can possibly have identical interests under all circumstances, except for possibly in the one case of being genetically identical. In sexually reproducing species, the interests of even the closest of genetic relatives therefore diverge, routinely creating conflict (Trivers, 1974). For instance, empirical data from humans indicates that there are inevitable and important clashes even between human mothers and the fetuses they gestate (Boyd & Silk, 1997; Hrdy, 1999). Given this constraint, we argue that an evolutionary explanation of behavior is only credible if it begins by assuming that natural selection favors selfish individuals and that any deviation from self-interested behavior must be specifically accounted for. As discussed in the next section, the phenomenon of communication itself is therefore potentially problematic, as it can be deemed a kind of reciprocal altruism in which one individual benefits another by producing informative signals. We are not arguing that this sort of helpful, cooperative behavior cannot evolve among unrelated individuals, but rather that it does so only if safeguards inherent to the system keep it stable in the face of countervailing selection pressure for exploitation and dishonesty.

ACCOUNTING FOR COMMUNICATION AMONG SELFISH INDIVIDUALS

The selfish-gene perspective thus puts the act of communication in an interesting light, as this phenomenon is in fact typically thought of as involving information sharing but also routinely occurs among unrelated individuals in many different species. This apparent contradiction has led some researchers to question not only whether signaling actually is an inherently cooperative event but also if it should be thought of in information transmission terms at all (Krebs & Dawkins, 1984; Owings & Morton, 1997; Owren & Rendall, 1997, in press). Because these issues are directly applicable to expressions of emotion in humans as well, we briefly review some of the main points that have arisen in studies of animal signaling.

Historical Trends in Animal Communication Theory

Both sharing and information were critical components of the communication theory developed in classical ethology (Krebs & Davies, 1981; Smith,

1977), an approach that has strongly influenced research and theory in human emotional expression (Fridlund, 1997; Grammer, 1990). Classical ethologists proposed that signals evolve from inadvertent behaviors or cues to upcoming behavior that probably occur in any kind of social interaction among animals. For instance, one could argue that a dog in a conflict situation bares its teeth as a threat gesture because ancestral dogs retracted their lips before biting an opponent. If these adversaries responded to such "intention" movements as predictive events, such conflicts could be resolved with minimal risk of physical damage to either party. Senders were thus selected to provide predictive cues about their upcoming behavior, while receivers who acted on such information were also able to do better in important interactions like courtship or intraspecific conflict over resources. Through a process of "ritualization," inadvertent cues became emancipated from their origins and were shaped as specialized communication signals by coevolution among senders and receivers (see D. Keltner & J. Haidt, Chapter 6, this volume, for a related discussion).

Selfish-gene theorists have viewed these issues quite differently. For instance, Krebs and Dawkins (1984; Dawkins & Krebs, 1978) argued that senders mostly attempt to manipulate receivers rather than to inform them. Because the receiver's well-being is irrelevant to the sender except as the latter can also benefit, the selfish-gene perspective suggests that communication is best described as an attempt to exert an influence on others by any means possible using signaling. In Krebs and Dawkins's view, it is more likely that senders will manipulate or persuade others by producing large numbers of salient but minimally informative signals. In most cases, senders would not in fact benefit by providing highly reliable indicators of their own upcoming behavior to receivers. The more frequent outcome should be that signals to unrelated receivers are just informative enough to be attended to, but will be more strongly selected to influence through bluffing than by being authentic and predictive. Selfish-gene logic therefore predicts that animal signals should be exaggerated in form and repetitious in use, as they are primarily designed to influence rather than to inform. Many animal signals indeed appear to be exactly like that, with "communication" often seeming to be more competitive than cooperative. In contrast, in cases of truly cooperative signaling, the exchange of information should be much more subtle, with both parties benefiting from producing brief, discrete signals that do not inadvertently provide important information to third-party competitors (see Hauser, 1996, for a further discussion).

Taking this argument a step further, a number of investigators have suggested that "communication" evolves for reasons other than signaling value (reviewed by Owings & Morton, 1998). For instance, younger, more helpless animals in many species produce noxious shrieking and screaming when under threat from others. While often characterized as cries for help that carry representational information to potential allies (Gouzoules, Gouzoules, & Marler, 1984), the vocalizations in question are often markedly aversive and in addition are typically repeated many times. According to Krebs and Dawkins's (1984) reasoning, these properties suggest a primary function of dissuading the attacking animal from its aggression rather than informing distant allies. Furthermore, these shrieks and screams are extremely variable in their acoustic features and thus poorly suited to conveying specific information either about caller identity or some representational content (Owren & Rendall, 1997, in press). Other forms of competitive rather than cooperative communication strategies have also been suggested (Owings & Morton, 1998), potentially replacing the more traditional account.

The Interplay of Honesty and Cheating in Animal Signaling

This general question of function in communication is particularly important because of its implications for the selection history that must underlie each signal that can now be observed in an extant animal species. An important but often overlooked implication of the information-sharing view in particular is that there must be a history of selection pressure acting on senders and receivers to produce complementary "matching" encoding and decoding processes in the two parties. Because a form of cooperative coevolution would be involved, this general characterization cannot serve as general model for animal communication without directly contradicting the spirit of the selfish-gene approach. For example, while communication among genetically related individuals may have an inherently cooperative foundation, animal signals are more prominently used between unrelated individuals who do not have closely allied interests. The evolutionary history implied in these cases must therefore involve a more intricate interplay of selection pressures. For example, if senders are selected for their ability to influence receivers regardless of whether information is being transmitted or is honest, then receivers will often be selected for resisting detrimental signaling rather than becoming more responsive to it. While such resistance may force senders to produce honest and informative signals some proportion of the time, selection pressure for cheating or alternative avenues of influence will always be present.

Again, however, senders who can use signals to manipulate receivers create the very selection pressure that ultimately makes their conspecifics less likely to be such dupes. This insight has led to one of the basic principles of contemporary communication theory, namely, that honest signaling can arise through competitive coevolution. For example, courtship signals produced by males in species where females can select among multiple possible partners are thought over time to necessarily become reliable. Honest signaling must eventually arise because reproductive success of females depends directly on their ability to discriminate the relative quality of their potential mates. Females who happen to be responsive to signal features that are predictive of high inherent genetic quality in males ultimately also produce higher-quality offspring. Thus, the conspicuous ornamentation and intricate courtship displays of males in a wide variety of species are now routinely being found to provide reliable cues to traits like fighting ability, current and past nutritional condition, and overall vigor and health (Zahavi & Zahavi, 1997).

But this elaborate ornamentation and courtship behavior is not beneficial to the males themselves except with respect to mate attraction. The selection pressure exerted by female choice thus becomes very costly, significantly increasing the energetic investment males must make in developing and maintaining the large, colorful structures and intricate, finely controlled motor patterns that females attend to when choosing a mate. Those attributes are in fact informative to females precisely because they are challenging and therefore provide a reliable index of male condition. Peafowl provide a ready example of this effect in the heavy, highly ornamented tail that characterizes adult males. Here, the larger and more exquisitely decorated the structure, the greater is the guarantee of high gene quality. When a peahen encounters a peacock who has dragged such a tail around throughout its adult life, she is inherently assured that this particular male has genes promoting not only good development and pathogen resistance but also effective foraging and skillful predator evasion. Because of the cost to males, there is always selection pressure for cheating—developing signals that are not as costly to produce but are nonetheless effective in swaying female choice. However, as successful dishonesty by males simply selects for females that are more discerning, mate-attraction signals inevitably gravitate toward stable forms that are necessarily honest. The safeguard in such cases is the cost of the signal itself, which represents a "handicap" imposed on males by selection pressure exerted by female mate choice (Zahavi, 1975; Zahavi & Zahavi, 1997). In other words, the costs inherent in effective courtship signaling are a hindrance to the male's success in other domains of its life, thereby guaranteeing that females will be choosing among the males whose unfakeable signals show that they can bear these costs.

Looking toward Humans

Together, these are the themes we return to below when considering human smiling and laughter: first, that one must take account of the relentless pressure favoring selfishness in any social behavior, including communication; second, that communication is fundamentally an attempt to influence others rather than to specifically inform them, thereby giving rise to a variety of both competitive as well as cooperative communication strategies; third, that successful competitive signaling by senders necessarily creates selection pressure on receivers, with evolutionary effects that eventually must also feed back to reshape the signaling behavior itself; fourth and finally, that if a signaling system is honest, then in one way or another it must include inherent safeguards against cheating. In competitive situations, dishonesty is prevented by the inherent cost of signaling. However, safeguards also necessarily exist in situations that are truly cooperative, involving mutual benefit and possible information sharing. For genetically unrelated senders and receivers, in fact, it becomes virtually impossible to imagine how a cooperative system could emerge except in an inherently protected form. Cooperative behavior shown by senders inevitably makes them vulnerable to exploitation unless the system is itself resistant to the selection pressure favoring selfish behavior in those individuals.

We believe human laughter and smiling to be such a system, as it has characteristics that point to a history of cooperative coevolution. One compelling clue is that human senders can use smiles and laughs to elicit positive emotional responses in others. Evidence from work on spontaneous smiling, for instance, shows that humans experience positive affect when exposed to the signal and adopt a more positive emotional stance toward people who display it (Fox & Davidson, 1988; Keltner & Bonanno, 1997; Messinger, 1994). The case of laughter is arguably even more clear-cut, for example, as shown by the power that laugh tracks have to enhance viewer enjoyment of television comedy shows and the commercial success of novelty items that do little more than present bouts of laughter (Provine, 1996). From the selfish-gene perspective, such vulnerability to emotional influence points to a history of selection on ancestral receivers for genes promoting tendencies to respond positively to smile-like facial expressions and laugh-like vocalizations. If so, receivers were thereby "cooperating" with senders and becoming "matched" to them. Such matching could not emerge as a stable evolutionary strategy if receivers were harmed more than benefited. Their interests must therefore have been importantly aligned with those of senders as far smiling and laughing are concerned.

If so, according to the reasoning we discussed, the coevolutionary process must have included some safeguard, and we must now ask how it worked. Furthermore, if smiling and laughter did emerge among some hominid species after divergence from our common ancestor with chimpanzees, the circumstances that created such selection pressure for hominids must be explained. Evidence of possible homologies between humans and nonhuman primates may indicate that the substrate from which smiles and laughs originated was widespread taxonomically, but does not account for why these signals evidently emerged only among the hominids. Leaving the question of safeguards to a later section, we first examine some critical aspects of primate evolution to attempt to account for the uniquely human nature of these signals.

IMPORTANT FEATURES OF PRIMATE AND HOMINID EVOLUTION

There are more than 200 extant primate species, all of whom likely evolved from an insectivorous squirrel- or shrew-like arboreal mammal that existed approximately 65 million years ago (Fleagle, 1999, provides a detailed but accessible discussion of primate evolution, which is the source of much of the information presented here). Modern humans stand out among these many species in a variety of ways, but for present purposes it is particularly important that our species is able to reproduce at significantly higher rates than our closest great-ape relatives. Chimpanzees, gorillas, and orangutans reproduce very slowly precisely because offspring in these species require a great deal of time, energy, and individual attention from their mothers. Yet, humans are able to combine an even higher level of parental investment with a shorter interbirth interval and faster overall reproductive rate. This paradoxical outcome is more understandable if seen in the larger context of primate evolution, where it becomes evident that while the ape strategy was at first highly successful, it also left these animals extremely vulnerable to the global climate changes and habitat losses that eventually followed. Modern humans are descendants of the particular apes that were able to adapt to these dramatically changing conditions, where the overwhelming majority of animals in this taxonomic group instead became extinct. Later in the chapter, we will propose that smiling and laughter played an important role in that success as an effective means of fostering cooperative relationships among genetically unrelated individuals. Here we set the stage for that argument by examining the unfortunate circumstances that befell the apes.

"K-Selection" and Extinction among the Apes

A characterization used to help understand how evolution shapes particular traits is whether the species in question is relatively "K-selected" or more "r-selected." These terms refer to selection pressure on reproductive rate resulting from overall habitat stability and associated fluctuations in food supply. On the one hand, when a species' ecological circumstances are relatively predictable and constant, population size tends to remain at or near a stable maximum. Resulting K-selection favors production of relatively few, slowly developing and carefully nurtured offspring. On the other hand, when conditions are inherently variable and food supplies are more transient, recurring fluctuations in overall population size produce r-selection. In this case, individuals do better if they are able to reproduce at high rates whenever possible, producing rapidly developing offspring, each requiring relatively little parental investment.

Although all mammals are considered to be K-selected relative to other animal groups, reproductive rate and degree of parental care nonetheless varies significantly within this class. In Norway rats, for instance, mothers produce two or three litters every year, each consisting of some 6–12 offspring. Gestation occurs over 21–26 days, and while pups are entirely dependent on their mother at birth, they develop quickly and disperse within a few months. Thus, while rodents are relatively K-selected compared to insects, amphibians, and reptiles, they are nonetheless strongly r-selected in relation to primates. In the latter, mothers characteristically give birth to single offspring, whose gestation requires several months or more in monkeys, and as much as almost 9 months in great apes. Offspring also depend on dedicated maternal care that lasts for periods ranging from months to years, which results in interbirth intervals of 1 to 2 years for many monkeys and as much as 5 years or more in the great apes. While thus dramatically slowing the overall reproductive rate, the outcome of these prolonged periods of gestation and postnatal care is a cognitively sophisticated adult animal that routinely exhibits a variety of much more complex behaviors than in r-selected species.

Similar variation in reproductive strategy is evident within the primate order as well. Compared to prosimians like lemurs and galagos, monkeys are relatively K-selected. However, the latter are thoroughly r-selected when compared to extant apes. Contrary to the popular notion that modern apes are more sophisticated descendants of Old World monkeys, these two lines diverged as much as 23 million years ago, with significant diversification subsequently occurring within each group. In fact, while only a handful of ape species now remain, these animals once were much more numerous and diverse than were monkeys. The period of greatest success for apes came shortly after their divergence from monkeys, which occurred in the early Miocene. However, after that point their numbers began to decline, while monkeys became increasingly successful. This reversal of fortunes in the two groups is often described as the apes losing out to the monkeys in competition over shared habitats. However, it is equally plausible that the apes were less able to adapt to the recurring and dramatic climatic changes that affected the earth over important periods of primate evolution. The global climate of the early Miocene was warmer and showed less seasonal variation than in any subsequent period, with subtropical conditions extending into significantly higher latitudes than today (Tattersall, Delson, & Van Couvering, 1988). Those conditions later changed dramatically as the continents drifted toward their current positions, ocean temperatures fell due to alterations in current patterns, and climatic conditions eventually began to show the oscillation that has marked recent geologic eras.

Whether climate changes were directly or indirectly to blame, by the time ancestral humans and apes diverged sometime between 4 and 6 million years ago, very few species remained of this once-flourishing group. A significant factor in the general demise of these animals is likely to have been that apes were strongly K-selected and unable to adapt to dramatic habitat changes. Each species filled its respective niche to the limit, with a low birthrate and slow, steady replacement, keeping the overall population stable and close to maximum levels. The slow development and high level of maternal care found in chimpanzees, orangutans, and gorillas, for instance, equip animals in each species with a detailed knowledge of their rich rainforest environments. The cognitive sophistication they bring to such learning is evident in other contexts, for instance in naturally occurring protocultural activities (Wrangham, McGrew, de Waal, & Heltne, 1994) and in the problem-solving and symbol-use tasks posed to them under laboratory conditions (reviewed by Tomasello & Call, 1997).

But while this cognitive sophistication allowed ancestral apes to maximize resource extraction from their stable and predictable environment, slowing of overall reproductive rate in these species also put them at risk. Subsequent glaciation periods brought dramatic fluctuations in both sea levels and mean temperatures, and ape species steadily disappeared as habitat conditions changed on a global scale. Today, apes are highly threatened and exist only in scattered groups around the world. The more r-selected Old World monkeys fared very well in comparison, adapting more readily to the new ecological opportunities as they became available. Higher reproductive rates and shorter generation times allowed monkeys to be much more responsive to new selection pressures and novel habitats. As a result, while many are also now threatened or endangered, monkey species remain much more numerous and widely distributed than are apes.

Increasing Reproduction through Cooperative Behavior

This perspective suggests that rather than viewing the eventual emergence of modern humans as the culmination of an inevitable climb up some evolutionary ladder, our species more accurately represents the last gasp of a dying line that has mostly "K-selected" itself out of existence (Gould, 1980). The eventual, dramatic success enjoyed by hominids and later humans stands as a remarkable and paradoxical exception to the fate that befell most apes, one that produced a unique and extreme level of K-selection in our species, in which continued escalation of parental investment has been combined with an increased birthrate and simultaneous rearing of multiple dependent offspring. This outcome has depended in part on the human ability to create stable, long-term cooperative relationships among genetically unrelated individuals, including not only the bonds that occur between mothers and fathers of common biological offspring but also the variety of both short- and long-term friendships and alliances that routinely allow two or more individuals to coordinate their activities for mutual benefit.

While other primates display cooperative behavior to varying degrees (Gouzoules & Gouzoules, 1986; de Waal, 1986; de Waal & Berger, 2000; Silk, 1986; Walters & Seyfarth, 1986), the level of behavioral coordination they exhibit is greatly exceeded by the everyday behaviors of humans. Although humans also exhibit strongly kin-based behavior, revealing the ever-present effects of kin selection (see Geary, 1998, for a recent review), routine and widespread reciprocal altruism among unrelated individuals is a particular hallmark of human behavior. Cooperation among both kin and nonkin alike help humans in subsistence-level hunter–gatherer societies to sustain a significantly higher reproductive rate than do the apes. For example, the interbirth interval of approximately 4 years shown by the !Kung of Botswana and Namibia (Blurton-Jones, 1993) is unusually long for humans (Boyd & Silk, 1997) but is still shorter than in chimpanzees.

This higher rate of reproduction is in part due to parental investment by human males—a behavioral innovation not found among chimpanzees, gorillas, orangutans, or the great majority of other primates. In addition, much of that resource investment does not lie in direct care of offspring, but rather through sharing of resources acquired outside the immediate family setting. Stable, cooperative relationships with both the children's mother and with other males in the larger social group are particularly critical if this strategy is to succeed. Such relationships play an equally important role in the reproductive success of females, whose long-term cooperative relationships with unrelated individuals also typically include a male partner as well as other females of the group.

However, simply noting the central role that such relationships play for humans of both sexes does not explain how they can occur. To reiterate an earlier caveat, while each party engaged in a coordinated, cooperative pursuit of common goals can benefit as a result, the short-term interests of the selfish individuals involved can nonetheless diverge at every turn. Defection and selfishness are extremely common in human relationships and are an unending source of interindividual conflict (Badcock, 1991; Frank, 1988). Although we humans have many admirable qualities, our behavior and sense of fairness is usually biased to favor ourselves in social transactions. That notion of ourselves can readily apply to kin as well but is more difficult to extend to nonkin. Self-interested decision making unmitigated by genetic kinship to the other party therefore poses an ongoing threat to the mutual affection and reciprocal trust that must exist in a cooperative relationship between unrelated individuals.

Honest Expressions of Positive Affect Are Key in Cooperative Relationships

The preceding discussions have highlighted the issues we think are crucial in understanding why humans routinely smile and laugh during the course of their interactions. One further assertion is necessary to fit the various pieces together, namely, that a person's internal emotional states are a critical causal factor in guiding behavior—especially in social relationships. In other words, an individual's positive or negative affective stance toward another plays an important role in determining what sort of treatment is shown that person, as reflected in the emotions that are typically experienced when in his/her presence. The consistency of those signals would be particularly important in providing prima facie evidence of an ongoing positive stance. If this outcome occurs consistently across repeated encounters, the receiver can thereby be ever more assured of receiving requisitely favorable treatment in joint endeavors.

However, the selfish-gene perspective stipulates that one cannot simply assume that each individual invariably benefits from revealing those feelings as they occur. In some cases, providing external cues to such states is probably quite useful to the sender, for instance, when presenting honest expressions of anger and aggression induces fear in an opponent. But even here, revealing one's emotions and likely behavior will not be the best strategy if signal receivers as a result become better able to exploit the sender in some fashion. Both observations are also applicable to honest expressions of positive emotions, with the caveat that the danger of exploitation is likely much higher when these signals provide reliable cues to sender cooperativeness. Accounting for the evolution of such signals therefore requires specific and separate consideration of each aspect—how senders benefit from producing such cues, why receivers allow themselves to be influenced, and how the interaction of each party's selfish interests have played out over the course of phylogenetic history.

Developing Cooperative Relationships among Unrelated Hominids

Our proposal begins with a claim that in early stages of hominid evolution, individuals who were able to form and maintain reciprocal, cooperative relationships with genetically unrelated conspecifics achieved greater reproductive success than did those less able to do so. While that assumption is unremarkable in and of itself, it is important to note that such relationships are generally rare among nonhumans. Of course, the circumstances of early hominid evolution were also unusual in that they involved highly intelligent and strongly K-selected apes that were facing unprecedented habitat loss. While the situation was devastating to many, changing ecologies also presented new opportunities to the species that could adapt to take advantage of the new niches that became available as a result.

Various monkeys were able to adapt by virtue of reproducing at rates that allowed relatively rapid evolutionary change. There were likely many different ways in which monkeys could change, and the resulting radiations ultimately filled a diversity of new ecological niches with a corresponding variety of well-adapted species. The situation was quite different for apes, who were strongly constrained by having become highly specialized for intelligent and efficient exploitation of a static rainforest environment. Due to low reproductive rates, the only chance these species had of adapting to new environments was arguably if quite modest genetic changes could produce effects with both rapid and far-reaching impact. Arguing post hoc, we suggest that the emerging hominid species were better able to invade new ecological niches because they became better able to form and maintain cooperative relationships. In other words, by greatly increasing the amount and quality of coordinated behavior between unrelated individuals of both sexes, hominids were able to significantly increase their birthrates. Ultimately, individual females were able to care for multiple dependent offspring simultaneously, for instance, by being able to rely in part on resources provided by a male mate. Reciprocal altruism among unrelated females as well as unrelated males would also have been a key element in successfully coping with the added investment burdens associated with a higher birthrate and correspondingly shorter interbirth interval.

Properties of the Signaling Mechanism

While individual hominids could probably all benefit from participating in cooperative long-term relationships, the constraints of selfish-gene evolution cannot be forgotten—any hominid that behaved favorably toward an unrelated conspecific ran the risk of being exploited in return. As high levels of reciprocal altruism developed in spite of this countervailing selection pressure, we are forced to conclude that even in its earliest form the mechanism underlying this new strategy of expressing positive affect must somehow have been protected from exploitation. Two characteristics in particular could provide this kind of safeguard. First, the expressions generated by this mechanism would have to be authentic indicators of positive affect that could not be produced by other means. Second, the mechanism would have to create a link both between positive affect and signal production and, conversely, between signal reception and affect production. Given these two properties, the nature of the adaptation itself would help shield hominids who had it from exploitation by those who did not, because the feedback loop facilitating growth of mutual positive affect between two individual would be created only when both parties had the new mechanism.

The "Green Beard" Effect

This latter, emergent property resembles Dawkins's (1989) hypothetical green beard effect, which is an argument that having a gene promoting true altruism can be a successful adaptation if that same allele also helps create an external mark that altruists can use to identify one another. While there is no evidence for this sort of gene, investigations of authentic smiling indicate that the mechanism underlying this signal does in fact exhibit the two antecedent properties we deem critical for a green-beard-like effect to occur. Investigations have shown, for instance, that spontaneous smiles that result from positive affect are distinguishable from smiles that a person produces upon request. The first, genuine form involves simultaneous retraction of the corners of the mouth and contraction of the muscles around the eyes (Ekman, Davidson, & Friesen, 1990). When smiling is not spontaneous, it is much less likely to include the latter. Responses to the forms also differ, with the genuine version being found to elicit significantly more positive affect in others (Frank, Ekman, & Friesen, 1993; Keltner & Bonanno, 1997). Thus, receivers experiencing spontaneous smiles from others are probably more likely to produce these expressions in response than when smiling is not spontaneous. Taken together, this evidence also argues that production and perception of smiling are integrated functions of a unitary mechanism, as we have surmised based on selfish-gene logic.

The logic of how hominids with this sort of mechanism would be protected by a green-beard-like effect is straightforwardly related to the feedback loop described earlier. While smiling senders were putting themselves at risk, the positive feedback in question could only occur if this signaling did in fact elicit positive affect and reciprocal smiling in another individual. Because the mechanism itself was being engaged, no feedback would occur if the receiver failed to smile in return. This absence of smiling would then mean that this particular receiver either did not have the mechanism or was not experiencing positive affect toward this particular sender. On the one hand, genuine, spontaneous smiling that was returned by another individual could trigger mutually reinforcing positive affect between the two parties. On the other hand, the adaptation itself would not put the sender at particularly great risk, because smiling could not yet occur dishonestly. Therefore the adaptation would be stable and protected even from the earliest stages of evolutionary emergence, as long as the mechanism only produced honest smiles and was in addition also responsive to these signals.

Two Caveats

Note that we are not suggesting that signals of positive affect have to involve this particular sort of mechanism. In fact, given the potential advantages that reciprocal altruism could likely provide to early hominids, a variety of mechanisms may have come and gone. Our argument is simply that if honest signaling was involved, the adaptation in question had to have either these two properties or some other safeguarding characteristics in order to be successful. Otherwise, even a slight tendency toward providing genuine signals of positive affective stance toward genetically unrelated conspecifics could be immediately exploited and the adaptation would not take hold.

Furthermore, we are also not proposing that the capacity to feel positive emotions toward unrelated individuals was itself part of the smiling-related adaptation. Based on evidence from monkeys and apes, we instead expect that even the earliest hominids were already capable of persistent positive feelings toward others. Among nonhuman primates, behaviors indicative of emotional bonding are prominent, particularly among kin. For example, related animals are much more likely than unrelated individuals to sit and sleep in proximity, groom one another, aid each other during agonistic encounters, forage together, stay in contact during group movements, handle one another's infants, and tolerate the antics of each other's young offspring. That strong kin bias in everyday behavior is one of the fundamental principles of contemporary behavioral primatology (see Smuts, Cheney, Seyfarth, Wrangham, & Struhsaker, 1986, for a variety of related reviews). Much less prominent but nonetheless documented in a variety of species are examples of alliances and friendships among unrelated individuals (Smuts, 1985; Smuts et al., 1986). In both cases, it is virtually impossible not to conclude that the very positive treatment individual nonhuman primates can show one another reflects an underlying foundation of affective bonding. The behaviors involved are markedly similar to those that typify positively toned human relationships, except for the striking lack of clear-cut facial and vocal displays of positive affect. We therefore conclude that it was these expressions that were the critical innovation for early hominids rather than the affect per se.

Dishonest Signaling Was Inevitable, Eventually

In this section, discussion has mainly focused on smiling as an early hominid adaptation. The last important piece of our proposal concerns events that occurred subsequent to such signaling and as a direct consequence of it. The argument again follows from selfish-gene logic, specifically from the observation that increased reproductive success due to an adaptation for honest smiling would in and of itself create selection pressure favoring dishonest, exploitative mimicry. In fact, even small increases in the prevalence of reciprocal altruism that occurred would up the payoff for being able to use smiling to foster positive regard in another person without actually having corresponding feelings oneself. This inherent relationship between the benefits to be gained from honest communication and corresponding advantages of then being able to use the same signals dishonestly probably guarantees that even a safeguarded system will sooner or later be circumvented. As a result, if smiling was necessarily honest in its initial protected form, facsimile versions that were not inherently tied to a positive emotional state would also be expected to eventually appear. Our inference is that these were chronologically separate events, with this dishonest smiling necessarily emerging later than the original version.

Emotion-Dependent versus "Volitional" Signaling

Continuing for the moment to focus specifically on smiling, we propose that the first form of this signal resulted from the operation of an automatic, unlearned motor program producing patterned activation of facial musculature and was not readily subject to conscious modulation. Because the function of such signaling was social influence, these "action patterns" would be triggered when a positive affective state was experienced while in the presence of others. In this view, these original emotion-dependent smiles resembled a "fixed-action pattern" as described by classical ethologists (Eibl-Eibesfeldt, 1989). Ethological theory proposes that all animal species show such adaptations, which are reflex-like but carefully sequenced motor behaviors narrowly specialized for use in performing important tasks. Classic examples include a stereotyped sequence of extending and retracting the neck that female greylag geese exhibit when retrieving an egg that has rolled out of the nest, and directed pecking motions that nestling herring gulls use to prompt food regurgitation from their caregivers when the latter return from a foraging trip. Such behaviors are argued to represent species-wide adaptations, with learning playing little or no role in their emergence. Rather, the associated brain circuitry is thought to become organized early in development, with the action pattern appearing in full-blown functional form the very first time an animal encounters the relevant circumstances.

While we do not endorse the baggage-laden terminology used to describe these kinds of action patterns, we are essentially proposing that emotion-dependent smiling shows similarities as an "innate" and "involuntary" signal. While oversimplified, such characterizations are arguably acceptable to the extent that the spontaneous smiles humans produce when experiencing positive internal states are consistent in form and emerge early in development in the absence of specific experience. The honest, safeguarded smiling mechanism we are proposing would have appeared in this kind of form, as a unique facial action pattern that was triggered by a positive affective state, producing a signal that could not be generated by other means and that elicited positive responses in others in the absence of specific learning effects.

The dishonest version of smiling that evolved specifically because of the effectiveness of the earlier signal would have to be significantly different. Although the form of the signal itself would necessarily be similar, the underlying mechanism involved would not be connected to positive affect and would probably require significant learning to be used effectively. Such smiles would be fundamentally volitional in nature, designed to be used manipulatively by senders attempting to further their own selfish interests. Those interests could be furthered by a sender who, without having to experience positive affect toward another, was nonetheless able to smile at key points in a social interaction and thereby elicit positive affect and concomitantly favorable treatment. Due to its inherent dishonesty, however, this volitional version would not be effective if used injudiciously. Rather, timing and placement of dishonest smiles would be quite important, with the impact of such a signal being inherently dependent on both the particular receiver involved and the dynamics of the social interaction unfolding with that individual. In other words, experience gained over a longer course of development and socialization with other group members would be virtually irrelevant to emotion-dependent smiling but would be central to using the same signal volitionally.

Competitive Coevolution Prompts Emergence of Laughter

The advent of a well-used dishonest version of smiling would necessarily have decreased the inherent reliability of the original, honest version. That devaluation would in turn produce two new selection pressures: (1) as the volitional signal could now be used in circumstances in which it might be costly to experience smile-induced positive affect toward a particular sender, receivers would do better if able to discriminate emotion-dependent from volitional smiling; (2) however, so long as the ability to form and maintain reciprocal, cooperative relationships continued to be advantageous, any decrease in the reliability of smiling would produce a requisite increase in the value of the honest signaling of positive affect. Conceivably, the effect of this second selection pressure could be to restore the reliability of the original signal by making it more distinguishable from the dishonest variety. As the latter was under volitional control, however, individual senders could simply modify this version to match the other form. Given the importance of the positive-affect mechanism to fundamental aspects of hominid social relationships, it is therefore more plausible that a new, more reliable form of such signaling emerged.

We must therefore surmise that the same selection pressures that earlier produced honest smiling as a species-typical expression of positive affect now selected for spontaneous, genuine laughter. This signal differs from emotion-dependent smiling in at least two important ways that are consistent with the proposed chronology. First, the motor activity itself is more complex than for smiling, at least when occurring in the song-like "ha-ha-ha" form resembling a series of vowel sounds. This song-like variety is considered to be the prototype version (Provine, 1996), although it is also clear that laughter is an acoustically variable signal (Bachorowski, Smoski, & Owren, forthcoming). Nonetheless, empirical experiments have recently shown that humans rate song-like laughter as being more positive, friendlier, sexier, a better choice for inclusion in a hypothetical laugh track, and more likely to make them interested in meeting the laugher than other acoustic forms (Bachorowski & Owren, in press). The second difference between emotion-dependent smiling and laughter is that the occurrence of the latter requires a higher degree of positive arousal. For example, while genuine laughter is typically accompanied by smiling, spontaneous smiles routinely occur in the absence of laughter. The latter begins as positive affect continues to increase, as illustrated by the "warm-up" effect that can routinely be observed through the course of an ongoing social interaction. Furthermore, whereas smile-related activity in facial muscles probably requires only very modest energetic effort, a variety of both facial and torso musculature is involved in producing song-like laughter (reviewed by Ruch, 1993). Laughter is thus much more demanding, to the point that some investigators characterize it as mild physical exercise that provides requisite cardiovascular health benefits (Fry, 1992).

These observations—that song-like laughter is a more complex action pattern than smiling, reflects a higher degree of positive arousal, and requires greater energy expenditure—are all consistent with the claim that laughter arose specifically in response to the declining reliability of smiling as a cue to positive affect. Other aspects of the emergence of this signal would arguably have been just as we described above in the case of emotion-dependent smiling. Specifically, we suggest that laughter would also have appeared due to a relatively simple genetic change and was triggered by positive emotions in the presence of others, and the mechanism involved inherently linked this affect to both production and perception components. Emotion-dependent laughter thus played exactly the same role as genuine, spontaneous smiling had before. In fact, we suggest that the changes involved occurred by elaborating the existing smile-related mechanism in some way rather than through emergence of a brand-new mechanism.

Summarizing the Hypothesis

To recapitulate, we are arguing that applying the basic tenets of selfish-gene selection to the evolution of communication in early hominids points to the emergence of honest signaling of positive affect as a valuable mechanism for forming and maintaining cooperative relationships. The same principles dictate that such signals must have emerged in an inherently safeguarded form that provided protection against exploitation by dishonest signalers. The first form would have been emotion-dependent smiling, produced by a brain mechanism that was instrumental both in producing smiling concomitantly with positive affect and in generating positive affect in response to experiencing this signal from others. An adaptation showing these properties could create a feedback loop that actively fostered growth of positive affect between two parties that both had this particular mechanism. This signaling system would have been inherently safeguarded because no such feedback effect would occur when the sender was interacting with a social partner who either lacked the adaptation or simply did not feel positive affect toward the sender. In both cases, the receiver would not produce smiles in response to the original sender's positive-affect signaling and would therefore not be able to better exploit that individual specifically because of the smiling-related adaptation being shown.

Emotion-dependent smiling was thus a key factor in fostering stable and reciprocal cooperative relationships because it provided a means by which genetically unrelated individuals could reliably gauge whether another person felt positively toward them. When detecting consistent evidence of a positive affective stance in a social partner, a given hominid could more accurately predict that this particular individual was likely to respond reciprocally to favorable, cooperative treatment. Given a unitary mechanism that linked both smile production and emotional responding to smiling, this single innovative adaptation could (1) foster growth of mutual positive affect between two unrelated individuals and (2) guide them to form such bonds only with conspecifics that had the crucial adaptation and showed evidence of at least some initial positive regard.

However, the very success of this innovative strategy created the selection pressure that eventually led to the emergence of a second, volitional form of the same signal. Here, a smile facsimile that was not inherently linked to positive affect in the sender could nonetheless be used to elicit this emotion in others. Using these mimicked smiles successfully would be more cognitively demanding, as the strategy would be effective only if the signal were used judiciously and in accordance with the other party's individual response characteristics. In the next two sections, we present a variety of empirical evidence about smiling and laughter that bears on a number of different aspects of these proposals.

EVIDENCE FROM EMPIRICAL STUDIES OF EMOTIONAL EXPRESSION

Central tenets of our proposal are (1) that honest, emotion-dependent smiling and laughter evolved in safeguarded form before dishonest versions appeared, and (2) that when cheating subsequently began, it occurred through volitional mimicry of the veridical forms. If the assumptions and reasoning involved are correct, then smiling and laughter in modern humans should each show evidence of two separable underlying production systems. Furthermore, while the volitional system should by definition operate quite flexibly, the emotion-dependent system should be fundamentally similar across individuals and produce requisitely consistent signals. In addition, our logic also forces the conclusion that in some way we cannot currently specify there is an inherent connection between brain circuitry involved in experiencing positive affect, producing facial and vocal expression of such states, and feeling positive emotional responses upon seeing or hearing these signals. We believe that there is important converging evidence that substantiates the first two claims, with at least indirect support for the third aspect as well.

Emotion-Dependent versus Volitional Affect Production

Smiling

There are several kinds of evidence that bear on the question of whether expressions of positive affect occur in two forms, one being emotion-dependent and the other being volitional. This general issue has actually been a prominent discussion point in affective science ever since Darwin (1872/1999) discussed such a hypothesis in the context of anatomist G. B. Duchenne de Boulogne's investigations of the facial musculature involved in producing emotional expressions. While we cannot hope to summarize even a small fraction of the relevant literature, some investigators at least argue very strongly that the distinction does exist for smiling. The work of Ekman and his colleagues in particular has suggested that spontaneous smiles are characterized by contraction of both zygomatic and orbicularis oculi muscles in the face. In other words, these "felt" (Ekman & Friesen, 1982), "enjoyment" (Ekman, 1989), or "Duchenne" (Ekman, 1989) smiles are the ones for which there is muscle activity around both the mouth and the eyes (Ekman et al., 1990). This form is contrasted with a variety of "voluntary" smiling patterns that may be "false," "masking," or "miserable," rather than being inherently connected to positive affect (Ekman, 1985; Ekman & Friesen, 1982).

Evidence from the neuropsychology of smiling supports the notion of two separable systems even more strongly. Rinn (1984), for instance, argues for distinguishing between "emotional" and "volitional" facial expressions based on dissociations observed in clinical neurology. His review of the evidence indicates that whereas volitional expressions have their origin in cortical motor circuitry and arrive at the face through the pyramidal tract, spontaneous emotional expressions originate in the phylogenetically older extrapyramidal motor system, which consists mostly of subcortical nuclei. Projections from this system arrive at the face through pathways other than the pyramidal tract.

This neuroanatomical distinction is consistent with the long-established diagnostic practice of distinguishing between an emotional and a volitional system. Unilateral lesions in the volitional system can, for example, produce partial paralysis, with the result that patients asked to retract the corners of their mouth are unable to do so on one side. However, the same patients often exhibit normal-looking spontaneous smiles, with full participation of the purportedly "paralyzed" musculature on the one side. Conversely, lesions that compromise the extrapyramidal motor system can eliminate spontaneous smiling while leaving voluntary movements unimpaired. This double dissociation is also illustrated in surgical interventions. In cases were both spontaneous and voluntary smiling has been lost due to damage to the facial nerve, surgeons have been able to restore the latter. In this procedure, motor nerves that normally innervate other structures are spliced into the distal "stump" of the facial nerve. After surgery, patients suffering from paralysis on one side of the face can regain volitional control of that musculature through nerves that, for instance, had originally innervated the shoulder. The patients' recovery involves learning to execute facial movements through the resectioned pathway separately from activity in the shoulder that is mediated through the remaining undisturbed nerve fibers. However, while sometimes able to regain voluntary control, these patients never again show spontaneous facial expressions on that side.

Additional evidence supporting the argument that spontaneous smiles are inherently different from volitional ones is provided both by studies showing that genuine smiling has greater power to elicit positive affect in others (Keltner & Bonanno, 1997) and that observers have some ability to distinguish the two types (Frank et al., 1993). On the other hand, the results of these studies also indicate that observers are far from perfect in differentiating emotion-dependent smiles from facsimile versions, as would be expected if volitional smiling arose as a form of dishonest signaling. If so, this turn of events would necessarily have decreased the reliability of smiling in general as an indicator of positive affect in senders. However, there is no reason to suspect that the payoff to be had from achieving reciprocal cooperative relationships showed any decline—either then or later.

Laughing

Less information is available about laughter than about smiling, but several kinds of relevant evidence are nonetheless available. Like smiling, laughter has been argued to exhibit at least one relatively stereotyped form—the regularly patterned series of vowel-like bursts we earlier described as song-like laughter (Provine & Yong, 1991; see also Provine, 1997). While no work has specifically addressed the question of whether this particular signal is inherently honest, it has figured prominently among the sounds recorded in studies eliciting spontaneous laughter from participants (Provine, 1996, 1997). As noted earlier, when these subjects were asked to laugh, they routinely reported being unable to do so on demand. Many then produced spontaneous song-like laughter in response to the silliness of the request. This particular sound has also been found to be effective in inducing positive affect in others, both under field conditions (Provine, 1996) and in a controlled laboratory setting (Bachorowski & Owren, in press). In the latter work, song-like laughter was consistently rated more positively than were other naturally occurring laugh sounds in five different experiments where participants were asked to judge either the laugh itself, one of several attributes of the laugher, or their own affective responses to the sound. The power of such laughter to induce positive affect is also demonstrated by the "contagious" nature of laughter, meaning that individuals who hear either live or prerecorded laugher become more likely to experience positive affect and laugh (Provine, 1992, 1996).

The evident difficulty of producing song-like laughter on demand may be particularly noteworthy (Provine, 1996), especially in comparison to the apparent ease of smiling in response to specific situational demands. We therefore suggest that the occurrence of emotion-dependent smiling prompted the eventual emergence of volitional smiling but that the emotion-dependent laughter that followed has as yet not been strongly compromised by an ability to produce convincing though dishonest song-like laugh sounds. The difficulty of producing this particular vocalization on demand suggests that the motor pattern involved in laughter is more complex than for smiling, that genuine laughter evolved more recently than did emotion-dependent smiling, or both.

Studies of monkeys and apes have independently provided evidence that the neural circuitry involved in laughter is different from that involved in volitional vocal behavior like speech. Deacon (1989) in particular argues this case, distinguishing between "vocalization" and "articulation" circuitry in the brain. Deacon proposes that the former controls production of "automatic" but uniquely human vocalizations like laughter and has access mainly to the respiratory system and larynx. The latter is involved in articulate speech production and therefore also has control over these components. However, this system can also produce a steady stream of complex supralaryngeal vocal-tract maneuvers, particularly involving the tongue. Based on neurophysiological evidence, Deacon argues that the circuitry involved in laughter and other emotion-dependent vocalizations is homologous to vocalization-related structures found in nonhuman primates. Speech, in contrast, makes use both of lower-level circuitry and purely cortical systems. Deacon thus proposes that laugh production originates in subcortical brain structures, much as we have earlier noted is the case for spontaneous smiling. He also infers that laughter itself emerged following the hominid divergence from other primates but likely preceded development of linguistically based vocal communication (Deacon, 1997).

Emotion-Dependent Signals Are Biologically Based

The evidence we have already reviewed also indicates that the emotion-dependent versions of both smiling and laughter have predictable forms that are similar across individuals. These relatively stereotyped signals have similar effects on observers and listeners no matter who produces them, indicating either that they are deeply rooted in basic human biology or that they emerge in response to formative developmental experiences with smiling and laughter that all humans tend to share. The first hypothesis is by far the more strongly supported, for instance with infant studies showing that spontaneous smiling and laughing both appear early in development (Sroufe & Waters, 1976). Very young infants typically produce their first smiles during sleep, with the mother's voice reliably eliciting active smiling in alert infants by the fourth week of life. Recognizable laughter is produced in response to vigorous physical stimulation by approximately 4 months of age and is thereafter reliably elicited by playful vocalizations, visual stimulation, and peekaboo games with caregivers. On the perceptual side, Haviland and Lelwicka (1987) have reported that by 10 weeks of age, infants responded differently to various facial and vocal expressions deliberately presented by their mothers. Not only did infants in this experiment mirror the facial expressions in question, but they also showed behavioral responses that were consistent with experiencing the associated emotion.

Both smiles and laughs can also appear even when an infant gets no experience with these expressions whatsoever. Although they never see others smiling, congenitally blind infants are nonetheless reported to produce readily identifiable smiles in appropriate circumstances (Freedman, 1964; Thompson, 1941). Deaf children have similarly been found to laugh, even when never hearing this sound either from others or from themselves (Goodenough, 1932). In fact, both signals have been shown to occur in children who are blind and deaf from birth (Eibl-Eibesfeldt, 1989). Taken together, this developmental evidence from both normal and impaired children indicates that spontaneous smiling and laughing are not behaviors that human infants learn from first observing them in others. Instead, both routinely appear in functional form with little or even no previous experience with these signals on the infants' part. Together with evidence that spontaneous smiling and laughter also show consistent form across individual humans, these results argue strongly that the neural circuitry involved in each is a basic component of species-typical biology.

Our Proposal Is Consistent with Basic Themes in Affective Science

While this brief review has been restricted to highlighting evidence that is consistent with our proposal, the findings described are in no way exceptional. On the contrary, these are oft-cited data addressing fundamental themes in research on emotion. It is therefore encouraging to our hypothesis that in this literature smiling has routinely been argued to occur in separable emotion-dependent and volitional forms, with laughter then showing less influence of voluntary control. The early emergence of the emotion-dependent versions of these signals in stereotyped, action-pattern-like form is also a mainstream finding, as is evidence of the differential impact of spontaneous versus purposefully produced smiles. Finally, we consider it noteworthy that the dissociated mechanisms that researchers have argued to be involved in the emotion-dependent and volitional versions of facial and vocal expressions exhibit the same chronology predicted by selfish-gene logic. In both cases, phylogenetically older circuitry is implicated in the honest, emotion-dependent form and involves neural pathways that are also found in nonhuman primates. Volitional versions, on the other hand, are mediated by cortical structures and associated tracts that show evidence of much greater, and hence chronologically later, change.

COMPARISONS TO OTHER HYPOTHESES

As noted, our conception has important points of overlap with a number of proposals concerning emotional expressions, in general, and displays of positive affect, in particular. However, there are some important differences as well, particularly in that we attempt to stick closely to the spirit of selfish-gene evolution. That has not been typical of previous theoretical work in the expression of emotion—for instance, in Ekman and colleagues' classic account of facial expression as involuntary and veridical "readouts" of internal state (Ekman, 1992; Izard, 1992), or in Fridlund's "behavioral ecology" perspective (Fridlund, 1994; see also Chovil, 1997, and Russell & Fernández-Dols, 1997).

Emotional Expressions Cannot Be Veridical Readouts of Internal State

Ekman's (1992) fundamental premise is that human emotional experience is grounded in a small set of basic, discretely organized emotions that occur as species-wide adaptations, including anger, disgust, fear, happiness, sadness, and surprise. These emotions are considered to occur in response to similar antecedent conditions for all humans, to trigger distinctive facial expressions, and to be innately organized and universally recognized. Thus, primary emphasis is on discrete facial expressions as veridical indicators of discretely organized emotional states. Although Ekman's approach does make clear that individual senders can modulate and inhibit their facial expressions in accordance with "display rules" that guide appropriate behavior in a given culture, overall facial expressions are thought to occur as a particular component of an integrated set of central and peripheral events that together form an adaptive response to important emotion-inducing circumstances. This approach differs from ours both in focusing almost exclusively on the sender and in making the implicit assumption that it is uniformly beneficial for senders to provide veridical representations of important internal states to receivers except when prohibited by culture-specific rules. There is no provision for the complex interplay of sender and receiver interests and resulting coevolutionary processes, nor any attempt to account for the existence of two physiologically distinct neural systems that are both involved in smiling.

Cheating Must be Considered

While a number of theorists have preceded us in suggesting that there can be direct links between emotional experience and expressions like smiling and laughter, Fridlund (1994) argues against this notion. Instead, he characterizes facial expressions as "social tools" that humans use to negotiate their encounters with others. As in the classical ethology approach, Fridlund proposes that these sorts of signals serve to share information with the receiver concerning the sender's likely upcoming behavior, thereby facilitating both parties' attainment of a mutually beneficial outcome. In contrast to the earlier ethological approach, however, Fridlund divorces the affect-related displays from underlying emotional processes, suggesting instead that they signify "motive" or "intent" (see also Chovil, 1997, and Russell, 1997). The approach is problematic, however, in that these are unobservable and arguably untestable constructs whose vague labels fail to illuminate their basic properties. As concepts like "motive" and "intent" have long been considered part of any given emotional experience, Fridlund's approach may be different mostly in attempting to shift the emphasis from affective to cognitive mechanisms.

However, doing so only compounds an error that Fridlund and other theorists writing about the evolutionary basis of emotional expressions routinely commit, namely, failing to recognize that senders and receivers have separate interests and that this divergence necessarily creates ongoing selection pressure for dishonest signaling. Furthermore, by freeing expressions like smiling and laughter from their mooring to internal emotional states, Fridlund is essentially arguing that these signals function either in symbolic fashion or as arbitrary predictors of upcoming behavior. In both cases, a history of cooperative coevolution between senders and receivers is implied, which raises the difficult evolutionary issues discussed earlier. Fridlund's proposals are therefore not viable unless they include convincing arguments that explain both how this coevolutionary process was sustained in the face of inherent selfishness, and how sender and receiver characteristics came to be matched in a shared system of arbitrarily defined signaling value.

Understanding Signal Form in Laughter

While those concerned with emotional expressions have frequently focused on the face, Provine (1992, 1996, 1997) has specifically examined the vocal form occurring as laughter. His work has emphasized description over explanation, but it does explicitly present laughter as a communicative signal whose function is to influence the behavior of others (see also Apte, 1985; Grammer, 1990; Grammer & Eibl-Eibesfeldt, 1990; and van Hooff, 1972). Provine's (1992) investigations of the contagious effects of laughter—meaning the power of even disembodied, prerecorded laugh sounds to elicit laughter and positive affect in listeners—led him to conclude that this signal is part of a cooperative, coevolved communication system, much as we have done here. Without presenting specific evidence about acoustic variability in laughter, Provine argues that it is a stereotyped, action-pattern-like signal (see Bachorowski & Owren, in press; Bachorowski, Smoski, & Owren, forthcoming). He also suggests that humans exhibit laughter-specific feature detectors, with a requisitely tight link between the production and perception of these sounds (Provine, 1996).

Here, we have incorporated the view that humans all appear to exhibit at least one consistently patterned form of laughing as part of their repertoire of such sounds, but we must also caution that much remains to be learned about acoustic variability in laughter, both within and among different individuals. Provine's work has emphasized proximate mechanisms rather than ultimate functions, and he implicitly accepts an information-sharing view of laughter without addressing the difficulties that are thereby raised. Thus the two approaches agree that song-like laughter at least has been shaped through natural selection and that receivers exhibit an enhanced affective response that must have evolved through an inherently cooperative coevolutionary process. However, stopping at that point raises more questions than are being answered, leaving the most difficult ones unaddressed. Here again, it is essential to account for the selfish interests of individual senders and receivers as an inherent part of explaining likely characteristics of laughter-related mechanisms. While Provine's mostly descriptive approach of examining proximate factors in isolation from functional questions is not unusual, it is nonetheless risky. The dangers are especially evident when the topic of interest is communication related, as noted in our earlier discussion of the temptation to view all signaling behavior as being inherently cooperative in nature.

CONCLUSIONS AND FUTURE DIRECTIONS

There are only a few aspects of our proposal that are truly new, as we hope to have acknowledged at various points. However, our proposal is fundamentally different from previous work on human emotional expression in being designed to reflect the principles and reasoning of the selfish-gene approach as much as possible. Whether or not its particular arguments turn out to have merit, we strongly believe that adopting a selfish-gene perspective will be a key factor in eventually understanding the evolution of smiling, laughter, and other emotional expressions, and we hope at least to have demonstrated that sort of thought process.

The crucial element is to recognize that selfish-gene evolution is both an entirely mechanical and a relentlessly tyrannical process. In the popular conception, evolution through natural selection involves an ongoing struggle to survive, with each generation thereby becoming ever better designed for tasks like procuring resources, fending off predators, finding mates, and rearing offspring. While natural selection has in fact shaped all animal species in exactly this way, evolutionary biology of the last several decades has increasingly emphasized that individuals in every species are also engaged in a never-ending struggle with others of their kind. It is in fact conspecifics who need the same resources, flee from the same predators, court the same potential mates, and work hard to provide for their own offspring at the potential expense of others. This form of competition does not create "better" designs, at least in the popular sense. There are no winners in the zero-sum game of within-species competition, because each new and successful strategy that emerges in the battle among conspecifics also undermines itself by inherently creating a countervailing selection pressure. This is the "Red Queen" aspect of evolution, a notion Van Valen (1973) borrowed from Lewis Carroll's *Through the Looking-Glass and What Alice Found There*. In this not-so-hypothetical domain, the monarch's every motion is matched by corresponding movement of the landscape, requiring her to run at maximum speed just to stay in the same place.

One cannot expect sensible or pretty outcomes from such an evolutionary process. It is instead unruly and nonlinear, with each adaptation producing new selection pressures, driving a species' traits this way and that, and creating interlocking but opposing forces that can give rise to ongoing change that plays out chaotic trajectories over time or even simply cycles back and forth. Seen in this light, human characteristics are extremely unlikely to constitute a "sensible," coherent package. For instance, scientific research on facial and vocal expressions of emotion has amply demonstrated that while some signals are spontaneous, involuntary, relatively stereotyped, and above all honest, others are none of those things. This confusingly inconsistent picture has contributed to polarization among investigators, who may erroneously be expecting to find a unitary underlying mechanism or process. That kind of outcome might occur if evolution were a linear process in which adaptations represent solutions to species-level problems. However, as we have attempted to illustrate, observable traits should instead be understood as improvised, stopgap solutions arising from the never-ending competition among individual species members as they jockey for any conceivable short-term reproductive advantage.

Thinking in these terms, one comes to always expect at least a bit of a hodgepodge of traits. In the hominid case, once honest signaling of positive emotions had emerged as a successful strategy for facilitating cooperation among unrelated individuals, it was necessarily only a matter of time before dishonesty and exploitation through mimicked, facsimile expressions also appeared. The best hope one has for being able to unravel this sort of tangle after the fact is to use the selfish-gene logic to trace the accumulation of strategies and counterstrategies that occurs in each species over time. The process is necessarily a cumulative one, meaning that subtle clues to the chronology involved should always be available in the behavior or anatomy of each species. Thus, our proposal that a newer system of volitional expression of positive affect arose as a result of the previous emergence of an honest system of emotion-dependent signaling may appear rather radical to an emotions theorist while seeming quite mundane to an evolutionary biologist.

By examining important issues in emotional communication from a selfish-gene perspective, we have brought to bear a different set of assumptions and logic than have others working on the same problems. Whether our particular proposals are right, partly right, or flat-out wrong, this difference from previous approaches has value if only in suggesting that further, hitherto unexplored possibilities must also exist. We also hope that our approach can be useful in stimulating fruitful empirical study, particularly with respect to the proposal that both smiling and laughter arise from coherently organized systems. This claim is of course central to our entire argument, as it forms the basis of the feedback loop hypothesized not only to have sparked the growth of positive affect among individual hominids who had the critical adaptation but also to have provided them inherent protection from exploitation. While the data we have reviewed support the existence of this sort of mechanism, none bear directly on the issue—perhaps because the question has not been posed in exactly this form before. The answer should nonetheless be of interest in emotions research regardless of whether our particular views are upheld, as either finding or failing to find the proposed link between production and perception of smiling and laughter would necessarily have important implications for understanding affective expressions in general. In writing this chapter, we thus hope at least to have encouraged others to also make use of the powerful conceptual tool that is selfish-gene logic, and thereby to have facilitated everyone in the joint effort to understand human emotional expressions.

REFERENCES

Apte, M. L. (1985). *Humor and laughter: An anthropological approach*. Ithaca, NY: Cornell University Press.

Axelrod, R., & Hamilton, W. D. (1981). The evolution of cooperation. *Science, 211,* 1390–1396.

Bachorowski, J.-A., & Owren, M. J. (in press). Not all laughs are alike: Voiced but not unvoiced laughter readily elicits positive affect. *Psychological Science.*

Bachorowski, J.-A., Smoski, M., & Owren, M. J. (2000). *Acoustic variability in laughter is associated with social context.* Manuscript in review.

Badcock, C. (1991). *Evolution and human behavior.* Oxford, UK: Blackwell.

Blurton-Jones, N. (1993). The lives of hunter–gatherer children: Effects of parental behavior and parental reproductive strategy. In M. E. Pereira & L. Fairbanks (Eds.), *Juvenile primates: Life history, development, and behavior* (pp. 309–326). New York: Oxford University Press.

Boyd, R., & Silk, J. B. (1997). *How humans evolved.* New York: Norton.

Chevalier-Skolnikoff, S. (1973). Facial expression of emotion in nonhuman primates. In P. Ekman (Ed.), *Darwin and facial expression: A century of research in review* (pp. 11–90). New York: Academic Press.

Chovil, N. (1997). Facing others: A social communicative perspective on facial displays. In J. A. Russell & J. M. Fernández-Dols (Eds.), *The psychology of facial expression* (pp. 321–333). New York: Cambridge University Press.

Darwin, C. (1999). *The expression of the emotions in man and animals* (Introduction by P. Ekman). London: HarperCollins. (Original work published 1872)

Dawkins, R. (1989). *The selfish gene* (2nd ed.). Oxford, UK: Oxford University Press.

Dawkins, R., & Krebs, J. R. (1978). Animal signals: Information or manipulation? In J. R. Krebs & N. B. Davies (Eds.), *Behavioural ecology: An evolutionary approach* (pp. 282–309). London: Blackwell.

Deacon, T. W. (1989). The neural circuitry underlying primate calls and human language. *Human Evolution, 4,* 367–401.

Deacon, T. W. (1997). *The symbolic species.* New York: Norton.

de Waal, F. B. M. (1986). Dynamics of social relationships. In B. B. Smuts, D. L. Cheney, R. M. Seyfarth, R. W. Wrangham, & T. T. Struhsaker (Eds.), *Primate societies* (pp. 421–429). Chicago: University of Chicago Press.

de Waal, F. B. M. (1988). The communicative repertoire of captive bonobos (*Pan paniscus*) compared to that of chimpanzees. *Behaviour, 106,* 183–251.

de Waal, F. B. M., & Berger, M. L. (2000). Payment for labour in monkeys. *Nature, 404,* 563.

Eibl-Eibesfeldt, I. (1989). *Human ethology.* New York: Aldine.

Ekman, P. (1985). *Telling lies.* New York: Norton.

Ekman, P. (1989). The argument and evidence about universals in facial expressions of emotion. In H. Wagner & A. Manstead (Eds.), *Handbook of psychophysiology: The biological psychology of emotions and social processes* (pp. 143–164). London: Wiley.

Ekman, P. (1992). An argument for basic emotions. *Cognition and Emotion, 6,* 169–200.

Ekman, P., Davidson, R. J., & Friesen, W. V. (1990). The Duchenne smile: Emotional expression and brain physiology. II. *Journal of Personality and Social Psychology, 58,* 342–353.

Ekman, P., & Friesen, W. V. (1982). Felt, false, and miserable smiles. *Journal of Nonverbal Behavior, 6,* 238–252.

Fleagle, J. G. (1999). *Primate adaptation and evolution* (2nd ed.). San Diego: Academic Press.

Fox, N. A., & Davidson, R. J. (1988). Patterns of brain electrical activity during facial signs of emotion in 10 month old infants. *Developmental Psychology, 24,* 230–236.

Frank, M. G., Ekman, P., & Friesen, W. V. (1993). Behavioral markers and recognizability of the smile of enjoyment. *Journal of Personality and Social Psychology, 64,* 83–93.

Frank, R. H. (1988). *Passions within reason: The strategic role of the emotions.* New York: Norton.

Freedman, D. G. (1964). Smiling in blind infants and the issue of innate vs. acquired. *Journal of Child Psychology and Psychiatry, 5,* 171–184.

Fridlund, A. J. (1994). *Human facial expression: An evolutionary view.* New York: Academic Press.

Fridlund, A. J. (1997). The new ethology of facial expressions. In J. A. Russell & J. M. Fernández-Dols (Eds.), *The psychology of facial expression* (pp. 103–129). New York: Cambridge University Press.

Fry, W. (1992). The physiological effects of humor, mirth, and laughter. *Journal of the American Medical Association, 267,* 1857–1858.

Geary, D. C. (1998). *Male, female: The evolution of human sex differences.* Washington, DC: American Psychological Association.

Goodenough, F. L. (1932). Expressions of the emotions in a blind-deaf child. *Journal of Abnormal and Social Psychology, 27,* 328–333.

Gould, S. J. (1980). *The panda's thumb.* New York: Norton.

Gouzoules, S., & Gouzoules, H. (1986). Kinship. In B. B. Smuts, D. L. Cheney, R. M. Seyfarth, R. W. Wrangham, & T. T. Struhsaker (Eds.), *Primate societies* (pp. 299–305). Chicago: University of Chicago Press.

Gouzoules, S., Gouzoules, H., & Marler, P. (1984). Rhesus monkey (*Macaca mulatta*) screams: Representational signaling in the recruitment of agonistic aid. *Animal Behaviour, 32,* 182–193.

Grammer, K. (1990). Strangers meet: Laughter and nonverbal signs of interest in opposite-sex encounters. *Journal of Nonverbal Behavior, 14,* 209–236.

Grammer, K., & Eibl-Eibesfeldt, I. (1990). The ritualisation of laughter. In *Naturlichkeit der Sprache und der Kultur: Acta colloqui.* Bochum, Germany: Brochmeyer.

Hamilton, W. D. (1964). The genetical evolution of social behaviour. *Journal of Theoretical Biology, 7,* 1–52.

Hauser, M. D. (1996). *The evolution of communication.* Cambridge, MA: Harvard University Press.

Haviland, J. M., & Lelwicka, M. (1987). The induced affect response: 10-week-old infants' responses to three emotion expressions. *Developmental Psychology, 23,* 97–104.

Hrdy, S. B. (1999). *Mother nature: A history of mothers, infants, and natural selection.* New York: Pantheon.

Izard, C. E. (1992). Basic emotions, relations among emotions, and emotion–cognition relations. *Psychological Review, 99,* 68–90.

Keltner, D., & Bonanno, G. A. (1997). A study of laughter and dissociation: Distinct correlates of laughter and smiling during bereavement. *Journal of Personality and Social Psychology, 73,* 687–702.

Krebs, J. R., & Davies, N. B. (1981). *An introduction to behavioural ecology.* Sunderland, MA: Sinauer.

Krebs, J. R., & Dawkins, R. (1984). Animal signals: Mind-reading and manipulation. In J. R. Krebs & N. B. Davies (Eds.), *Behavioural ecology: An evolutionary approach* (2nd ed., pp. 380–402). Oxford, UK: Blackwell.

Marler, P., & Tenaza, R. (1977). Signaling behavior of apes with special reference to vocalization. In T. A. Sebeok (Ed.), *How animals communicate* (pp. 965–1033). Bloomington: Indiana University Press.

Messinger, D. S. (1994). *The development of smiling: A dynamic systems approach.* Unpublished doctoral dissertation, University of Utah, Salt Lake City.

Owings, D. H., & Morton, E. S. (1997). The role of information in communication: An assessment/management approach. In D. H. Owings, M. D. Beecher, & N. S. Thompson (Eds.), *Perspectives in ethology: Vol. 12. Communication* (pp. 359–390). New York: Plenum Press.

Owings, D. H., & Morton, E. S. (1998). *Animal vocal communication: A new approach.* Cambridge, UK: Cambridge University Press.

Owren, M. J., & Rendall, D. (1997). An affect-conditioning model of nonhuman primate vocal signaling. In D. H. Owings, M. D. Beecher, & N. S. Thompson (Eds.), *Perspectives in ethology: Vol. 12. Communication* (pp. 299–346). New York: Plenum Press.

Owren, M. J., & Rendall, D. (in press). Sound on the rebound: Bringing form and function back to the forefront in understanding nonhuman primate vocal signaling. *Evolutionary Anthropology.*

Preuschoft, S. (1992). "Laughter" and "smile" in barbary macaques (*Macaca sylvanus*). *Ethology, 91,* 220–236.

Preuschoft, S., & van Hooff, J. A. R. A. M. (1995). Homologizing primate facial displays: A critical review of methods. *Folia Primatologica, 65,* 121–137.

Provine, R. R. (1992). Contagious laughter: Laughter is a sufficient stimulus for laughs and smiles. *Bulletin of the Psychonomic Society, 30,* 1–4.

Provine, R. R. (1996). Laughter. *American Scientist, 84,* 38–45.

Provine, R. R. (1997). Yawns, laughs, smiles, tickles, and talking: Naturalistic and laboratory studies of facial action and social communication. In J. A. Russell & J. M. Fernández-Dols (Eds.), *The psychology of facial expression* (pp. 158–175). New York: Cambridge University Press.

Provine, R. R., & Yong, Y. L. (1991). Laughter: A stereotyped human vocalization. *Ethology, 89,* 115–124.

Redican, W. K. (1975). Facial expressions in nonhuman primates. In L. A. Rosenblum (Ed.), *Primate behavior: Vol. 4. Developments in field and laboratory research* (pp. 103–194). New York: Academic Press.

Rinn, W. E. (1984). The neuropsychology of facial expression. *Psychological Bulletin, 95,* 52–77.

Ruch, W. (1993). Exhilaration and humor. In M. Lewis & J. M. Haviland (Eds.), *Handbook of emotions* (pp. 605–616). New York: Guilford Press.

Russell, J. A. (1997). Reading emotions from and into faces: Resurrecting a dimensional–contextual perspective. In J. A. Russell & J. M. Fernández-Dols (Eds.), *The psychology of facial expression* (pp. 295–320). New York: Cambridge University Press.

Russell, J. A., & Fernández-Dols, J. M. (1997). What does a facial expression mean? In J. A. Russell & J. M. Fernández-Dols (Eds.), *The psychology of facial expression* (pp. 3–30). New York: Cambridge University Press.

Savage-Rumbaugh, S., & Lewin, R. (1994). *Kanzi: The ape at the brink of the human mind.* New York: Wiley.

Silk, J. B. (1986). Social behavior in evolutionary perspective. In B. B. Smuts, D. L. Cheney, R. M. Seyfarth, R. W. Wrangham, & T. T. Struhsaker (Eds.), *Primate societies* (pp. 318–329). Chicago: University of Chicago Press.

Smith, W. J. (1977). *The behavior of communicating: An ethological approach.* Cambridge, MA: Harvard University Press.

Smuts, B. B. (1985). *Sex and friendship in baboons.* Hawthorne, NY: Aldine.

Smuts, B. B., Cheney, D. L., Seyfarth, P. M., Wrangham, R. W., & Struhsaker, T. T. (Eds.). (1986). *Primate societies.* Chicago: University of Chicago Press.

Sroufe, L. A., & Waters, E. (1976). The ontogenesis of smiling and laughter: A perspective on the organization of development in infancy. *Psychological Review, 83,* 173–189.

Tattersall, I., Delson, E., & Van Couvering, J. (1988). *Encyclopedia of human evolution and prehistory.* New York: Garland.

Thompson, J. (1941). Development of facial expression of emotion in blind and seeing children. *Archives of Psychology in New York, 264,* 1–47.

Tomasello, M., & Call, J. (1997). *Primate cognition.* New York: Oxford University Press.

Trivers, R. (1971). The evolution of reciprocal altruism. *Quarterly Review of Biology, 46*, 35–57.

Trivers, R. (1974). Parent–offspring conflict. *American Naturalist, 14*, 249–264.

van Hooff, J. A. R. A. M. (1967). The facial displays of the catarrhine monkeys and apes. In D. Morris (Ed.), *Primate ethology* (pp. 9–88). Chicago: Aldine.

van Hooff, J. A. R. A. M. (1972). The phylogeny of laughter and smiling. In R. Hinde (Ed.), *Nonverbal behaviour* (pp. 209–241). Cambridge, UK: Cambridge University Press.

Van Valen, L. (1973). A new evolutionary law. *Evolutionary Theory, 1*, 1–30.

Walters, J. R., & Seyfarth, R. M. (1986). Conflict and cooperation. In B. B. Smuts, D. L. Cheney, R. M. Seyfarth, R. W. Wrangham, & T. T. Struhsaker (Eds.), *Primate societies* (pp. 306–317). Chicago: University of Chicago Press.

Williams, G. C. (1966). *Adaptation and natural selection: A critique of some current evolutionary thought*. Princeton, NJ: Princeton University Press.

Wrangham, R. W., McGrew, W. C., de Waal, F. B. M., & Heltne, P. G. (1994). *Chimpanzee cultures*. Cambridge, MA: Harvard University Press.

Zahavi, A. (1975). Mate selection: A selection for a handicap. *Journal of Theoretical Biology, 53*, 205–214.

Zahavi, A., & Zahavi, A. (1997). *The handicap principle*. New York: Oxford University Press.

6

Social Functions of Emotions

DACHER KELTNER
JONATHAN HAIDT

> The primary function of emotion is to mobilize the organism
> to deal quickly with important interpersonal encounters.
> —EKMAN (1992, p. 171)

> Emotions are a primary idiom for defining and negotiating
> social relations of the self in a moral order.
> —LUTZ AND WHITE (1986, p. 417)

Emotion theorists disagree in many ways, but most share the assumption that emotions help humans solve many of the basic problems of social living. For evolutionary theorists, emotions are universal hard-wired affect programs that solve ancient, recurrent threats to survival (Ekman, 1992; Lazarus, 1991; Plutchik, 1980; Tomkins, 1984; Tooby & Cosmides, 1990). For social constructivists, emotions are socially learned responses constructed in the process of social discourse according to culturally specific concerns about identity, morality, and social structure (Averill, 1980; Lutz & White, 1986). These contrasting approaches conceive of the defining elements, origins, and study of emotions in strikingly different ways, but both ascribe social functions to emotion.

In this chapter we present a social functional account of emotions that attempts to integrate the relevant insights of evolutionary and social constructivist theorists. Our account can be summarized in three statements:

1. Social living presents social animals, including humans, with problems whose solutions are critical for individual survival.
2. Emotions have been designed in the course of evolution to solve these problems.
3. In humans, culture loosens the linkages between emotions and problems so that cultures find new ways to solve the problems for which emotions evolved, and cultures find new ways of using emotions.

In the first half of the chapter we synthesize the positions of diverse theorists in a taxonomy of problems of social living and then consider how evolution-based *primordial emotions* solve those problems by coordinating social interactions. In the second half of the chapter we discuss the specific processes according to which culture transforms primordial emotions and how culturally shaped *elaborated emotions* help solve the problems of social living.

PRIMORDIAL EMOTION

Evolutionary theorists concern themselves with universal, biologically based, genetically encoded emotion-related patterns of appraisals and responses observed across species and cultures, which we refer to throughout as *primordial emotions*. Primordial emotions are shaped by evolutionary forces, genetically encoded, embedded in the human psyche, linked to biological maturation, and they involve coordinated physiological, perceptual, communicative, and behavioral processes that are meant to produce specific changes in the environment. They occur most typically within the context of immediate face-to-face interactions, and they are brief, lasting seconds to perhaps minutes, but not hours or days (Ekman, 1992).

Although functional analyses have been a mainstay of evolutionary theorizing about emotion (see, e.g., Campos, Campos, & Barrett, 1989; Darwin, 1872/1999; Izard, 1977; Plutchik, 1980), it is only recently that theorists have begun to systematically link specific emotions to social functions. This recent theoretical development can be attributed to several sources (Barrett & Campos, 1987). Advances in ethology and behavioral ecology have illuminated the specific advantages and problems posed by group living (Krebs & Davies, 1993). Working within different traditions, theorists have begun to characterize the connections between specific emotions and attachment (see, e.g., Shaver & Hazan, 1988), mate selection and protection (Buss, 1992), game theoretical characterizations of altruism, cooperation, competition, and interpersonal commitment (Frank, 1988;

Nesse, 1990; Trivers, 1971), and dominance and submissiveness (see, e.g., Keltner & Buswell, 1997; Ohman, 1986).

We believe these recent developments can be summarized in a social functional approach to emotion (Frijda & Mesquita, 1994; Keltner & Haidt, 1999; Keltner & Kring, 1998). Social functional accounts operate at multiple levels of analysis, specifying the social benefits emotions bring about for the individual, dyad, group, and culture. Across diverse methods and levels of analysis, social functional accounts share certain assumptions. Most notably, social functional accounts assume that group living, which has been characteristic of humans and other species for millions of years, confers many advantages over solitary living. These advantages include more proficient food gathering, responses to predation, and raising of offspring. Group living also creates new problems requiring the coordination of group members.

To meet these problems and opportunities, humans have evolved a variety of complex systems. Each system is organized according to a specific goal (e.g., to protect offspring or maintain cooperative alliances) that is served by multiple subsystems. These include specific perceptual processes, higher-order cognition, central and autonomic nervous system activity, as well behavioral responses, both intentional and reflex-like. For example, theorists have observed that humans form reproductive relationships with the help of an attachment system (see, e.g., Bowlby, 1969; Shaver & Hazan, 1988). The attachment system involves perceptual sensitivities to potential mates, representations of relationships, autonomic and hormonal activity related to affiliative, sexual, and intimate behavior, behavioral routines such as flirtation, courtship, and soothing, and specific emotions (discussed below).

Within each system, primordial emotions serve two general functions (see also Johnson-Laird & Oatley, 1992). First, primordial emotions signal that action is necessary, either because of a deviation from an ideal state of social relations or because an opportunity presents itself. Primordial emotions therefore involve perceptual, appraisal, and experiential processes that monitor the conditions of ongoing relations, detecting disturbances (e.g., an infant's distress) or opportunities (a potential mate). Once activated, emotion-related perception and experience interrupt ongoing cognitive processes and direct information processing to features of the social environment that allow for the restoration or establishment of desirable social relations (Clore, 1994; Lazarus, 1991; Lerner & Keltner, 2000; Schwarz, 1990). Second, primordial emotions motivate behavior that establishes (or reestablishes) more ideal conditions of social relations. Primordial emotions involve autonomic, hormonal, and central nervous system activities that are tailored to specific social actions, such as fighting, copulating, offering comfort, and signaling dominance (Davidson, 1993; Frijda, 1986; LeDoux,

1996; Levenson, 1994; Porges, 1995; Sapolsky, 1989). Primordial emotions also involve vocal, facial, and postural communication that provide quick and reliably identified information to others (Ekman, 1984, 1993; Izard, 1977; Scherer, 1986), which shapes social interactions in ways we detail in a subsequent section. We now consider how different emotions might help solve the different problems of group living.

THE PROBLEMS OF GROUP LIVING AND PRIMORDIAL EMOTIONS

Functional accounts begin with an analysis of the problems emotions were presumably designed to solve, either by evolution or cultural construction (Keltner & Gross, 1999). Our review of the theorizing on the social functions of emotion identifies three classes of problems related to group living to which emotions are intimately linked and, we would argue, have been designed to solve. Table 6.1 summarizes the nature of these problems, the general systems that have evolved to meet these problems, as well as related emotions and their specific functions. We note that Table 6.1 does not include all states we consider emotions (e.g., amusement does not fit neatly into the taxonomy); rather, it lists the emotions that seem well suited to solving specific social problems. Additionally, although Table 6.1 describes how emotions are linked to prototypical social objects (e.g., sympathy for vulnerable family members), we believe emotions generalize to related social objects (e.g., sympathy for downtrodden members of society). Several theorists have commented on the flexibility of the associations between emotions and their intentional objects (see, e.g., Tomkins, 1984), which we discuss in an ensuing section.

The Problems of Physical Survival

First, individuals must solve the problems of physical survival, including avoiding death by predation, violence, and disease. Fear is the primordial emotion at the heart of the "fight–flight" system (Ohman, 1986), which helps individuals avoid death by predation or other physical attacks. Much is understood about the physiology of fear (LeDoux, 1996). On the appraisal side, the amygdala contains specialized areas that scan incoming sensory information for patterns that have been associated with danger. The amygdala can trigger a fear response even before the incoming information has been sent to the occipital cortex for full processing, and even before an individual knows what an object is (LeDoux, 1996; see K. N. Ochsner & L. Feldman Barrett, Chapter 2, this volume, for further elaboration). On the output side, primordial fear involves triggering the hypothalamic–

TABLE 6.1. A Taxonomy of Problems and the Functional Systems and Emotions That Solve Them

Problem	Functional systems	Emotions	Specific Functions
Problems of physical survival			
Predation	Fight–flight	Fear	Avoidance of threat to self
		Rage	Removal of threat to self
Disease	Food selection	Disgust	Avoid microbes/parasites
		Interest	Learn about new foods/resources
Problems of reproduction			
Finding a mate	Attachment	Desire	Increase likelihood of sexual contact
		Romantic love	Commit to long-term bond
		Sadness	Replace loss of mate
Keeping mate	Mate protection	Jealousy	Protect mate from rivals
Protecting vulnerable children	Caregiving	Filial love	Increase bond between parent and offspring
		Sympathy	Reduce distress of vulnerable individuals
Problems of group governance			
Cooperation and defection	Reciprocal altruism	Guilt	Repair own transgression of reciprocity
		Moral anger	Motivate other to repair transgression
		Gratitude	Signal and reward cooperative bond
		Envy	Reduce unfair differences in equality
Group organization	Dominance–submissiveness	Shame and embarrassment	Pacify likely aggressor
		Contempt	Reduce status of undeserving other
		Awe	Endow entity greater than self with status

pituitary–adrenocortical axis, which pumps a quick dose of cortisol and other stress hormones into the bloodstream to ready the organism for fight or for flight. Primordial fear can be seen as the heart of a system that includes a variety of cognitive and behavioral mechanisms that make it more effective, for example, vicarious learning and the preparedness of animal phobias (Mineka & Cook, 1988).

Disgust can similarly be seen as the primordial emotion at the heart of the "food-selection" system (Rozin, 1976b), which helps humans choose a balanced and safe diet. Unlike fear, disgust is not found in other animals; only a simpler precursor, distaste, can be seen in rats and other generalist animals. Coevolving with the tremendous expansion of cognitive ability in humans, the distaste response has expanded to become the disgust response

(Rozin, Haidt, & McCauley, 2000). In humans, food rejections are not based primarily on the sensory properties of the object, but rather on a knowledge of what it is or what it has touched (Rozin & Fallon, 1987). Potential foods elicit disgust if they resemble or have come in contact with certain powerful elicitors of disgust, such as feces and decaying animal bodies. The food selection system is further expanded by the addition of learning mechanisms, such as one-trial learning for nausea-inducing foods (Seligman, 1971), and by cultural mechanisms, such as cuisine, which marks prepared foods with a reassuringly familiar blend of spices or flavors (Rozin, 1996).

The Problems of Reproduction

Evolutionary and attachment theorists have speculated how a variety of emotions solve the problems of reproduction, which include procreation and the raising of offspring to the age of reproduction. The problems of finding and keeping a mate are in part met by emotions of romantic love and desire, which facilitate the identification, establishment, and maintenance of reproductive relations. These emotions involve appraisals, perceptions, and experiences that are sensitive to cues related to potential mate value. These include beauty, fertility, chastity, social status, and character (Buss, 1992; Ellis, 1992), expressive behaviors that signal interest and commitment (Frank, 1988) and evoke desire and love, and hormonal and autonomic responses that facilitate sexual behavior. In Table 6.1 we also contend that the experience and display of emotions related to the loss of a partner provoke succorance in others and eventually help individuals establish bonds with new mates. We label this emotion "sadness" (for similar analysis of distress, see Dunn, 1977; for analysis of grief, see Lazarus, 1991).

The protection of potential mates from competitors is equally critical. Jealousy, the literature shows, relates to mate protection, and is triggered by cues that signal potential threats to the relationship, such as possible sexual or emotional involvement of the mate with others (Buss, 1992). Jealousy motivates possessive and threat behaviors that discourage competitors and prevent sexual opportunities for the mate (Wilson & Daly, 1996).

Mammalian neonates are extremely dependent and vulnerable to predation, and continue to be so for much longer periods of time compared to other species. As a consequence, social species have evolved caregiving-related emotions of parental and child love and sympathy, which facilitate protective relations between parent and offspring (Bowlby, 1969; Shaver & Hazan, 1988). The caregiving system involves perceptions and experiences that sensitize parents to infantile cues (e.g., of baby-faced features, distress) and infants to vocal and visual cues of parenthood (Fernald, 1992). Filial love and sympathy are characterized by experiences and expressive behavior such as mutual smiles and gaze patterns. These are elements of interactions that strengthen loving bonds and physiological responses that help caretakers respond to others' distress (see, e.g., Eisenberg et al., 1989).

The Problems of Group Governance

Finally, theorists have argued that emotions help solve two subclasses of problems related to group governance, which arise in several contexts, including the allocation of resources and distribution of work (Fiske, 1991). First, to avoid the problems of cheating and defection and to encourage cooperation, in particular among nonkin, humans reciprocate cooperative and noncooperative acts toward one another (Trivers, 1971). Reciprocity is a universal social norm (Gouldner, 1960) and is evident in gift giving, eye-for-an-eye punishment, quid pro quo behavior in other species (de Waal, 1996), and a tit-for-tat strategy (Axelrod, 1984). Several emotions signal when reciprocity has been violated and motivate reparative behavior (de Waal, 1996; Frank, 1988; Nesse, 1990; Trivers, 1971). Guilt occurs following violations of reciprocity and is expressed in apologetic, remedial behavior that reestablishes reciprocity (Keltner & Buswell, 1996; Tangney, 1991). Moral anger motivates the punishment of individuals who have violated rules of reciprocity and is defined by a sensitivity to issues of justice and unfairness (Keltner, Ellsworth, & Edwards, 1993). Gratitude at others' altruistic acts is a reward for adherence to the contract of reciprocity (Trivers, 1971). Envy motivates individuals to derogate others whose favorable status is unjustified, thus preserving equal relations (Fiske, 1991).

Second, humans must solve the problem of group organization. Status hierarchies provide heuristic solutions to the problems of distributing resources, such as mates, food, and social attention, and the labor required of collective endeavors (de Waal, 1986, 1988; Fiske, 1990). Hierarchies are dynamic processes and require continual negotiation and redefinition. The establishment, maintenance, and preservation of status hierarchies is in part accomplished by emotions related to dominance and submission (de Waal, 1996; Ohman, 1986). Embarrassment and shame appease dominant individuals and signal submissiveness (Keltner & Buswell, 1996; Miller & Leary, 1992), whereas contempt is defined by feelings of superiority and dominance vis-à-vis inferior others. Awe tends to be associated with the experience of being in the presence of an entity greater than the self (Keltner & Loew, 1996). In some cases, awe is elicited by nature or art (Shin, Keltner, Shiota, & Haidt, 2000). In other instances, awe is elicited by the presence of higher-status others, thereby endowing such higher-status individuals with respect and authority (Fiske, 1991; Weber, 1957).

PRIMORDIAL EMOTIONS AND SOCIAL INTERACTION

We believe that emotions most typically solve the problems of social living in the context of ongoing face-to-face interactions (see, e.g., Frijda & Mesquita, 1994; Keltner & Kring, 1998). This view has typically been espoused by those who argue that emotions are constructed within social relationships and, by implication, are not biologically based or universal (see, e.g., Lutz & Abu-Lughod, 1990). Evolutionary theorists, however, have long suggested that humans evolved adaptive responses to the emotional responses of others (see, e.g., Darwin, 1872/1999; Ohman & Dimberg, 1978), consistent with the claim that communicative behavior of senders and receivers coevolved (Eibl-Eibesfeldt, 1989; Hauser, 1996). From this perspective, one individual's emotional expression serves as a "social affordance" which evokes "prepared" responses in others. Primordial emotions structure social interactions in at least three ways:

First, emotional displays evoke complementary emotional responses in others (for a more complete review, see Keltner & Kring, 1998). These complementary emotions are core elements of interactions such as courtship, bonding, appeasement, and reconciliation (Eibl-Eibesfeldt, 1989). Thus, soothing interactions involve sympathetic responses to another's distress. Some socialization interactions involve angry responses to another's transgression, followed by a shamed or guilty response to the anger (Ausubel, 1955; Gibbard, 1990). Appeasement interactions involve displays of submissive emotions, such as embarrassment and shame, which evoke reconciliation-related emotions in the observer, such as amusement (in the case of embarrassment) and sympathy (in the case of shame) (Keltner, Young, & Buswell, 1997). Displays of love and desire coordinate the flirtatious interactions of potential romantic partners (Eibl-Eibesfeldt, 1989).

Second, emotional communication conveys information about the sender's mental states, intentions, and dispositions, which are critical to social interactions (Fridlund, 1992). The empirical literature suggests that emotional displays provide rapid, fairly reliable cues of the sender's emotion, intentions, and disposition (for a review, see Keltner & Kring, 1998). Contagious emotional responses provide a more direct route to the understanding of others' mental states, leading individuals to experience similar responses to objects or events in the environment, resulting in coordination of individuals' perception and action (Hatfield, Cacioppo, & Rapson, 1994).

Third, emotions serve as incentives for others' social behavior. An individual's expression and experience of emotion may reinforce another individual's social behavior within ongoing interactions (see, e.g., Klinnert, Campos, Sorce, Emde, & Svejda, 1983). For example, the display of positive emotion by both parents and children rewards desired behaviors and shifts in attention, thus increasing the frequency of those behaviors (see, e.g., Tronick, 1989). The literature on social referencing indicates that displays of more negative emotions deter others from engaging in undesirable behavior (Klinnert et al., 1983).

To summarize, we have argued that group living presents humans with the problems of physical survival, reproduction, and group governance. Humans have evolved complex systems to meet these problems and opportunities, and emotions serve important functions within these systems by signaling that problems or opportunities exist and by coordinating the actions of interacting individuals. We now consider how culture elaborates upon primordial emotions.

CULTURE AND THE SOCIAL FUNCTIONS OF ELABORATED EMOTIONS

Evolutionary perspectives on emotion have always included a role for culture. Darwin begins *The Expression of the Emotions in Man and Animals* (1872/1999) with a description of a cross-cultural study in which he sent questionnaires to missionaries around the world asking them to comment on the facial and bodily expressions of emotions shown by non-Western people. He concluded that some expressions are highly universal whereas others are more variable, a conclusion that has withstood the test of time (Haidt & Keltner, 1999). Ekman has also always included an important role for culture in his "neuro-cultural" theory of emotions (1972). Ekman built on Tomkins's (1963) notion of universal "affect programs," suggesting that culture plays its role as a modulator of both inputs (what counts as an insult or a loss?) and outputs (display rules about which emotions can be expressed in which circumstances).

While Ekman's critics have often ignored his writings about culture (see, e.g., Ekman, 1972), they have also pointed out ways in which culture may play a more profound role in human emotional life. Impressed by how culture and language give humans flexibility and creativity in designing their lives and societies, social constructivists concern themselves with the total package of meanings, social practices, norms, and institutions that are built up around emotions in human societies (Lutz, 1988; Lutz & Abu-Lughod, 1990; Shweder & Haidt, 2000; White, 1990). We refer to these complex meanings as *elaborated emotions*. Elaborated emotions are shaped by social discourse and interaction, and by concepts of the self, morality, and social order (Markus & Kitayama, 1991; Shweder & Haidt, 2000). Elaborated emotions vary across cultures, cannot be experienced by infants, and can last for years or centuries. For example, the hatred felt toward a historical enemy, although at any moment in time composed brief emotional experiences, is made up of values, beliefs, images, action tendencies, and affective dispositions or sentiments that can pass from one generation to the next and last for extended periods of time.[1]

In human beings, culture alters the use and expression of many evolved traits or systems, including primordial emotions, in several ways. Childhood instruction, culturally specific environmental conditions, and personal experiences determine culture-specific elicitors of emotions and shape the manner in which primordial emotions develop and are expressed. We will now analyze cultural variation in emotion by applying our functionalist perspective to the sorts of objects that anthropologists and social constructivists are concerned with: meaning systems and emergent social phenomena such as institutions and practices.

Modern approaches to culture often focus on how humans create the symbolic and material worlds that then shape and constrain them and enable them to function effectively; as in Shweder's (1990) succinct formulation, "culture and psyche make each other up." Cultures draw on many sources to create their symbolic worlds, including the human body and the phenomenological experiences it provides (Geertz, 1973; Lakoff, 1987, 1996). All cultures have noticed that people experience hunger, fatigue, illness, and sexual arousal, and all cultures have developed ethnotheories, customs, and practices that explain the origins and govern the interpretation of these experiences. Primordial emotions, we propose, provide universally available patterns of perception, experience, and action that cultures work into their ethnotheories, values, practices, and institutions. The primordial emotion of anger, for example, might be elaborated into a codified defense of the social–moral order, linked to satisfying feelings of righteousness, and valued as a prosocial force (e.g., the Ifaluk emotion of *song*; see Lutz, 1988). Conversely, anger might be elaborated as a childish and destructive response whose expression is suppressed, leading to the use of other methods to solve interpersonal disputes (Briggs, 1970).

Culture and the elaboration process loosen the link between a primordial emotion and the social problem it was designed to solve in two ways (as we elaborate in the following subsections). First, cultures find new solutions to the ancient problems that emotions were designed to solve. Second, cultures find new uses for old emotions that have little to do with their "original" function. Once this loosening is recognized it becomes easier to reconcile evolutionary approaches (which focus on primordial emotions and therefore find universality) and social constructionist approaches (which focus on elaborated emotions and therefore find cultural variation).

New Solutions to Old Problems: Artifacts and Institutions

Humans have developed an enormous variety of artifacts and technological solutions to the problems of survival, reproduction, and group governance. Cole (1995, p. 32) writes that "the basic function of these artifacts is to co-ordinate human beings with the environment and each other." For example, the invention of weaponry, walls, and towns largely solves the problem of predator avoidance and reduces the need for primordial fear reactions toward nonhuman animals, although such technological developments may then create new reasons to fear other people. Social institutions are a re-lated means by which humans solve ancient problems.

How do evolved artifacts, institutions, social structures, and technolo-gies change the emotional profile of a culture? We perceive at least two pos-sibilities. First, social institutions may work together with emotional sys-tems, formalizing their functions and extending them into new domains. For example, the institution of marriage can build upon sexual and attach-ment-related emotions in cultures that practice love-based marriage, to cre-ate stable environments for child rearing. Or marriage can build upon the emotions of the reciprocal altruism system in cultures that practice ar-ranged marriages, to bind families together that trade daughters. Other so-cial institutions formalize the functions of emotions. For example, Moore (1993) has observed how court-related mediations between defendant and victim formalize exchanges of shame and forgiveness, and forge bonds fol-lowing transgressions. Goffman (1967) likewise observed how group-based status rituals that revolve around social practices, such as teasing and man-ners of dress and diction, ritualize displays of embarrassment and pride. In these circumstances, emotions may serve their original social functions in more pronounced, consistent, and consciously recognized ways.

Second, innovations in technology, social structure, or social institu-tions may bypass certain emotional mechanisms, making those emotions less prevalent in a society. For example, cultures must address the prob-lem that young women can become pregnant in their midteens and that men who are not bound by marriage often do not help to raise their off-spring. Many cultures therefore make girls marry right after their first menses. But another common solution is to delay female sexual activity by making a virtue of chastity and by linking female sexuality outside of marriage to shame. This linkage was clearly in place in the United States until recently. The word "modesty" used to connote a feminine virtue in which properly socialized women felt shame when confronted by issues of sexuality, particularly their own. In this way American women experi-enced deferential, modesty-related feelings such as embarrassment and shame that are comparable to the experience of *lajya* of Oriya women (Menon & Shweder, 1994) and *hasham* of Awlad-Ali women (Abu-

Lughod, 1986). But new technology (birth control), new social and economic facts (women working and reducing the power differential with men), and new institutions (women's groups and magazines) have greatly reduced the association of sexuality with shame. We cannot be certain, but it seems quite likely that the frequency of sexual shame/modesty experiences has greatly diminished for American women, as has the link between shame/modesty and appeasement or submissiveness functions in the context of sexuality.

New Problems for Old Solutions: Preadaptation and the Creativity of Culture

In the course of evolution physical structures and behavioral patterns evolve under selection pressures for one purpose but often are serviceable for a different purpose (Mayr, 1960; Rozin, 1976a). For example, the human tongue evolved as a mechanism to select and handle food, but it was preadapted to play a role in speech production, which has affected its current form. If the reuse of such a preadapted feature gives an advantage to certain individuals, the new use will become more common in succeeding generations, guided by a new set of selection pressures. This process can happen in biological evolution over the course of thousands of generations or in cultural evolution over the course of a few years or decades.

The process of cultural preadaptation is visible in the transition from primordial emotions to their elaborated forms. As a general principle, we suggest that primordial emotions will be recruited for new uses when features of their antecedents, appraisal patterns, or behavioral patterns match characteristics of the new domain where a solution to a similar social problem is needed. Certain emotion-related appraisals can be extended into new domains with slight changes. For example, because ideas can spread quickly from person to person, like germs, primordial disgust and its defense against microbial contagion is easily recruited and elaborated into a defense against ideological contagion, such as communist infiltration during the Cold War. Once ideas are seen as "contaminating," the solution to the problem is clear—infected individuals must be isolated or expelled from the community. (See Lakoff, 1987, 1996, for more on the importance of metaphor in human thought.) Thus, the food rejection of primordial disgust (or core disgust; see Rozin et al., 2000) is easily adaptable to social rejection, and most cultures seem to have some form of social–moral disgust in response to certain classes of "offensive" social violations (Haidt, Rozin, McCauley, & Imada, 1997).

Preadaptation can occur at the level of emotion-related behavior as well, according to similar principles of similarity and generalization. Thus, many contexts requiring politeness, such as more formal interactions or those involving strangers, resemble those involving individuals in social hierarchies—the interactions are defined by potential threat. Theorists have argued that appeasement-related behaviors, including submissive displays and embarrassment, have been elaborated into more complex politeness and deference rituals (Eibl-Eibesfeldt, 1989; Visser, 1991). As one example, negotiating locations of limited space (e.g., doorways) often involves polite smiles, gaze aversion, and specific gestures (head bows in other cultures) that draw upon the nonverbal cues of embarrassment. Emotion-related displays can be extended into new domains, thereby developing new uses. It will be important for future research to establish the extent to which the different components of primordial emotion are activated when one component of emotion (appraisals, display behavior) are generalized to a new domain.

In sum, primordial emotions are universal, biologically based, coordinated response systems that have evolved to enable humans to meet the problems of physical survival, reproduction, and group governance. The creative process of culture, however, loosens the link between the primordial emotions and their functions, finding new solutions to old problems and new uses for old emotions. Evolutionary theorists are therefore right when they document high degrees of cross-cultural similarity in (primordial) emotion and emotion-based preferences, interactions, and practices (see, e.g., Buss, 1992; Eibl-Eibesfeldt, 1989; Ekman, 1992). Social constructivists are also right when they document striking cultural variation in the uses and functions of (elaborated) emotions in human societies. We now apply this framework to a discussion of the biologically and culturally determined social functions of two specific emotions, disgust and embarrassment.

TWO CASE STUDIES OF PRIMORDIAL AND ELABORATED EMOTION

Disgust

The dangers of parasites and bacteria are particularly acute for humans, who live in close quarters and eat a great variety of potentially dangerous foods. Humans are aided by a variety of food-related emotions, strategies, and learning mechanisms, which work together as a functional system to achieve the right balance between exploration of new foods and the avoidance of dangerous foods (Rozin, 1996). Humans show neophobia, nibbling, and preparedness to associate nausea with new foods, even after a long delay (Rozin, 1996; Seligman, 1971). In humans, disgust is at the center of the food-selection system, having evolved from the more primitive reaction of distaste into a way of making people concerned about the contact history and nature of their potential foods, rather than just their sensory properties (Rozin et al., 2000). Disgust pushes against sensation seeking as part of the "omnivore's dilemma": the simultaneous interest in and fear of new foods (Rozin, 1976b).

Human societies have developed diverse ways to safeguard their food supplies and to minimize the threats of bacteria and parasites. These solutions include technological innovations (cooking or curing meat, boiling or filtering water), institutions (government food inspectors), and cultural norms and food taboos whose violation triggers disgust or outrage. More recently, newspaper columns and television reports offer consumers advice from experts on what foods to eat and how to prepare them.

Perhaps because it has been partially freed from its original mission—as a guardian of the mouth against dangerous foods—disgust has been put to a variety of new uses. Its eliciting conditions have expanded so much that disgust may now be described as a social emotion whose function is to guard the social order against certain forms of deviance and to guard the soul against certain forms of debasement (Rozin et al., 2000). The link between material progress and the expansion of disgust in European history has been pointed out by Elias (1978). Disgust and its associated cognitions about contamination and purity are recruited into the maintenance of social groups with distinct boundaries (e.g., the Indian caste system, upper-class attitudes toward the lower class). Disgust is used in initiation rites (e.g., of American college fraternities) in which new members are forced to touch or eat the body products of others, thereby deliberately courting the risk of disease, yet simultaneously marking individuals as members of a communal sharing group.

Embarrassment

The establishment, maintenance, and preservation of status hierarchies is in part accomplished by dominant and submissive emotions (de Waal, 1996; Ohman, 1986). Embarrassment is a primary example. The primordial form of embarrassment involves submissive-related behavior (Keltner, 1995) much akin to the appeasement displays of other species (e.g., gaze aversion, head movements down, controlled smiles) and submissive phenomenology (e.g., feelings of smallness and weakness) (Keltner & Buswell, 1996; Miller & Leary, 1992). Empirical evidence indicates that displays of embarrassment appease dominant individuals by evoking affiliative emotion and forgiveness (Keltner & Buswell, 1997).

Several interactions that systematically recruit and revolve around embarrassment and other submissive emotions reinforce status hierarchies and status-based relations. Status-demarcating rituals, such as greeting and teasing, involve the ritualized display and elicitation of embarrassment (de Waal, 1986, 1988; Goffman, 1967; Keltner, Young, Heerey, Oemig, & Monarch, 1998), thus signaling the hierarchical relations between interacting individuals.

Culture has evolved several new solutions to the problem of coordinating hierarchies. These include class and caste systems, aristocracy, status arrangements in groups and organizations, status-signaling clothing (e.g., the length of a doctor's lab coat in medical hospitals), linguistic practices (Brown & Levinson, 1987), status-determinant role-related norms for women and men, and moral codes dictating the individual's place within a community (Shweder, Much, Mahapatra, & Park, 1997). Status-related emotions have also been coopted in several more recent human social practices. Politeness systems, including table manners and conversational pragmatics, incorporate submissive emotion and gesture (Brown & Levinson, 1987; Keltner et al., 1997). In many Hindu and Islamic cultures the expression of submissive emotions demonstrates feminine virtue (Abu-Lughod, 1986; Menon & Shweder, 1994). Flirtation and courtship involve submissive smiles of embarrassment (Eibl-Eibesfeldt, 1989) and dominant displays (Fisher, 1992).

CONCLUSIONS AND FUTURE PROSPECTS

We have argued that emotions are part of systems that solve problems related to physical survival, reproduction, and group governance. Biologically based, universal primordial emotions involve experience, perception, physiology, and communication that solve these problems in the context of ongoing social interactions. Elaborated emotions are the total package of meanings, behaviors, social practices, and norms that are built up around primordial emotions in actual human societies. This approach integrates the insights of evolutionary and social constructivist approaches and points to the systematic role of emotion in social interactions, relationships, and cultural practices.

We have intentionally focused on classes of emotions that solve specific social problems. Other emotions are likely to serve more context-general social functions: amusement may relate to the transformation of dangerous situations into safe ones (Keltner & Bonanno, 1997); interest may motivate general exploratory behavior and learning; happiness or contentment may signal to the individual his/her general level of social functioning (Nesse, 1990). These sorts of issues await further investigation.

Our hope in this chapter has been to prompt researchers to continue to examine the social functions of emotions, both in their universal and culturally elaborated forms. Toward this end, we make the following recommendations for future research.

First, researchers need to study emotion within theoretically relevant relationships. Many studies of emotion and social interaction have looked at strangers or, in more ambitious cases, friendships. We would suggest that the net needs to be cast more broadly, that researchers need to study emotion in different kinds of relationships. The study of embarrassment and shame may be most appropriate in interactions between superiors and subordinates. Love, desire, and jealousy are most fruitfully examined in interactions between actual or potential romantic partners. We further suggest, following our functional analysis, that empirical research may be most revealing when it focuses on the nature and consequences of emotions when relationship-relevant problems (e.g., the maintenance of reciprocity between friends) are most salient, say, when stances toward them are being established, negotiated, or changed. The functions of love and desire are likely to be most clearly documented during initial stages of courtship or when a romantic bond is threatened. The manner in which shame and embarrassment help define status-related roles is likely to be most illuminated when researchers are studying groups during dynamic times of status negotiation.

Our second recommendation follows quite closely from the first— namely, study emotion in the context of social interactions and practices. A great deal of the study of emotion, even of the more social nature of emotion, examines the individual's response to controlled stimuli. This sort of work is no doubt necessary; the understanding of emotion in social interaction rests upon the understanding of individual emotional response. Yet, given the advances in the study of emotion, it may be time to study social interactions and practices that revolve around emotions. In the course of this review we have identified ways that cultural practices elaborate upon more primordial emotions (e.g., appeasement rituals) and ways in which primordial emotions are generalized to new practices (e.g., disgust related to unsavory ideologies). These different social practices have begun to be and should continue to be a focus of emotion research. The emphasis on emotions within social practice raises difficult conceptual issues. In studies of emotion-related interactions, such as teasing, it will be necessary to treat the dyad or group as the unit of analysis (see comments below). Studies of how culture elaborates upon emotion will direct researchers to cultural objects and practices, such as etiquette manuals, religious texts, or institutions, which do not appear, from the traditional point of view, to involve emotion. Yet it is precisely in looking at these sorts of interactions and practices where one will find culturally elaborated emotion.

Finally, a functional approach suggests that it is important to study systematic consequences. The functions of a specific emotion will in part be revealed by its regular consequences (see, e.g., Keltner & Gross, 1999). This view shifts the emphasis from looking at emotion as an outcome or dependent measure to the view that emotions themselves have important outcomes. As a field we know all too little about the systematic consequences of emotions, and this remains a very important line of inquiry. Relevant research can proceed at multiple levels of analysis. At the individual level of analysis, one would expect the disposition to experience and express specific emotions (e.g., anger or the lack of embarrassment) to be associated with specific social consequences. In moving to the dyad as the unit of analysis, one might look at how patterns of emotional expression and experience lead to specific consequences for ongoing interactions. Thus, we would expect timely displays of love and desire to predict more interest and intimacy in ongoing interactions between potential romantic partners. One could look at the long-term consequences of patterns of emotional experience and expression for relationships. For example, following the analysis offered in this chapter, one might expect frequent displays of gratitude to predict the long-term sense of fairness in friendships. Finally, it will be important for researchers to document the consequences of emotion for groups and cultures. Ritualized displays and experiences of embarrassment may contribute to the stability of group hierarchy. The culturally elaborated experience of disgust may correlate at the cultural level with specific stereotypes and outgroup prejudices.

Emotion researchers have long moved across and around discipline-specific theoretical inclinations and methodological practices. This tradition has led to great debate in the study of emotion (is emotion universal or culturally specific?) and great advances. The study of the social functions of emotion, we contend, depends vitally on the integration of ideas and evidence from different disciplines.

NOTE

1. An example may clarify the distinction: Is motherhood universal? We might speak of primordial motherhood as a system of tightly coordinated physical and psychological processes (involving gestation, parturition, and hormones that increase attachment) that is universal to humans and similar to motherhood in many nonhuman species. On the other hand, many researchers have documented cross-cultural variation in elaborated motherhood, for example, single versus multiple mothering, breast versus bottle feeding, and valuation versus devaluation of the role of the mother (Kurtz, 1992).

REFERENCES

Abu-Lughod, L. (1986). *Veiled sentiments.* Berkeley: University of California Press.
Ausubel, D. P. (1955). Relationships between shame and guilt in the socializing process. *Psychological Review, 62,* 378–390.

Averill, J. R. (1980). A constructivist view of emotion. In R. Plutchik & H. Kellerman (Eds.), *Emotion: Theory, research, and experience* (pp. 305-339). New York: Academic Press.

Axelrod, R. (1984). *The evolution of cooperation.* New York: Basic Books.

Barrett, K. C., & Campos, J. J. (1987). Perspectives on emotional development II: A functionalist approach to emotions. In J. D. Osofsky (Ed.), *Handbook of infant development* (2nd ed., pp. 555–578). New York: Wiley-Interscience.

Bowlby, J. (1969). *Attachment.* New York: Basic Books.

Briggs, J. L. (1970). *Never in anger.* Cambridge, MA: Harvard University Press.

Brown, P., & Levinson, S. C. (1987). *Politeness.* New York: Cambridge University Press.

Buss, D. (1992). Male preference mechanisms: Consequences for partner choice and intrasexual competition. In J. H. Barkow, L. Cosmides, & J. Tooby (Eds.), *The adapted mind* (pp. 267–288). New York: Oxford University Press.

Campos, J. J., Campos, R. G., & Barrett, K. C. (1989). Emergent themes in the study of emotional development and emotion regulation. *Developmental Psychology, 25,* 394–402.

Clore, G. (1994). Why emotions are felt. In P. Ekman & R. J. Davidson (Eds.), *The nature of emotion* (pp. 103–111). New York: Cambridge University Press.

Cole, M. (1995). Culture and cognitive development: From cross-cultural research to creating systems of cultural mediation. *Culture and Psychology, 1,* 24–54.

Darwin, C. (1999). *The expression of the emotions in man and animals* (Introduction by P. Ekman). London: HarperCollins. (Original work published 1872)

Davidson, R. J. (1993). Parsing affective space: Perspectives from neuropsychology and psychophysiology. *Neuropsychology, 7,* 464–475.

de Waal, F. B. M. (1986). The integration of dominance and social bonding in primates. *Quarterly Review of Biology, 61,* 459–479.

de Waal, F. B. M. (1988). The reconciled hierarchy. In M. R. A. Chance (Ed.), *Social fabrics of the mind* (pp. 105–136). Hillsdale, NJ: Erlbaum.

de Waal, F. B. M. (1996). *Good natured.* Cambridge, MA: Harvard University Press.

Dunn, J. (1977). *Distress and comfort.* Cambridge, MA: Harvard University Press.

Eibl-Eibesfeldt, I. (1989). *Human ethology.* New York: Aldine de Gruyter Press.

Eisenberg, N., Fabes, R. A., Miller, P. A., Fultz, J., Shell, R., Mathy, R. M., & Reno, R. R. (1989). Relation of sympathy and distress to prosocial behavior: A multimethod study. *Journal of Personality and Social Psychology, 57,* 55–66.

Ekman, P. (1972). Universals and cultural differences in facial expressions of emotion. In J. K. Cole (Ed.), *Nebraska Symposium on Motivation* (Vol. 19, pp. 207–283). Lincoln: University of Nebraska Press.

Ekman, P. (1984). Expression and the nature of emotion. In K. R. Scherer & P. Ekman (Eds.), *Approaches to emotion* (pp. 319–344). Hillsdale NJ: Erlbaum.

Ekman, P. (1992). An argument for basic emotions. *Cognition and Emotion, 6,* 169–200.

Ekman, P. (1993). Facial expression and emotion. *American Psychologist, 48,* 384–392.

Elias, N. (1978). *The history of manners.* New York: Pantheon.

Ellis, B. (1992). The evolution of sexual attraction: Evaluative mechanisms in women. In J. H. Barkow, L. Cosmides, & J. Tooby (Eds.), *The adapted mind* (pp. 267–288). New York: Oxford University Press.

Fernald, A. (1992). Human maternal vocalizations to infants as biologically relevant signals: An evolutionary perspective. In J. H. Barkow, L. Cosmides, & J. Tooby (Eds.), *The adapted mind* (pp. 391–428). New York: Oxford University Press.

Fisher, H. E. (1992). *Anatomy of love*. New York: Norton.

Fiske, A. P. (1990). Relativity within Moose culture: Four incommensurable models for social relationships. *Ethos, 18*, 180–204.

Fiske, A. P. (1991). *Structures of social life*. New York: Free Press.

Frank, R. H. (1988). *Passions within reason*. New York: Norton.

Fridlund, A. J. (1992). The behavioral ecology and sociality of human faces. In M. S. Clark (Ed.), *Emotion*. Newbury Park, CA: Sage.

Frijda, N. (1986). *The emotions*. Cambridge: Cambridge University Press.

Frijda, N. H., & Mesquita, B. (1994). The social roles and functions of emotions. In S. Kitayama & H. Marcus (Eds.), *Emotion and culture: Empirical studies of mutual influenced* (pp. 51–87). Washington, DC: American Psychological Association.

Geertz, C. (1973). *The interpretation of cultures*. New York: Basic Books.

Gibbard, A. (1990). *Wise choices, apt feelings*. Cambridge, MA: Harvard University Press.

Goffman, E. (1967). *Interaction ritual: Essays on face-to-face behavior*. Garden City, NY: Anchor.

Gouldner, A. W. (1960). The norm of reciprocity: A preliminary statement. *American Sociological Review, 25*, 161–178.

Haidt, J., & Keltner, D. (1999). Culture and facial expression: Open ended methods find more faces and a gradient of recognition. *Cognition and Emotion, 13*, 225–266.

Haidt, J., Koller, S., & Dias, M. (1993). Affect, culture, and morality, or is it wrong to eat your dog? *Journal of Personality and Social Psychology, 65*, 613–628.

Haidt, J., Rozin, P., McCauley, C. R., & Imada, S. (1997). Body, psyche, and culture: The relationship between disgust and morality. *Psychology and Developing Societies, 9*, 107–131.

Hatfield, E., Cacioppo, J. T., & Rapson, R. L. (1994). *Emotional contagion*. New York: Cambridge University Press.

Hauser, M. D. (1996). *The evolution of communication*. Cambridge, MA: MIT Press.

Izard, C. E. (1977). *Human emotions*. New York: Plenum Press.

Johnson-Laird, P. N., & Oatley, K. (1992). Basic emotions, rationality, and folk theory. *Cognition and Emotion, 6*, 201-223.

Keltner, D. (1995). The signs of appeasement: Evidence for the distinct displays of embarrassment, amusement, and shame. *Journal of Personality and Social Psychology, 68*, 441–454.

Keltner, D., & Bonanno, G. A. (1997). A study of laughter and dissociation: Distinct correlates of laughter and smiling during bereavement. *Journal of Personality and Social Psychology, 73*, 687–702.

Keltner, D., & Buswell, B. (1996). Evidence for the distinctness of embarrassment, shame, and guilt: A study of recalled antecedents and facial expressions of emotion. *Cognition and Emotion, 10*(2), 155–172.

Keltner, D., & Buswell, B. N. (1997). Embarrassment: Its distinct form and appeasement functions. *Psychological Bulletin, 122*, 250–270.

Keltner, D., Ellsworth, P. C., & Edwards, K. (1993). Beyond simple pessimism: Effects of sadness and anger on social perception. *Journal of Personality and Social Psychology, 64,* 740–752.

Keltner, D., & Gross, J. J. (1999). Functional accounts of emotion. *Cognition and Emotion, 13*(5), 467–480.

Keltner, D., & Haidt, J. (1999). Social functions of emotions at multiple levels of analysis. *Cognition and Emotion, 13*(5), 505–522.

Keltner, D., & Kring, A. (1998). Emotion, social function, and psychopathology. *Review of General Psychology, 2,* 320–342.

Keltner, D., & Loew, D. (1996). *The structure of awe.* Unpublished manuscript, University of California, Berkeley.

Keltner, D., Young, R., & Buswell, B. N. (1997). Appeasement in human emotion, personality, and social practice. *Aggressive Behavior, 23,* 359–374.

Keltner, D., Young, R. C., Heerey, E., Oemig, C., & Monarch, N. D. (1998). Teasing in hierarchical and intimate relations. *Journal of Personality and Social Psychology, 75,* 1231–1247.

Klinnert, M., Campos, J., Sorce, J., Emde, R., & Svejda, M. (1983). Emotions as behavior regulators: Social referencing in infants. In R. Plutchik & H. Kellerman (Eds.), *Emotion theory, research, and experience: Vol. 2. Emotions in early development* (pp. 57–68). New York: Academic Press.

Krebs, J. R., & Davies, N. B. (1993). *An introduction to behavioural ecology.* Oxford, UK: Blackwell.

Kurtz, S. (1992). *All the mothers are one.* New York: Columbia University Press.

Lakoff, G. (1987). *Women, fire, and dangerous things.* Chicago: University of Chicago Press.

Lakoff, G. (1996). *Moral politics: What conservatives know that liberals don't.* Chicago: University of Chicago Press.

Lazarus, R. S. (1991). *Emotion and adaptation.* New York: Oxford University Press.

LeDoux, J. (1996). *The emotional brain.* New York: Simon & Schuster.

Lerner, J. S., & Keltner, D. (2000). Beyond valence: Toward a model of emotion specific influences on judgment and choice. *Cognition and Emotion, 14,* 473–493.

Levenson, R. W. (1994). Human emotions: A functional view. In P. Ekman & R. J. Davidson (Eds.), *The nature of emotion* (pp. 123–126). Oxford, UK: Oxford University Press.

Lutz, C. A. (1988). *Unnatural emotions.* Chicago: University of Chicago Press.

Lutz, C. A., & Abu-Lughod, L. (1990). Introduction: Emotion, discourse, and the politics of everyday life. In C. A. Lutz & L. Abu-Lughod (Eds.), *Language and the politics of emotion* (pp. 1–23). New York: Cambridge University Press.

Lutz, C. A., & White, G. (1986). The anthropology of emotion. *Annual Review of Anthropology, 15,* 405–436.

Markus, H. R., & Kitayama, S. (1991). Culture and the self: Implications for cognition, emotion, and motivation. *Psychological Review, 98,* 224–253.

Mayr, E. (1960). The emergence of evolutionary novelties. In S. Tax (Ed.), *Evolution after Darwin: Vol. 1. The evolution of life* (pp. 349–380). Chicago: University of Chicago Press.

Menon, U., & Shweder, R. A. (1994). Kali's tongue: Cultural psychology, cultural consensus and the meaning of "shame" in Orissa, India. In H. Markus & S.

Kitayama (Eds.), *Culture and the emotions* (pp. 241–284). Washington, DC: American Psychological Association.

Miller, R. S., & Leary, M. R. (1992). Social sources and interactive functions of embarrassment. In M. S. Clark (Ed.), *Emotion and social behavior* (pp. 332–339). Newbury Park, CA: Sage.

Mineka, S., & Cook, M. (1988). Social learning and the acquisition of snake fear in monkeys. In T. R. Zentall & J. B. G. Galef (Eds.), *Social learning: Psychological and biological perspectives* (pp. 51–74). Hillsdale, NJ: Erlbaum.

Moore, D. B. (1993). Shame, forgiveness, and juvenile justice. *Criminal Justice Ethics, 12,* 3–25.

Nesse, R. (1990). Evolutionary explanations of emotions. *Human Nature, 1,* 261–289.

Ohman, A. (1986). Face the beast and fear the face: Animal and social fears as prototypes for evolutionary analysis of emotion. *Psychophysiology, 23,* 123–145.

Ohman, A., & Dimberg, U. (1978). Facial expressions as conditioned stimuli for electrodermal responses: A case of "preparedness"? *Journal of Personality and Social Psychology, 36,* 1251–1258.

Plutchik, R. (1980). *Emotion: A psychobioevolutionary synthesis.* New York: Harper & Row.

Porges, S. P. (1995). Orienting in a defensive world: Mammalian modifications of our evolutionary heritage. A polyvagal theory. *Psychophysiology, 32,* 301–317.

Rozin, P. (1976a). The evolution of intelligence and access to the cognitive unconscious. In J. A. Sprague & A. N. Epstein (Eds.), *Progress in psychobiology and physiological psychology* (Vol. 6, pp. 245–280). New York: Academic Press.

Rozin, P. (1976b). The selection of food by rats, humans, and other animals. In R. A. Hinde, C. Beer, & E. Shaw (Eds.), *Advances in the study of behavior* (Vol. 6, pp. 21–76). New York: Academic Press.

Rozin, P. (1996). Towards a psychology of food and eating: From motivation to module to model to marker, morality, meaning, and metaphor. *Current Directions in Psychological Science, 5,* 18–24.

Rozin, P., & Fallon, A. (1987). A perspective on disgust. *Psychological Review, 94,* 23–41.

Rozin, P., Haidt, J., & McCauley, C. R. (2000). Disgust. In M. Lewis & J. M. Haviland-Jones (Eds.), *Handbook of emotions* (2nd ed., pp. 637–653). New York: Guilford Press.

Sapolsky, R. M. (1989). Hypercortisolism among socially subordinate wild baboons. *Archives of General Psychiatry, 46,* 1047–1051.

Scherer, K. R. (1986). Vocal affect expression: A review and a model for future research. *Psychological Bulletin, 99,* 143–165.

Schwarz, N. (1990). Feelings as information: Informational and motivational functions of affective states. In E. T. Higgins & R. M. Sorrentino (Eds.), *Handbook of motivation and cognition* (Vol. 2, pp. 527–561). New York: Guilford Press.

Seligman, M. E. P. (1971). Phobias and preparedness. *Behavior Therapy, 2,* 307–320.

Shaver, P., & Hazan, C. (1988). A biased overview of the study of love. *Journal of Social and Personal Relationships, 5,* 473–501.

Shin, M., Keltner, D., Shiota, L., & Haidt, J. (2000). *The realm of positive emotion: Studies of lexicon and narrative.* Manuscript in preparation.

Shweder, R. (1990). Cultural psychology: What is it? In J. W. Stigler, R. A. Shweder, & G. Herdt (Eds.), *Cultural psychology: Essays on comparative human development* (pp. 1–43). New York: Cambridge University Press.

Shweder, R. A., & Haidt, J. (2000). The cultural psychology of the emotions: Ancient and new. In M. Lewis & J. M. Haviland-Jones (Eds.), *Handbook of emotions* (2nd ed., 397–414). New York: Guilford Press.

Shweder, R. S., Much, N. C., Mahapatra, M., & Park, L. (1997). The "big three" of morality (autonomy, community, and divinity), and the "big three" explanations of suffering, as well. In A. M. Brandt & P. Rozin (Eds.), *Morality and health* (pp. 119–169). New York: Routledge.

Tangney, J. P. (1991). Moral affect: The good, the bad, and the ugly. *Journal of Personality and Social Psychology, 61,* 598–607.

Tomkins, S. S. (1963). *Affect, imagery, and consciousness: Vol. II. The negative affects.* New York: Springer-Verlag.

Tomkins, S. S. (1984). Affect theory. In K. Scherer & P. Ekman (Eds), *Approaches to emotion* (pp. 163–195). Hillsdale, NJ: Erlbaum.

Tooby, J., & Cosmides, L. (1990). The past explains the present: Emotional adaptations and the structure of ancestral environments. *Ethology and Sociobiology, 11,* 375–424.

Trivers, R. L. (1971). The evolution of reciprocal altruism. *Quarterly Review of Biology, 46,* 35–57.

Tronick, E. Z. (1989). Emotions and emotional communication in infants. *American Psychologist, 44,* 112–119.

Visser, M. (1991). *The rituals of dinner.* New York: Grove Weidenfeld.

Weber, M. (1957). *The theory of social and economic organization.* New York: Free Press.

White, G. M. (1990). Moral discourse and the rhetoric of emotions. In C. A. Lutz & L. Abu-Lughod (Eds.), *Language and the politics of emotion* (pp. 46–68). New York: Cambridge University Press.

Wilson, M. I., & Daly, M. (1996). Male sexual proprietariness and violence against wives. *Current Directions in Psychological Science, 5,* 2–6.

7

Culture and Emotion
Different Approaches to the Question

BATJA MESQUITA

Do people in different cultures experience similar emotions, or are the emotions of people in different cultures different? This is the basic question addressed in the research on culture and emotions. It has important practical implications. For example, how sure are we that we can judge what veiling, polygamy, or circumcision means to women in other cultures (see Shweder, 1999)? Can we judge the affective tone of parent–child relations in other cultures? Do we understand the emotional expressions of our non-Western business partners correctly when we are at the negotiation table with them? Is it possible to counsel people from other cultures? Are we able to interpret the aggressive threats or the populist emotional addresses of the leaders of antagonistic countries in other parts of the world? Or, perhaps more importantly, do we know how to increase the likelihood that those leaders will agree to negotiate peaceful solutions? The question of the cross-cultural diversity of emotions is thus important in the light of any social relations across cultures.

Straightforward as the question on the cross-cultural variation of emotions may seem, it has been understood in markedly different ways. This chapter reviews the different approaches to the field of culture and emotions. Its goal is not so much to define the views of particular researchers in great detail as to frame the research questions that have driven research on culture and emotions. We will see that the focus on a particular research question has had implications for the kinds of emotional phenomena studied, the research designs, and even the definition of cross-cultural similarities and differences. We will also see that the majority of research was really designed to find cross-cultural similarities and that, in order to establish cultural differences in emotions, a different kind of paradigm needs to be adopted and developed than the majority of research has used so far. In our discussion of the literature, we will distinguish between three paradigmatic approaches—each starting from a distinct interpretation of the question on cross-cultural variability of emotional phenomena.

A lot of contemporary research on culture and emotion has focused on the question of universal emotions. Studies were designed either to show that a number of emotions could be found cross-culturally or to challenge that idea by providing evidence for the absence of certain emotions in other cultures. Either way, the assumption was that emotions come as packages, consisting of invariant patterns of emotion-specific responses, whose presence or absence in different cultures needed to be established. The question addressed by this type of research was thus a dichotomous one: Is emotion X present or absent in culture A?

In the last decade, componential theories of emotions have questioned the idea of emotions as unitary wholes. The assumption that emotions, if they occurred, consisted of cross-culturally invariant configurations of responses was turned into a central empirical issue: To what extent is emotion X cross-culturally characterized by the same pattern of responses, and to what extent are there differences in the responses associated with emotion X? Generalizing across emotions, componential approaches also tried to identify the components of emotion that were most and least susceptible to cultural influence. Most importantly, the focus of this type of research shifted from the dichotomous question of universality to the question of the degree of cultural similarities and differences in the components of emotions.

More recent yet is the cultural approach to research on culture and emotion. In some ways, this approach focuses on a different level of phenomena than the other two. The focus is on the distinct patterns of emotional responses found in different sociocultural contexts, rather than on the particular responses by emotion. The question is thus: Which are the prevalent or focal emotional responses in culture A versus culture B, and which emotional responses are rare in culture A versus culture B? In another way, the cultural approach is a step beyond the previous two: It promises to develop a theory of cultural differences in emotions. Cultural differences in the patterns of emotions are understood as a function of the difference in the culture at large. Thus, the cultural approach tries to understand how the tendency of people in culture A to respond in certain emotional ways relates to cultural ideas and practices.

The research motivated by each approach has advanced our insight into the role of culture in emotion. Each approach also has important limitations that will be summarized at the end of each section below. It will be argued that neither the quest for universal emotions nor the multicomponential approach has been designed to reveal cultural *differences* in emotions. Therefore, the overwhelming evidence for cross-cultural similarities in emotions should, at least in part, be attributed to research questions and methods that focused on the detection of cross-cultural similarities. More research is needed that theoretically predicts cultural differences in emotions and thus allows for their assessment.

THE QUEST FOR UNIVERSAL EMOTIONS

Many studies on culture and emotion can be constructed as attempts to prove or disprove the hypothesis of universal emotions. This section reviews the research that seemed to address the question of universality. We first review research in the tradition of basic emotions theories, followed by lexical research.

Basic Emotions Theories

Basic emotions theories (Ekman, 1992a, 1992b; Izard, 1980, 1992, 1994) have proposed the existence of a set of basic emotions. Although the precise number of basic emotions postulated varies across different theories, basic emotion theories have in common that they propose a limited set of emotions as part of the human potential and thus as universal. Each basic emotion is assumed to have unique experiential qualities that are unanalyzable (Izard, 1977; Johnson-Laird & Oatley, 1989; Oatley & Johnson-Laird, 1987). The emotion is a signal that is "evolutionarily old and simple. It has no internal structure, and in this sense it is not propositional: It does not carry semantic information. . . . The phenomenological experience of the signal is a distinctive feeling of happiness, sadness, anger, or some other emotional state" (Oatley & Johnson-Laird, 1996, p. 363). Each unique experience of emotion is postulated to be linked to certain other responses of emotions, such as specific facial expressions, particular patterns of physiology, and particular cognitive modes. Basic emotion theories thus predict the universal occurrence of a small number of emotions and postulate specific and unique patterns of responses for each of the presumably universal basic emotions. This specificity is particularly expected to hold for the motor response and the neurophysiological modalities.

Research on Basic Emotions

Facial Expression

The most well-known line of research in support of the notion of basic emotions focused on the facial motor responses. It consisted of the facial recognition studies by Ekman and colleagues (Ekman, Friezen, & Ells-worth, 1982) and Izard (1971). The paradigm used in recognition studies was simple and elegant. Respondents were asked to associate a picture of a face showing a given expression with one emotion word from a list. The list consisted of the words for basic emotions (e.g., happiness, anger) and thus differed somewhat according to the specific theory represented in the research. One conclusion from the recognition studies is clear: People from very different cultures recognized the facial expressions above chance. This was even true for people and cultures with minimal exposure to the West, such as the Fore in New Guinea (Ekman & Friesen, 1971). Later research even reported cross-cultural convergence in the intensity ratings of each expression (Ekman et al., 1987).

The evidence for universal facial expressions is indirect in that it is almost entirely based on the recognition of posed pictures, but there is at least one exception. Ekman and colleagues (1982) studied the production of emotional expressions in a standardized test. They videotaped the facial expressions produced by New Guineans who were asked "to show how their face would appear if they were the person described in one of the emotion stories used in the judgement task" (p. 136). American students who viewed the videotaped expressions recognized four out of six expressions (happiness, anger, disgust, and sadness) above chance. This study thus yielded evidence for universal production of the same facial expressions.

There is consensus that the cross-cultural studies on facial expression have shown the existence of a universal modes of communication of emotion or certain emotion components (see, e.g., Mesquita, Frijda, & Scherer, 1987; Russell, 1994) and have thus made a significant contribution to the research on culture and emotion. However, the conclusion that these studies provide evidence for basic emotions has been challenged for at least three reasons:

1. There are considerable cultural differences in the rates of recognition of facial expressions, even though the recognition in all cultures is above chance. The focus on recognition above chance defines the question as a dichotomous one—consistent with the dichotomous question of universality versus nonuniversality. Yet this may not be the only relevant framing of the evidence. The differences in the rates of recognition may be equally interesting. What does it mean if respondents from Western cultures recognize the facial expressions more "accurately" than respondents from non-Western cultures? Cultural differences in recognition rates are not easily explained by the notion of basic emotions.

2. The results do not show that the emotions cross-culturally associated with facial expressions are in fact the same. The words used in different languages as the equivalents of the English words *happiness, sadness, fear, anger, disgust,* and *surprise* may in fact not have been entirely similar

in meaning. Of course, they would not be chosen as translations for each other if they did not have some common core of emotional meaning. Yet, to what extent the supposedly equivalent words in other languages are equivalent in all respects is an empirical question not addressed by the facial expression studies. In fact, psychological and linguistic studies that do address this question have found that the meanings associated with "basic" emotion words in different languages differ importantly (Wierzbicka, 1992).

3. Yet another possibility is that facial expressions are recognized not on the basis of their correspondence to discrete emotions but rather on the basis of their position on bipolar dimensions of emotional experience, on the basis of the action readiness mode that they present, or on the basis of situational meanings that they represent (Russell, 1994). The results of facial recognition studies definitely suggest that across cultures people infer some psychological state from facial expression, just as they can from anything else that a person does, but it is unclear whether emotions are spontaneously inferred by people across the world (Russell & Fernández-Dols, 1997).

Vocal Expression

Most research on vocal expression was modeled after facial recognition studies. Respondents from different cultures were asked to identify the vocal expressions of emotions in either a nonsensical phrase in one language (Davitz, 1969; Van Bezooijen, Otto, & Heenan, 1983) or content-filtered speech (Albas, McCluskey, & Albas, 1976). In all studies respondents selected the most appropriate word from a list of emotion words in their own language. Recognition of vocal expressions was cross-culturally above chance (Albas, McCluskey, & Albas, 1976; Van Bezooijen et al., 1983). One study found that, in all cultures, the recognition of vocal expression was best for the same emotions (Davitz, 1969), implying that some emotions have more vocal signature than others and that the emotions with unique vocal expressions were cross-culturally the same. Japanese and American respondents recognized anger best, then sadness, pride, love, nervousness, and jealousy, in that order. The Israeli participants deviated only by recognizing the sad tone of voice better than the angry one. Both results point to universality of the vocal expressions associated with particular emotions. Van Bezooijen (1984) found that the activation level of an emotion is one of the major aspects conveyed by voice intonation. It seems logical, therefore, that anger and sadness—both emotions that are importantly defined by their activation level—would be universally well recognized from vocal expression.

However, universality of vocal recognition has been challenged by other findings. Van Bezooijen and colleagues (1983) found cultural differences in the emotions best recognized by vocal expression, suggesting that the vocal signature of particular emotions differs by culture. Consistent with the latter finding, several studies yielded a better recognition of vocal expression in the listeners' own language (Albas et al., 1976; Van Bezooijen et al., 1983). There are several explanations for the poorer recognition of vocal expressions from a different culture (Mesquita & Frijda, 1992). First, emotional expression might be composed of both universal and culture-specific components (Davitz, 1964). Second, the general tone of a given language may suggest expressive content to a foreigner that play in with the expressive content of individual utterances. Third, the emotion words considered as equivalents in different languages again may very well differ in important aspects, such as implied activation level.

Focusing on the dichotomous question of universality would again lead to the conclusion that vocal expressions of certain emotions are cross-culturally similar. However, the research on the vocal expressions of emotion also points to cultural differences in degree. Finally, the criticism that the emotion words from different languages used in the research may not be fully equivalent may well affect the conclusions on vocal expression research just as it has affected the conclusions on facial expression research (Mesquita & Frijda, 1992).

Autonomic Nervous System Activity

Central to the notion of basic emotions is the hypothesis that typical physiological response patterns in the autonomous nervous system (ANS) associated with the basic emotions are universal (see, e.g., Levenson, 1994). Due to difficulties in experimentally inducing strong emotions as well as in obtaining reliable physiological measurements outside of laboratories, there is little research measuring ANS responses accompanying cross-culturally comparable emotional states. An exception is research by Levenson and colleagues among young Minangkabau men in West Sumatra (Levenson, Ekman, Heider, & Friesen, 1992). The study made use of the *directed facial action task,* in which subjects were instructed to move specific muscles in their faces in configurations assumed to signal basic emotions. The physiological measures included heart rate, finger temperature, skin conductance, finger pulse transmission time, finger pulse amplitude, respiratory period, and respiratory depth. The study with the Minangkabau men was a replication of earlier research among American college students. The results of the two studies were compared. While the results in the Minangkabau group did not completely replicate earlier findings with the American students, there was sufficient overlap in ANS responses to allow the authors to claim support for the existence of pancultural physiological differentiation between the basic emotions. However, cultural differences emerged in reports of subjective experience: Minangkabau reported experiencing less emotion than did the American college students. The authors attributed the difference in self-experienced emotion to the Minangkabau's greater emphasis on emotions as parts of interpersonal relationships. Several criticisms have been aimed at this study. First, the Minangkabau and American groups differed significantly on two out of the seven ANS responses (heart rate and skin conductance) (Mesquita et al., 1997). Therefore, it is quite possible to conclude that there are cultural differences in addition to similarities in ANS patterns. Second, the failure of many studies to establish stable and specific response patterns differentiating between the basic emotions in Western samples casts doubt on the stability of the results found in this particular study (Cacioppo, Klein, Berntson & Hatfield, 1993; Stemmler, 1989; Zajonc & McIntosh, 1992). Finally, whether the patterns of ANS responses in fact reflected different emotions has been questioned on two completely different grounds. Boiten (1996) has argued that Levenson's reported ANS changes are a function of the metabolic demands associated with making the various facial expressions, rather than of basic emotions elicited by the task. Markus and Kitayama (1994) have challenged the assumption that the directed facial action task induced emotions in both cultures; they argued that the failure of Minangkabau men to recognize emotions outside of an interpersonal context meant that

> in contrast with the Americans, the activity of the autonomic nervous system stemming from the configuration of the facial musculature did not constitute an emotion. . . . Americans and Minangkabaus define emotions differently, and . . . they have different expectations about when and why an emotion will be experienced. (p. 103)

Markus and Kitayama thus challenged the idea of basic emotions as a culture-free concept.

Conclusion

In sum, basic emotions theory has fostered research that searched for unique patterns of responses universally characteristic of the basic emotions. Research on facial and vocal expressions, and ANS response patterns has suggested that there are pancultural patterns of responses associated with the same classes of emotions. Although research in this area underemphasizes the cultural variability of the phenomena, the results show some cross-cultural differences. Therefore, even the quest for universal emotions has produced evidence that challenges the idea of invariant basic emotions.

Cultural Differences in Emotions: Display Rules

In order to explain cultural differences in the observed emotions, basic emotions theory has coined the notion of cultural display rules. Display rules are culture-specific proscriptions about who can show which emotions, to whom, and when. Ekman explicitly "postulated display rules . . . to explain how cultural differences may conceal universality in expression" (1992a, p. 384).

Although the concept has often been posited to explain cultural differences in emotional phenomena (see, e.g., Matsumoto & Ekman, 1989), to our knowledge only one study has been done with the intention of measuring cross-cultural differences in display rules. In this study, the facial expressions of American and Japanese students were recorded while they were watching a stress-producing movie. The students were either in the condition in which they were led to believe that they were alone or in the condition in which they were interviewed about their feelings by a member of their own culture. Facial expressions were measured by the Facial Action Coding System (Ekman & Friesen, 1978). The facial expressions of American and Japanese students did not differ in the alone condition but differed markedly in the social condition. Japanese students in the latter condition exhibited more positive expressions, supposedly to mask the original negative expression; the American subjects showed signs of negative affect.

One assumption of this study is that the real basic emotion takes place in the alone condition and that the different responses of the Japanese subjects in the social condition should thus be interpreted as a result of emotion regulation. The display rule supposedly says, "Do not show negative emotions in the presence of other people." Alternative explanations are possible, however. For example, the social condition may in fact have had positive meaning to the Japanese, outweighing the negative impact that the movie might have had when the students were alone. Whether or not the results of the alone condition show that we fundamentally share the same emotions with other cultures is thus still open to debate.

Other studies in East Asian cultures, supposedly sharing the display rule of emotion moderation in the presence of others, have not confirmed the findings of Ekman and Friesen. Tsai, Levenson, and McCoy (1999) failed to find a similar pattern of display rules in a study comparing Chinese American and European American couples in conflict situations. In this study couples discussed relational problems, either in the presence of an authority figure—the "public" condition—or by themselves—the "private" condition. Chinese American couples displayed less positive emotional expression but did not differ from the European American couples with respect to the expression of negative emotions.

Emotion Lexicon

Basic emotions theory has predicted the pancultural occurrence of certain words (e.g., angry, happy) reflecting universal experiences (see, e.g., Boucher, 1979; Plutchik, 1980). Consequentially, it was predicted that the prevalent emotion words in all languages would be those referring to basic emotions.

Russell (1991), reviewing the evidence on emotion lexicons, found that by far most languages had words for the basic emotions. Also, Agnoli, Kirson, Wu, and Shaver (1989) found that the basic level of organization of the American English, Italian, and Mandarin Chinese emotion lexicons was constituted largely by words for similar emotions. In this latter study, respondents from the three cultures were asked to classify emotion words into groups of "emotions that go together" (Agnoli et al., 1989, p. 4). The co-occurrence matrices were aggregated and subjected to hierarchical cluster analyses. There was a substantial cross-cultural overlap of the words found at a basic level of hierarchical organization, the level that represents the most psychologically salient phenomena (Rosch, 1978). Words roughly corresponding with happiness, sadness, anger, and fear were basic (in the Roschian sense) in all three languages.

However, the universality of basic concepts of emotions may be challenged on a number of grounds. Agnoli and colleagues (1989) found cultural variations in the basic level concepts in addition to similarities. For example, the concept of shame was a basic level concept in Chinese but not in the other two languages. These authors argue that the cultural salience of shame in China might have moved that emotion concept up to a basic emotion category in that culture.

Furthermore, some ethnographic work on emotion words has challenged the idea of universality of the most salient emotion concepts. Russell (1991) distinguished two types of claims coming from this type of work. The first is that important words in other languages are without an equivalent in English. The Japanese emotion of *amae* (see, e.g., Doi, 1973), a pleasant feeling of dependence, is a good example. A second claim is that some English words have no equivalent in some other language. Some cultures appear to lack distinctions that are made in English between several basic emotions. For example, Levy (1973) reported that the Tahitians have no words for guilt and sadness. Leff (1973) pointed out that some African languages do not make the distinction between anger and sadness. Rosaldo's (1980) account of the indigenous word *liget* among the Philippine Ilongot suggests the same blurring between anger and sadness (this point has also been made by Russell, 1991). *Liget* is translated as angry and has overtones of activation, yet one of the emotions that it reflects is grief.

Russell (1991) concluded on the basis of this and other research that people in different cultures categorize emotions somewhat differently. Most problematic for the thesis of basic emotions was that fact that certain languages lack words for supposedly fundamental experiences. As Russell put it, "It is puzzling why a language would fail to provide a single word for an important, salient, discrete, and possibly innate category of experience—if such exists" (1991, p. 440).

The linguist Anna Wierzbicka (1986) remarks on such differences in lexicons:

> One of the most interesting and provocative ideas that have been put forward in the relevant literature is the possibility of identifying a set of fundamental human emotions, universal, discrete and presumably innate. . . . I experience a certain unease when reading claims of this kind. . . . How is it that these emotions are all so neatly identified by means of English words? For example, Polish does not have a word exactly corresponding to the English word *disgust*. What if psychologists working on the "fundamental human emotions" happened to be native speakers of Polish rather than English. (p. 584)

Whereas most languages thus seem to have words that correspond to the English words for alleged basic emotions, some languages are lacking a specific word for some of those emotions, and others name prevalent "fundamental" experiences for which English lacks a word. Even if words were the perfect indicators of emotional experiences, which there is ample reason to doubt (see Mesquita & Frijda, 1992; Russell, 1991; Wierzbicka, 1992; Zammuner & Frijda, 1994) lexical research does not provide univocal evidence for the idea of basic emotions. In the next subsection we will see that there are cross-cultural differences in the precise meanings of the words roughly referring to emotions like happiness and anger.

Limitations of the Basic Emotions Approach

The theory of basic emotions has thus been influential in shaping contemporary cross-cultural psychology of emotions. Although the approach has motivated a host of informative studies, it has also limited the research on culture and emotion in a number of ways (Mesquita et al., 1997).

1. The notion of basic emotions has limited the focus of research to the question of whether or not emotions are cross-culturally similar. The possibility that emotions can be similar in some aspects yet different in others has been largely overlooked. Thus, for example, research has focused on the question of whether anger can be found across cultures, rather than questioning to what extent emotions in the class of anger are cross-culturally similar.

2. The focus on the search for basic emotions has furthered a conceptualization of emotions as intraindividual states rather than as processes unfolding in a social context. Since basic emotions were assumed to be invariant across contexts, inclusion of the context in research was typically not deemed necessary. For example, the basic emotions approach has promoted the search for the patterns of physiological responses and facial movement (generally associated with a state of anger), rather than looking for the ways in which certain contexts afford particular patterns of responses.

3. The basic emotions approach has fostered interest in cross-cultural research on the potential for emotions, rather than on their actual prevalence or significance. For example, studies on facial expression have shown that people from different cultures recognize facial expressions in similar ways. Investigators have thus obtained evidence that a broad variety of people have the ability to manifest emotions through certain facial expressions, rather than determining the ecology, the actual occurrence, or the frequency of occurrence of these facial expressions.

In sum, for some time the notion of basic emotions has dominated cross-cultural research on emotions. As a consequence: (1) universality and cultural specificity of emotions have been treated as mutually exclusive, also defining the statistical questions asked; (2) emotions have been treated as intraindividual states rather than processes unfolding in a social context, fostering decontextualized research; and (3) the potential for emotional responses has been emphasized in cross-cultural research at the expense of attention to emotional practice.

THE QUEST FOR CULTURAL VARIATIONS IN THE COMPONENTS OF EMOTIONS

Componential Theories of Emotion

Many investigators no longer consider emotions as unitary, elementary entities but rather as multicomponential phenomena (Frijda, 1986; Lang, 1977; Lazarus, 1991; Levenson, 1994; Ortony & Turner, 1990; Scherer, 1984). These so-called componential approaches define the emotion process as a complex of changes in the various components. The emotion process, according to componential views, generally includes the following components:

- An antecedent event
- Appraisal, defined as the evaluation of the relevance of an emotional situation to an individual's well-being and his/her possibilities for coping with the event

- Physiological change
- Change in action readiness, consisting of impulses to establish, maintain, or disrupt the individual's relationship with an object and of more or less general states of enhanced or diminished activation
- Behavior
- Change in cognitive functioning and beliefs
- Regulatory processes that may occur at any of those stages (see G. A. Bonanno, Chapter 8, and L. Feldmann-Barrett & J. J. Gross, Chapter 9, this volume)

Most instances of emotion are thought to involve all of these components. In most cases, an emotionally charged event starts the emotion process, yet each component has its particular determinants as well. In an emotion, the components are thus thought to change somewhat independently of each other, although their mutual influence is assumed as well.

Much of the theorizing and research in the relatively new tradition of componential emotions is concentrated on the experience of emotion. Different from basic emotions approaches, componential models postulate that it is possible to analyze emotional experience (see, e.g., Frijda, 1986). Emotional experience is thought to be contingent on the particular appraisal of the emotion antecedent (Ellsworth, 1994; Scherer, 1997b) or, alternatively, on appraisal and the changes in action readiness combined (Frijda, Kuipers, & Terschure, 1989). Appraisal may be conscious, but more often than not it is supposed to be automatic. Both cortical and subcortical processes may be involved in appraisal (see LeDoux, 1997; Scherer & Schorr, in press)

Componential approaches do not presuppose universality of emotions. Emotions in different cultures are assumed to be similar only to the extent that they are characterized by similar patterns of appraisal and emotional response. The combined similarities and differences in emotion components are thought to shape the emotion. The extent to which emotions vary across cultures is considered an empirical question.

Changes in the Research on Culture and Emotion

The componential approach of emotions has shaped the interest of the cross-cultural field in several ways:

1. Componential models have changed the working assumption of cross-cultural research on emotions. One cross-culturally invariant component was no longer taken to imply the universality of the emotion as a whole. The cross-cultural variability of each component had to be studied

individually. Several studies studied the cross-cultural variability of each of a number of different components independently.

2. The componential approach has also changed the research question from a dichotomous into a gradual one. The focus thus has become to what extent emotions are similar (or different) across cultures, rather than whether or not an emotion is cross-culturally similar. The change in research question entailed a change in statistical criteria as well. Rather than above-chance rates of occurrence, the variance explained by "emotion" and "culture" became the relevant statistical criterion. Componential approaches have not engendered a systematic search for cultural differences, but both the design and statistical methods of the studies they motivated have allowed for the establishment of cultural differences.

3. Finally, componential approaches have motivated the empirical study of emotional *experience* across cultures. In practice, this generally meant cross-cultural research of the appraisals and action readiness modes associated with certain emotions. Questionnaire research became the most prevalent technique, since "two important components of the total emotion process, cognitive appraisal of emotion-antecedent situations and subjective feeling state [and one could add changes in action readiness], are accessible only through self-report" (Scherer & Wallbott, 1994, p. 312).

Componential Research on the Cross-Cultural Variation of Emotions

Different Components Compared Alongside

Most cross-cultural studies that were based on the componential approach concentrated on the core components of emotional experience: appraisal and action readiness. We review those studies in the next two subsections.

Only a small number of studies have actually endeavored to compare multiple components of emotions simultaneously. The most important study was a large-scale questionnaire by Scherer and his colleagues motivated by a componential view of emotions (Scherer & Wallbott, 1994; Scherer, Wallbott, Matsumoto, & Kudoh, 1988; Scherer, Wallbott, & Summerfield, 1986). In its final form this study compared the emotions of college students from 37 countries distributed over six geopolitical regions with regard to a large number of emotion components. The degrees of cross-cultural variation and convergence were established for each component separately and with respect to several different aspects of each component.

The method used in this study, and one adopted by most other componential studies, was to have respondents report a situation that had elicited a particular emotion (in Scherer and colleagues' study, joy, anger, sadness, fear, shame, guilt, or disgust). After the respondents described the antecedent event, they were asked to answer a large number of questions referring to different aspects of the event and the subsequent emotion (Scherer & Wallbott, 1994). Published results from the 37-country study pertained to appraisal, subjective experience, physiological symptoms, and expressive behavior. The appraisal outcomes will be discussed below. Aspects of subjective experience were the time past since the emotional instance took place ("time duration"), the duration of the emotion, the emotional intensity, efforts to control the emotion, and any effects on relationships the emotion might have had. Physiological symptoms were measured by questions on ergotropic symptoms (e.g., increased heart beat and tensed muscles), trophotropic symptoms (e.g., stomach trouble and a lump in the throat), and temperature changes. Expressive behavior consisted of an approach–avoidance dimension, nonverbal behavior (e.g., smiling), paralinguistic behavior (e.g., speech melody change), and verbal behavior (e.g., ranging from silence to lengthy utterance).

The study yielded a large degree of cross-cultural convergence in the patterns of responses associated with the seven emotions being studied (with etas—i.e., standardized effect sizes—for emotions varying between .7 and .8). However, cultural differences were found as well: Both country main effects and country–emotion interaction effects were found, though those effects were generally small to medium (etas for country ranging between .2 and .4; etas for the emotion by country interactions, between .2 and .3). Cultures differed the most with respect to the average frequency of particular emotions ("time duration"), their duration, and their level of intensity, as well as with respect to the amount of verbal behavior associated with emotions (or possibly the amount of verbal behavior generally). Yet, the relative position of different emotions on these dimensions was the same across cultures. The eta for the cross-product of country and emotion was highest for perceived relationship effects, meaning that the relative positions of different emotions on this dimension was different across cultures. It is conceivable that, for example, in some cultures the relationship effects of shame might have been perceived as particularly powerful, whereas in other cultures anger was perceived as having more impact on relationships (the example is imaginary).

The study has provided a rich collection of emotion data, more inclusive than ever collected before. By comparing many components of emotions, a much more complete idea has been obtained about the various response modes of emotions, in general, and these seven emotions, in particular. As Scherer and Wallbott (1994) concluded, the cultural effects were small in comparison to the emotion-specific effects, and an extreme position of cultural relativism is not warranted by the data. Yet, exactly how much the emotional experience in different cultures varies is not easily inferred from this study. It is very problematic to compare the main effects of emotion with the main effects of culture (cf. Reise & Flannery, 1996). The reason is that the emotions included in the study may be a better representation of the emotion domain than the cultures included are of the culture domain. If the cultures studied were not representative of the cultures of the world, the cultural effects may have been underestimated. Scherer and Wallbott contest that: "One can argue that 37 countries from all continents can be considered a reasonably representative sample of all countries in the world" (1994, p. 316). Yet, some parts of the world appear to have been better represented in the large-scale questionnaire than others. Moreover, the exclusive use of college students in this study is likely to have reduced the variance in cultural background substantially. These factors may have biased the results in the direction of similarities.

Another criticism (which we address more extensively below in the section on cultural approaches) is that the methodology of the study did not allow for the full range of differences in emotional experience. First, the study started from the translations of English emotion words in the different languages. These translations were chosen on the basis of their similarity to the English words. An alternative method, one that would possibly have allowed for more cultural differences in emotions, would have been to start from the most prevalent emotions in each culture. Actually, the finding of a medium-sized main effect of culture on the time elapsed since the reported instance of emotion occurred may point to cultural differences in the prevalence of the seven emotions selected for research. Second, the dimensions of comparison may not have lent themselves to the finding of cultural differences. Different dimensions, selected to be particularly salient in other cultures, may have revealed more cultural differences in the patterns of emotional responses.

Research on Emotional Experience

Most of the research motivated by the componential approach has been on a core element of emotional experience: appraisal. Appraisal is usually conceived of as the combination of a series of evaluations on a limited number of dimensions, such as novelty, pleasantness, control, certainty, agency, and compatibility with personal or social values (Frijda, 1986; Roseman, 1984; Scherer, 1984; Smith & Ellsworth, 1985). The assumption underlying appraisal research is that emotional experience is contingent on appraisal. The appraisal–emotion association, rather than either appraisal or emotion, has been considered universal (Mesquita & Ellsworth, in press).

In several studies using cross-cultural questionnaires, participants from different cultures were asked to report instances of specific emotions from their past. In all studies, the participants were subsequently asked to answer questions about how they appraised these emotional events. The largest study was the one just reported in the previous subsection. As noted, it included students from 37 different countries, which for the analysis of the appraisal outcomes were grouped into six geopolitical regions (addressing the problem of the differential sampling density in different parts of the world): countries of northern and central Europe, Mediterranean countries, Anglo-American countries of the New World, Latin American countries, Asian countries, and African countries (Scherer, 1997a, 1997b). Other studies have compared students from the United States, Hong Kong, Japan, and the People's Republic of China (Mauro, Sato, & Tucker, 1992); students from the United States and India (Roseman, Dhawan, Rettek, Naidu, & Thapa, 1995); students from the Netherlands, Indonesia, and Japan (Frijda, Markam, Sato, & Wiers, 1995); and Dutch, Surinamese, and Turkish community samples in the Netherlands (Mesquita, 2000). The emotions as well as the appraisal dimensions studied differed somewhat in the different studies.

The research generally supports the hypothesis that equivalent emotions in different cultures are characterized by similar appraisal patterns. Scherer (1997b) found similar appraisal patterns across cultures for joy, fear, anger, sadness, disgust, shame, and guilt. For example, joyful situations were cross-culturally characterized as expected, very pleasant, requiring no action, and enhancing self-esteem. Across cultures, the situations that produced fear were conceived of as unpleasant, obstructing goals, and hard to cope with. Anger was provoked in situations that were seen as unexpected, unpleasant, obstructing goals, unfair, and caused by other people.

However, Scherer (1997b) also found cultural differences in appraisal. In comparison to other geopolitical regions, African countries appraised the antecedents of all negative emotions as significantly higher on unfairness, external causation, and immorality, while Latin American countries gave them lower ratings of immorality than the countries in other geopolitical regions.

Similar results were obtained by Frijda and colleagues (1995), Mesquita (2000), and Roseman and colleagues (1995), who included different emotions than those chosen by Scherer and slightly different sets of appraisal dimensions. Despite these methodological differences, the results were comparable in that equivalent emotions in different cultures shared a core of similar appraisals but were also different on some other appraisals.

A slightly different way of representing the appraisal–emotion relationship was adopted by Mauro and colleagues (1992), who asked people to remember times when they had felt each of 16 different emotions and to rate each of the eliciting situations on several appraisal dimensions. The researchers then compared the absolute and relative positions of the 16 emotion episodes in four cultures on the dimensions of appraisal. They found no significant cultural differences in the positions of emotions on the appraisal dimensions of attentional activity, certainty, coping ability, or norm/self compatibility. They found cultural differences in the absolute but not in the relative positions of emotions on the pleasantness, legitimacy, and control dimensions. On the dimensions of anticipated effort, control, and responsibility the results from different cultures were substantially different. Again, the evidence supported the hypothesis of a cross-culturally similar experiential core of "equivalent" emotions, but there are cultural variations in the appraisal–emotion relationship as well. Taken together, these studies show that there are important cross-cultural similarities in appraisal–emotion relationships. However, each of these studies also suggests that the relationship between appraisals and emotions is subject to cultural influence.

If emotional experience is contingent on appraisal, one should also expect that cultural *differences* in the appraisals have implications for the subsequent emotional experience. Roseman and colleagues (1995) tested whether cultural differences in emotional intensity reported by Indian and American college students were mediated by differences in appraisal. Compared to the American respondents, the Indians reported lower overall intensity for both emotions. Cultural differences in emotion intensity were accounted for by greater perceived motive consistency (one of Roseman and colleagues' appraisal dimensions) in Indians than in Americans. This suggests that the more consistent an emotional event is with a person's motives, the less intense the person's feelings of sadness and anger. Cultural differences in emotional intensity were completely mediated by appraisal differences: After the effect of perceived motive consistency was taken into account, no direct effect of culture on emotional intensity was left. Based on the results of this single study, we may thus tentatively conclude that cultural differences in appraisal make a difference in people's actual emotional experience.

Finally, several studies have addressed the question of to what extent the same appraisal dimensions cross-culturally explain the variance in emotions. The variance of emotions explained by appraisal has not exceeded 40% in any of the studies cited here (Frijda et al.,1995; Mauro et al., 1992; Scherer, 1997a).The same appraisals cross-culturally predicted emotional variance to the same degree. Scherer (1997a) found that across all emotions, the appraisal profiles of different cultures were intercorrelated at $r = .80$, implying that the relative contribution of each appraisal dimension must be largely similar across cultures and across emotions. However, he also established sizable differences between the intercultural correlations of appraisal profiles for individual emotions. On average, joy profiles were most correlated across cultures ($r = .99$), and disgust profiles least ($r = .61$). This leaves some room for cross-cultural differences in the relative contributions of particular appraisal dimensions to emotional experiences of a kind.

Frijda and colleagues (1995) also found that appraisals explained approximately 40% of the variance in emotions in all three groups of study. However, the percentage of variance explained by particular appraisals appeared different across cultures, although no test of significance was reported. For example, valence explained 23% of the variance in the Dutch emotion words, 30% in the Indonesian words, and 15% in the Japanese words. Therefore, although the combined appraisal dimensions explained similar levels of variance cross-culturally, the independent impact of each appraisal seemed to differ to some extent across cultures, again raising the possibility that the association between appraisal and emotion is not entirely universal.

In summary, the research has provided support for similarities in the relationship between appraisal and emotional experience. The emotional variance explained does not exceed 40%, however, which is far removed from a contingency relationship. The research has also supported the notion that the same set of appraisal dimensions predicts considerable variance in emotions within many different cultures. However, slight variations in the relative contribution of appraisal dimensions in different cultures are suggested as well. One reason for the differences found may be that emotion lexicons in different languages do not perfectly map onto each other. Differences in appraisals may be due to differences in the exact meaning of supposedly equivalent emotion words in different languages. Alternatively, the relation between appraisal and experience may be somewhat different in different cultures.

Action Readiness

Two studies have cross-culturally compared the action readiness modes associated with certain emotions (Frijda et al., 1995; Mesquita, 2000), based on the idea that action readiness is an important component of emotional experience as well. Both studies started from emotion words that were prevalent in the cultures of study. Both studies found that similar emotions are cross-culturally characterized by a core of similar action readiness modes. Mesquita, for example, found that words in the category of shame were characterized by the desire not to be seen or noticed. Furthermore, Frijda and colleagues (1995) found that, across cultures, the same set of action readiness modes contributed significantly to the explained variance in emotions and that it added to the variance explained by appraisal. Together, action readiness predicted 55% of the differentiation in Dutch emotion words correctly, 40% of the Indonesian emotion words, and 41% of the Japanese emotion words.

However, differences in action readiness were established as well. Mesquita (2000) found that Surinamese shame words were characterized by some angry action readiness modes, such as boiling inwardly, and the tendency to verbal and physical aggression, whereas Dutch shame words were not. Surinamese shame is often felt when an intimate other fails the individual, hence the angry components.

More importantly, Frijda and colleagues (1995) reported that it was impossible to find a common factor structure for action readiness modes in the three cultural groups. This result can be taken to show that the structure of emotional action readiness is quite different across cultures. However, Frijda and colleagues attribute the failure to find a cross-culturally similar factor structure of action readiness to cultural differences in the precise meanings of behaviors. The specific items of action readiness grouped together differently across cultures, yet the general meaning of some of the factors was argued to be similar. The first five factors of action readiness in each cultural group could be named: moving away, moving toward, moving against, wanting help, and submission. These authors conclude, therefore, that the relational aims of emotional behaviors are largely similar across cultures but that the same relational aims are achieved by means of culturally differential behaviors.

Action readiness factors also differed across cultures with respect to their relative significance (Frijda et al., 1995). *Moving away* explained 28% of the variance in emotions in the Dutch group, but only 6% in the Indonesian group and 10% in the Japanese group. On the other hand, *moving toward* was much more important in differentiating the Indonesian and Japanese emotion vocabularies (31% and 27%, respectively) than it was for the Dutch (12%). These differences may reflect the different cultural values attached to seeking social distance and independence versus seeking social closeness.

The few studies on action readiness thus suggest both cross-cultural similarities and differences. In support of universality it was found that (1) similar emotions are characterized by a similar core of action readiness, (2) the same set of action readiness modes explains a significant part of the variance in emotions, and (3) the action readiness modes group together into factors that can be thought to represent similar relational aims. In support of differences, it was found that (1) emotions in different languages tend to have a culture-specific action readiness profile in addition to a similar core, (2) it was impossible to find a common factor structure for the different cultures, and (3) the relative contribution of different action readiness factors to the explained variance of emotions varied across cultures.

Limitations of the Componential Approach

Some limitations of the componential approach have less to do with the approach as such as with its instantiation in research. First, the exclusive reliance on retrospective self-report studies makes the approach vulnerable.

We may wonder what it is exactly that we learn from these studies: Is it the ways people in different cultures think about their emotions, or is it the ways in which emotions actually differ? It may be argued that emotional experience does not happen independently from the way people think about it and that self-reports provide a window on this experience that cannot be obtained in any other way. Still, the use of convergent methods would have great advantages over the single-method approach that has been adopted so far.

Another limitation of the research is that it has compartmentalized the study of emotion. The focus on individual components has been at the expense of attention to process characteristics of emotions and attention to the coherence between the components. Despite the insight that emotions are processes that unfold over time and in interaction with social context, none of the cross-cultural studies have paid attention to similarities and differences in process characteristics or, for that matter, the differential context variables that contribute to the unfolding of emotion.

A serious problem with the methodology used in componential studies of emotion is that it relies on emotion words in different languages that were established equivalents, at least to the extent that they are conceived as each others' translations. Similarities in appraisal, action readiness, or any other component of emotion may have been the very basis of translation, and it is therefore not surprising to find similarity in one of the components. It would be more meaningful if words that were translations of each other on the basis of, say, similarity in appraisal would also be found associated with similar patterns of action readiness or physiological changes— or, alternatively, with differences in those components (Mesquita & Frijda, 1992).

Finally, componential models have allowed for accidental findings of cultural differences, but they have not given any direction to the search for cultural differences in emotions. Research in the componential paradigm started from clear expectations for similarities in emotions but did not formulate any hypotheses with regard to cultural differences (except perhaps implicitly that their occurrence would be rare and would affect content rather than process). Cultural differences were hit upon and not sought for. Cultural approaches, discussed in the next section, have a complementary focus on the systematic description and understanding of cultural differences in emotions.

THE QUEST FOR CULTURE-SPECIFIC PATTERNS OF EMOTIONS

Cultural Theories of Emotion

Cultural approaches to emotions focus on the ways emotion and culture make each other up (Shweder, 1991). That is, "emotions observed in everyday life seem to depend on the dominant cultural frame in which specific social situations are constructed and, therefore, cannot be separated from culture-specific patterns of thinking, acting, and interacting" (Kitayama & Markus, 1994, p. 4). Emotions are understood from the sociocultural contexts in which emotions occur. In turn, emotions are assumed to play a significant role in the production and reproduction of cultural practices and patterns of relating (Lutz & Abu-Lughod, 1990; White, 1994). Cultural approaches thus share the insight that emotions—however conceived—cannot be meaningfully studied without taking their sociocultural context into account.

Typically, the focus in cultural studies is on cultural differences rather than similarities. Ethnographic work on emotions has described emotional phenomena as they occur in a particular cultural context. Comparative studies, commonly undertaken by those who are psychologists by training, have addressed differences in the degree to which certain emotional phenomena prevail in different cultures. Furthermore, these comparative approaches have focused on phenomena known to be relevant or salient in the cultures of study and have explained these relevant emotional phenomena from the specific cultural context in which they occur. In comparative cultural studies, statistical differences in the degree to which emotional phenomena occur have been tested. This is in contrast with the statistical criteria used in the other paradigms: above-chance occurrence in the quest for universal emotions, and degree of explained variance in many componential studies.

The cultural approach thus focuses on cultural specificity or difference, in contrast to the basic emotions and componential approaches. Needless to say, both differences and similarities are worth studying. However, the claim made by other approaches that emotions are basically universal has been challenged by cultural approaches. In recent years, the methods and statistical analyses adopted by cultural studies have allowed researchers to establish many cultural differences in emotions.

No Natural Category

Cultural approaches have challenged the idea that emotions form a natural category and have put the category of emotion itself on the research agenda (see, e.g., Lutz, 1988; Shweder, 1993). The idea is that emotions, rather than being ready-made phenomena out in reality, are constructed culturally. Cultural approaches do not deny that many of the components of emotions may be hard-wired, but they contend that by themselves those components would not make for emotions. "Rather the components may be combined and afforded their divergent functions and forms through social and cultural process. . . . Through [the] pursuit of adaptation and adjustment to one's cultural and social environment, the component processes are organized and enabled to become emotions" (Kitayama & Markus, 1994, pp. 1–2). This idea is quite different from both basic emotions and componential approaches, which assume—to different degrees of explicitness—that certain component processes naturally combine into the phenomenon of emotion.

The idea is, therefore, that emotional experience is differently construed across different cultures. This may be reflected in the way "emotion" is defined. Differences in the category of emotion were suggested by Lutz (1987, 1988), who argued that the category of emotion does not have the same structure for the Ifaluk (people living on an atoll in the Western Pacific) as it does in American culture. Her analysis of Ifaluk emotion concepts suggests that emotions in that culture are identified on the basis of the eliciting (social) situations as well as behavioral and social consequences. The links between emotion, on the one hand, and social conditions or consequences, on the other, are not probabilistic as they would be in the West. Rather, the social situations and the behavioral or social consequences are defining of the emotion. Therefore, the Ifaluk category of emotions appears to be grounded in particular events and relationships. Emotional experience appears to be constructed on the basis of relational events rather than feelings.

The Ifaluk ethnotheory of emotion appears to have some similarity with the ways the Minangkabau of West Sumatra, Indonesia, conceive of emotion. In the study by Levenson and colleagues (1992) that was described earlier, the Minangkabau failed to report emotions after they had been exposed to the *directed facial action task*. In contrast, American respondents did report emotions in those same conditions. Differences in the conception of what it is to have an emotion have been suggested to underlie the differences in reported experience (Markus & Kitayama, 1994; see the earlier discussion). Levenson and colleagues suggest that the respondents may have had difficulty describing their emotional states because they were alone, since emotions are typically experienced in the presence of someone else. Thus the Minangkabau category of emotion is grounded in social and interpersonal situations.

A similar discrepancy between the cultural differences in experience and those in physiology was found by Tsai and Levenson (1997). In their experiment, Chinese American and European American couples had a 15-minute discussion on an issue that they had identified as a source of conflict in their relationship. On-line physiological measures were taken during this discussion. Immediately after the conversation, the partners each watched a video of the conflict and indicated at each moment how they had felt. The affect ratings were continuous, as the participants were asked to move a rating dial that traversed a 180° arc according to what they felt at that moment (from very negative to very positive). The authors calculated the mean change of affect from a baseline recorded during a preconversation period, the variability, and the number of periods of positive as well as negative affect.

Very little physiological differences were found between the cultures. No cultural differences were found in the mean levels of change of physiological responding, and the variability of responding was different only for two out of seven physiological measures. However, cultural differences were found in the affect ratings. Although the mean level of change of affect did not differ between the cultures, Chinese American couples' rating dial responses were less variable and less positive than those of European American couples. There were no cultural differences in the periods of reported negative affect (Tsai & Levenson, 1997). Therefore, the differences in emotional experience were not accompanied by differences in physiology.

Results from a recent experience-sampling study comparing the emotions of Japanese and American students also pointed to cultural differences in the structure of emotional experience (Mesquita & Karasawa, in press). Students from the different cultures were asked to report their emotional experiences four times a day (every 3 hours during the day and evening) for a week. They rated the last emotional experience in the preceding 3-hour time interval with respect to a number of appraisal dimensions. The appraisal dimensions commonly found in the literature (such as pleasantness, control, self-esteem, goal conduciveness) were supplemented by some appraisal dimensions thought to be particularly relevant to the Japanese group. Some examples were loss of face, social engagement, and the hurtful or immoral behavior of another person. Emotional experience (pleasant or unpleasant) was construed differently in Japan and the United States. In comparison with the American group, pleasantness in the Japanese group was more associated with social engagement, and more negatively correlated with loss of face and the immoral behavior of another person. The Japanese results converge with earlier research by Markus and Kitayama (1991), who found that Japanese emotion words were defined by, among other things, their position on the dimension of engaged in versus disengaged from an interpersonal relationship. In the American group, social appraisals were as important in predicting pleasantness as were appraisals of self-esteem, coping, and control. To the extent that emotional experience is constituted by appraisals, the differential association of pleasantness with independent appraisals, on the one hand, and interdependent appraisals, on the other, will affect the nature of the emotion.

Therefore, the results of different studies—using different research methodologies—are convergent. In all the Asian or Pacific cultures discussed above, emotions tended to be grounded in relationships. An experience was more likely to be constructed as emotional on the basis of its relational relevance, rather than on the basis of inner feelings. Of course, Western emotion theories have emphasized the relational character of emotions as well (Frijda, 1986; Sartre, 1934/1965). However, the emotion is thought to take place within the subject and to be directed to a social object of emotions. From the Asian/Pacific point of view, emotions tend to be part of the social relationships themselves. The difference goes beyond the mere way people talk about emotions. At the very least, there is a difference in the circumstances under which people experience emotions. To a Japanese it is a funny idea, for example, that one can have emotions all by themselves (M. Karasawa, personal communication, August 1999). A relational setting is what makes an experience recognizable as an emotional one.

The different cultural definitions of emotion have some tangible consequences for emotion research. In our recent open interviews on emotions with different cultural groups (Mesquita, Karasawa, Haire, & Kobara, 2000), Japanese students proved unable to answer questions on the intensity of the emotion, a question commonly and habitually asked in research in an American context. Information about internal feelings may not have been a salient characteristic of the Japanese emotional experience and may therefore not have been available or as readily accessible to the Japanese students. This is not to say that Japanese cannot quantify the magnitude of the emotional episode, but indicators different from internal feelings seem to be salient in the assessment of such magnitude.

Several ethnographers have suggested differences in the definition of emotional experience beyond the dimension just reviewed. For example, emotions and thought might not be distinguished in the same way (see, e.g., Lutz, 1987, 1988), nor might emotions and the (experiential) qualities of the outward environment be so distinguished (see, e.g., Rosaldo, 1980). It is typical for cultural approaches to assume that these differences in conceptualization are reflected in experience. Certainly, the described failure of people to recognize emotions under certain conditions and their failure to answer certain questions about the quality of their experience suggest this.

Culture-Specific Response Tendencies

Cultural research has yielded cultural differences in emotional response tendencies. Many of those different response propensities can be linked to characteristics of the larger cultural frame.

Tsai and colleagues (1999) monitored Chinese American and European American couples as they discussed a domain of conflict in their relationships. Chinese Americans reported that they felt fewer positive emotions while watching a video of the conflict discussion, and they displayed less positive expressive behaviors than did European Americans. No differences were found with respect to negative and self-conscious emotions (the above authors distinguish between these three groups of behavior). The same authors suggest that the suppressed positive emotionality is constituted by the Chinese norm of emotional moderation.

Mesquita (in press) compared emotions in individualist and collectivist contexts. The particular cultures were indigenous Dutch, known to be individualist, and Surinamese and Turkish immigrant groups in the Netherlands, known to be collectivist in orientation. The study compared the emotional response tendencies to six event types that, in previous research, had been established as reasonably frequent in all three cultures (e.g., success, offense by an intimate other). All respondents reported some emotional incidents from their past that met the event type described to them. They then answered questions about the appraisal/concerns, action readiness, social sharing, and belief changes they had experienced in the incident reported.

Collectivist and individualist cultures were expected to frame emotions differently and therefore produce different response propensities. Emotions in collectivist cultures were expected to derive their meaning from their role in and effect on relationships and to highlight the self as an interdependent identity. In contrast, emotions in individualist cultures were expected to highlight the self as an independent identity, bounded and separate from the environment.

Collectivist emotions were found to highlight the interdependent self in a number of different ways. First, they were actually more grounded in the relationships in which they occurred than were emotions occurring in an individualist context. As compared to individualist emotions, collectivist emotions were significantly more based on shifts in the person's own social worth as well as that of the ingroup. They occurred when a situation was assessed relevant to respectability, status, or ingroup respectability. Consistently, appraisal of the impact of emotional situations on one's relative social position was an important part of emotions in collectivist cultures. Emotions arose when another person was assessed to gain power or status at the expense of the individual's own status (e.g., "He humiliated me in front of others") or, to the contrary, when the individual him/herself gained status relative to or at the expense of others (e.g., "Other people were jealous because I was selected to sing a solo"). Appraisals in individualist cultures were lacking such a social focus.

Emotions in an individualist culture seem to emphasize and reinforce the subjectivity of emotions (as opposed to objective reality). However, the boundaries between subjectivity and reality were less clear in the collectivist context. Respondents in the collectivist cultures judged the emotion to be more obvious than did respondents in the individualist culture. They thus assumed that their feelings and thoughts were dictated by and interdependent with the features of the event, rather than an effect of subjective interpretation. Respondents from the individualist culture, by contrast, perceived a distinction between the actual event and its subjective interpretation, and maintained that the relationship between the two can be different. In the individualist culture a clear distinction was made between subjectivity and objectivity, whereas the collectivist cultures seemed to endorse the principle of a subjective reality. Consistent with the view that culture and emotion are mutual constituents, we may assume that the sources of these cultural differences in obviousness will lie both in the individual and in the environment. In individualist cultures there may be objectively more room for subjective interpretation than in collectivist cultures, where meaning tends to be established socially. At the same time, the psychological tendencies will emerge from this reality and reinforce it (see the following subsection on mutual constitution).

Consistently, respondents in the collectivist cultures reported more belief changes than did those in the individualist culture. This result speaks to the same issue of subjectivity–objectivity versus subjective reality. Belief changes transform the emotion from a subjective evaluation of an event into a belief about the external world. Once the belief is formed, the distinction between subjectivity and the objective environment is abandoned. At that point, one perceives the world as one feels about it. Thus respondents in the collectivist cultures, who reported a high readiness to belief changes, appeared to assume that they experienced the reality. Respondents in the individualist culture, on the other hand, did not as readily form belief changes and can thus be said to adhere to the boundaries between subjective evaluation and objective reality. Whereas emotions in the collectivist cultures tended to emphasize the relatedness of individuals and their social environment, emotions in individualist cultures appeared to underline the disparity of self and others. The results on action readiness and social sharing constituted relevant examples.

Across event types, a higher level of action readiness was found in collectivist than in individualist cultures. Thus, under emotional circumstances, respondents in the collectivist cultures reported a greater impulse to interact with their environment and to change the relationship with that environment than did respondents from the individualist culture. Most, though not all, action readiness factors represented social acts. Therefore, a high level of action readiness suggests that emotions are occasions to enter self–other relationships, and more so in the collectivist than in the individualist cultures.

Differences in the practice of social sharing of emotions were another case in point of the different self–other relationship in collectivist and individualist cultures. In collectivist cultures the concern with emotions seems to be shared with others from the beginning: Respondents of the collectivist cultures perceived the people with whom they shared the emotion (to be called "sharing partners") to be more personally concerned with the emotional event than respondents of the individualist Dutch culture perceived their sharing partners to be. Furthermore, more involvement was solicited as well as obtained from the sharing partners in collectivist than in individualist cultures. Whereas the practice of social sharing in the collectivist groups thus underlined the shared concern with emotions and their antecedents, the practice in the individualist groups rather stressed the distinction between the self as the one emotionally affected and others as relative outsiders.

In sum, the cultural differences in emotions yielded by this study were consistent with the respective value orientations of the cultures in which they occurred. As compared to emotions in the individualist culture, emotions in collectivist cultures—

1. Were more grounded in assessments of social worth and of shifts in relative social worth (e.g., appraisals of respect).
2. Were to a large extent taken to reflect reality, rather than the inner world of the individual (e.g., belief changes).
3. Belonged to the self–other relationship, rather than being confined to the subjectivity of the self (e.g., social sharing) (Mesquita, in press).

The Mutual Constitution of Culture and Emotion

One of the hallmarks of many cultural studies is that they focus on the bidirectionality of culture and emotion: Not only does culture afford the psychological tendencies to have certain emotions, but emotions also reinforce and promote culturally important concerns.

In a recent study, Kitayama, Markus, Matsumoto, and Norasakkunkit (1997) asked groups of Japanese and American students to rate success and failure situations that were previously generated by American and Japanese groups of subjects. Cultural differences were found with respect to the tendencies to appraise situations as either self-enhancing or self-criticizing. Overall, Japanese were more likely to perceive failure situations than success situations as relevant to their self-esteem. In the American group it was found to be the other way around. Success situations were considered more relevant to self-esteem than were failure situations. Furthermore, Americans judged that their self-esteem would increase more in success situations than it would decrease in failure situations. By contrast, the Japanese students judged that their self-esteem would decrease more in the failure situations than it would increase in success situations. Thus, the propensity to appraise events as either negative or positive to the self is subject to cultural variation.

Furthermore, American situations were generally recognized as more self-enhancing and Japanese situations as more conducive to self-criticism (Kitayama et al., 1997). Moreover, the tendency of Americans to appraise situations as self-enhancing was particularly strong for situations that were generated by Americans. On the other hand, the tendency of Japanese for self-criticism was particularly strong for situations that were generated by Japanese. Cultures amplified the culture-specific psychological tendencies. Therefore, culture appeared to provide opportunities for the culturally desired emotional responses; in turn, the psychological tendencies as constituted by the culture were tailored to taking those opportunities and reinforcing the desired practice.

Appraisal differences have been explained from the different self-goals (Kitayama et al., 1997). Americans would be motivated to maintain and enhance a positive evaluation of the self, as positive self-esteem is conditional to healthy independence. On the other hand, the Japanese cultural system would be rooted in the importance of maintaining, affirming, and becoming part of social relationships. In order to be and stay a good member of the social unit, the individual has to constantly reflect on and improve his/her shortcomings. The tendencies of self-enhancement and self-criticism were thus hypothesized to be part of the general cultural frames of independence and interdependence, respectively.

In a different fashion, a series of studies by Nissbett and Cohen and their colleagues on honor in the U.S. South illustrates this point as well (Cohen & Nisbett, 1995, 1996; Cohen, Nisbett, Bowdle, & Schwarz, 1996; Nissbett & Cohen, 1996). Nissbett and Cohen tested the hypothesis that the culture of honor was responsible for the higher incidence of murders in the U.S. South, as compared to the North. Central to the culture of honor is that a man's status is defined in terms of his power to enforce his will on others. This power is undermined in insult situations, since an insult implies that the target is weak enough to be bullied. Since a reputation for strength is the essence of a culture of honor, the individual who insults someone must be forced to retract, if necessary with violence or even threat of death.

In a laboratory experiment Nissbett and Cohen showed that Southerners who were insulted looked more angry and less amused, and completed vignettes in a more aggressive way than Northerners. After insults, Southerners also had higher levels of testosterone and cortisol, and did not yield as quickly as did Northerners to a person approaching from the other direction. None of these differences were found in the control situation, where the subjects were not insulted. Therefore, Southerners had a larger propensity to angry, assertive, and aggressive responses than Northerners in honor-related situations only.

The emotional propensities found in Southerners appeared to be reinforced or even amplified by cultural practices. Southerners had much more favorable opinions about violent behavior committed in the context of threats to honor. One of the field experiments by Nissbett and Cohen showed that Southern employers were much more cooperative and forgiving after receiving a letter from an applicant who had been convicted of an honor-related crime than were Northern employers. No such differences were found if the conviction regarded a similar crime that was not honor related, however. Generally, survey research showed that Southerners, compared to Northerners, were more likely to justify violence in honor-related contexts. Therefore, the cultural climate is conducive to the propensity of angry and aggressive responses to threats of honor, and is likely to reinforce and amplify those responses.

Together, these studies suggest that the responses in different emotional components—appraisal, cognitive modes, physiological responses, and behavior—tend to be afforded by positive cultural concerns. Responses that are conducive to fulfillment of central cultural goals tend to be the ones most common in a given culture.

Discussion and Limitations of the Cultural Approach

The cultural approach has clearly suggested that theoretically driven research of cultural differences in emotions is likely to yield those differences. Thus, in order to establish culture-specific emotional patterns, one has to start from the central cultural models of self, relationship, and emotion. It is in the context of those cultural models that emotional differences become interesting and predictable.

The cultural approach is new, and not many studies have been done that shed light on the exact cultural differences in emotions. Most, if not all, studies have focused on the emotional experience of people from different cultures, as appears from retrospective self-reports and concurrent evaluations. Hardly any research has been done that studies cultural differences in other components of emotions and in the relationship between physiology or behavior and self-reported experience. Multicomponential and multimethod approaches starting from theory on cultural differences in emotion would be very informative.

If descriptive research on cross-cultural differences in emotional phenomena is scarce, research on the processes underlying the cultural constitution of emotions is absent. There is hardly any systematic comparative research of the development of emotions across cultures or of emotion socialization processes. And neither is there research on the ways in which cultural practices and meanings afford and limit emotional experience and expression of adults on a daily basis. At this point, the idea of the "mutual constitution" of emotion and culture is no more than an idea that can be made plausible by very suggestive examples from the starting research in this area.

Another limitation of the cultural approach is that it is guided by those phenomena that in each culture are salient. By focusing on culturally salient practices, cultural differences in emotions have become the object of study. The cultural approach has not tried to map the cultural similarities in emotions as well. Clearly, both the basic emotions approach and the componential approach have covered the universal aspects of emotions better. Eventually, a meaningful integration of universal and culture-specific aspects of emotions will be called for.

CONCLUSIONS AND FUTURE DIRECTIONS

The quest for universal emotions, the quest for cultural variations in the components of emotion, and the quest for culture specificity in emotions have resulted in different objects of study, different research designs, and even diverse definitions of similarities and differences. Throughout this chapter we have emphasized that these three quests vary in the degree to which they assume and look for cross-cultural universality and difference in the emotion domain. Clearly, the quest for universal emotions is on one end of the dimension of cultural similarities and differences, whereas the quest for cultural specificity is on the other end.

Another way of contrasting the three quests is by assessing to what extent each of them focuses on the potential versus the practice of emotions (Mesquita et al., 1997). The quest for universal emotions has focused on the potential of emotions—the capacities and constraints of having and expressing emotions. Cultural approaches have been almost exclusively interested in emotional practices, the emotions that people actually experience in concrete social settings. Componential approaches may be placed somewhere in between. On the one hand, componential approaches assume (and test) the existence of a potential for certain universal appraisal dimensions and modes of action readiness. On the other, they compare the degree to which these components of experience are in fact relevant in different cultural contexts, and thus allow for differences in the practice or use of these components. Both the potential and the practice of emotions are valid objects of study. However, the study of emotion potential is more likely to yield cross-cultural similarities, whereas the study of emotional practice is more likely to yield differences. To some extent, the three quests can therefore be seen as merely addressing different questions in the field of culture and emotions.

One conclusion to be drawn from this review is that the quest for universality has not led to the detection of interesting and interpretable cultural differences in emotions. In fact, the field has seemed to collectively suffer from a "confirmation bias" (Wason & Johnson-Laird, 1972): Evidence that could confirm the universality of emotions has been looked for; evidence for differences has been ignored. Universality in emotions does not rule out the possibility of differences, however. In order to meaningfully establish, predict, and understand cultural differences, one needs to start from a cultural theory of emotions.

It should also be noted that cultural differences or similarities in emotional phenomena do not justify any conclusions about their source. Cultural differences in emotional phenomena have often been explained as an effect of differences in cultural meanings and practices, but it cannot be ruled out that some of the differences in emotional phenomena have a physiological or genetic background. For example, Lewis and Rosenblum (1978), explaining why Japanese babies tend not to cry when given inoculations whereas American babies do, argues that Japanese culture has promoted the selection of low emotional reactivity genes. Because Japanese culture places a value on low emotional reactivity, it would have promoted the selection of low-reactivity partners, thus leading to the natural selection of a "low-reactivity" gene pool. On the other hand, cross-cultural similarities in emotional phenomena may have been due to universal contingencies in the organization of social life (Frijda, 1994; Lazarus, 1994). Universality in emotional responses does not necessarily imply that emotions are innate or biologically preprogrammed. The biological or cultural constitution of emotions is a question that cannot be answered by the convergence or diversity of emotional phenomena alone but that needs to be separately addressed. Most researchers in the field believe that both biology and culture contribute to emotions. The question is, how and how much?

This is exactly the question that future research will have to address. First, we need a better assessment of the cultural differences in emotions. Multicomponential studies will have to reveal how physiological, cognitive, and behavioral responses are differentiated in different cultures and how these responses in other modalities relate to emotional experience. Second, research that reveals the mechanisms by which culture affects emotions is called for. What aspects of culture function to create different experiences and possibly different responses in other emotional modalities? Third, we will need a clearer understanding of how cultures incorporate the universal elements of emotions into culture-specific patterns.

Finally, let's return to the question of understanding emotions across cultures. Can I be a counselor to people of other cultures? Can the U.S. government trust its own assumptions about Saddam Hussein's motives, emotions, and plausible future actions? Can we judge the emotional impact that such foreign practices as veiling have on the women who participate in them? None of the aforementioned approaches would answer these questions with an unconditional yes. Yet, different approaches would be likely to define the conditions of cross-cultural understanding of emotions differently. According to the basic emotions approach, the most important emotions are similar across cultures. This approach would assume that one can understand the emotions of people in other cultures, provided that one knows the display rules of expression and behavior. From the perspective of componential models, one can understand the emotions in other cultures, provided that one knows how certain situations are appraised in other cultures. Finally, cultural approaches would maintain that one has to know and understand major cultural concerns, meanings, and relational practices in order to have any sense of the emotional experience in another culture. Although none of these approaches would thus say that understanding emotions across cultures is an easy job, cultural approaches define the job as most involved whereas basic emotions approaches view it as least involved.

REFERENCES

Agnoli, A., Kirson, D., Wu, S., & Shaver, P. R. (1989, April). *Hierarchical analysis of the emotion lexicon in English, Italian, and Chinese.* Paper presented at the annual meeting of the International Society for Research of Emotion, Paris.

Albas, D., McCluskey, K. W., & Albas, C. A. (1976). Perception of the emotional content of speech: A comparison of two Canadian groups. *Journal of Cross-Cultural Psychology, 7,* 481–489.

Boiten, F. (1996). Autonomic response patterns during voluntary facial action. *Psychophysiology, 33*(2), 123–131.

Boucher, J. D. (1979). Culture and emotion. In A. J. Marsella, R. G. Tharp, & T. V. Ciborowski (Eds.), *Perspectives on cross-cultural psychology* (pp. 159–178). San Diego, CA: Academic Press.

Cacioppo, J. T., Klein, D. J., Berntson, G. G., & Hatfield, E. (1993). The psychophysiology of emotion. In M. Lewis & J. M. Haviland (Eds.), *Handbook of emotions* (pp. 119–142). New York: Guilford Press.

Cohen, D., & Nisbett, R. E. (1995). Self-protection and the culture of honor: Explaining southern violence. *Personality and Social Psychology Bulletin 20*(5), 551–567.

Cohen, D., & Nisbett, R. E. (1996). Insult, aggression, and the Southern culture of honor: An "experimental ethnography." *Journal of Personality and Social Psychology 70*(5), 945–960.

Cohen, D., & Nisbett, R. E. (1997). Field experiments examining the culture of honor: The role of institutions in perpetuating norms about violence. *Personality and Social Psychology Bulletin, 23*(11), 1188–1199.

Cohen, D., Nisbett, R., Bowdle, B., & Schwarz, N. (1996). Insult, aggression, and the southern culture of honor: An "experimental ethnography." *Journal of Personality and Social Psychology, 70,* 945–960.

Davitz, J. R. (1964). Minor studies and some hypotheses. In J. R. Davitz (Ed.), *The communication of emotional meaning* (pp. 143–156). New York: McGraw-Hill.

Davitz, J. R. (1969). *The language of emotion.* San Diego, CA: Academic Press.

Doi, T. (1973). *The anatomy of dependence.* Tokyo: Kodansha.

Ekman, P. (1992a). Are there basic emotions?: A reply to Ortony and Turner [1990]. *Psychological Review, 99,* 550–553.

Ekman, P. (1992b). An argument for basic emotions. *Cognition and Emotion, 6*(3–4), 169–200.

Ekman, P. (1994). Strong evidence for universals in facial expression: A reply to Russell's mistaken critique [1994]. *Psychological Bulletin, 115,* 268–287.

Ekman, P., & Friesen, W. V. (1971). Constants across cultures in the face and emotion. *Journal of Personality and Social Psychology, 17,* 124–129.

Ekman, P., & Friesen, W. V. (1978). *The facial action coding system.* Palo Alto, CA: Consulting Psychologists Press.

Ekman, P., Friesen, W. V., & Ellsworth, P. (1982). What are the similarities and differences in facial behavior across cultures? In P. Ekman (Ed.), *Emotion in the human face* (pp. 128–146). Cambridge, UK: Cambridge University Press.

Ekman, P., Friesen, W. V., O'Sullivan, M., Diacoayanni-Tarlatzis, O., Krause, R., Pitcairn, T., Scherer, K., Chan, A., Heider, K., Ayan LeCompte, W., Ricci-Bitti, P. E., & Tomita, M. (1987). Universals and cultural differences in the judgements of facial expressions of emotion. *Journal of Personality and Social Psychology, 53,* 712–717.

Ellsworth, P. (1994). Sense, culture and sensibility. In S. Kitayama & M. R. Markus (Eds.), *Emotion and culture: Empirical studies of mutual influence* (pp. 23–50). Washington, DC: American Psychological Association.

Frijda, N. H. (1986). *The emotions.* Cambridge, UK: Cambridge University Press.

Frijda, N. H. (1994). Universal antecedents exist, and are interesting. In P. Ekman & R. J. Davidson (Eds.), *The nature of emotion: Fundamental questions* (pp. 155–162). New York: Oxford University Press.

Frijda, N. H., Kuipers, P., & Terschure, E. (1989). Relations between emotion, appraisal, and emotional action readiness. *Journal of Personality and Social Psychology, 57,* 212–228.

Frijda, N. H., Markam, S., Sato, K., & Wiers, R. (1995). Emotions and emotion words. In J. A. Russell, A. S. R. Manstead, J. C. Wellenkamp, & J. M. Fernández-Dols (Eds.), *Everday conceptions of emotion: An introduction to the psychology, anthropology and linguistics of emotion* (pp. 121–143). Dordrecht, Netherlands: Kluwer.

Izard, C. E. (1971). *The face of emotion.* New York: Appleton-Century-Crofts.

Izard, C. E. (1977). *Human emotions.* New York: Plenum Press.

Izard, C. E. (1980). Cross-cultural perspectives on emotion and emotion communication. In H. C. Triandis & W. Lonner (Eds.), *Handbook of cross-cultural psychology* (Vol. 3, pp. 185–221). Boston: Allyn & Bacon.

Izard, C. E. (1992). Basic emotions, relations among emotions, and emotion–cognition relations. *Psychological Review, 99*(3), 561–565.

Izard, C. E. (1994). Innate and universal facial expressions: Evidence from development and cross-cultural research. *Psychological Bulletin, 115,* 288–299.

Johnson-Laird, P. N., & Oatley, K. (1989). The language of emotions: An analysis of a semantic field. *Cognition and Emotion, 3,* 81–123.

Kitayama, S., & Markus, M. R. (Eds.). (1994). *Emotion and culture: Empirical studies of mutual influence.* Washington, DC: American Psychological Association.

Kitayama, S., Markus, H. R., Matsumoto, H., & Norasakkunkuit, V. (1997). Individual and collective processes in the construction of the self: Self-enhancement in the United States and self-criticism in Japan. *Journal of Personality and Social Psychology, 72,* 1245–1267.

Lang, P. J. (1977). Psychological assessment of anxiety and fear. In J. D. Cone & R. P. Hawkins (Eds.), *Behavioral assessment: New directions in clinical psychology* (pp. 178–195). New York: Brunner/Mazel.

Lazarus, R. S. (1991). *Emotion and adaptation.* New York: Oxford University Press.

Lazarus, R. S. (1994). Universal antecedents of the emotions. *The nature of emotion: Fundamental questions* (pp. 163–171). New York: Oxford University Press

LeDoux, J. E. (1997). *The emotional brain: The mysterious underpinnings of emotional life.* New York: Simon & Schuster.

Leff, J. P. (1973). Culture and the differentiation of emotional states. *British Journal of Psychiatry, 123,* 299–306.

Levy, R. I. (1973). *Tahitians: Mind and experience in the Society Islands.* Chicago: University of Chicago Press.

Lewis, M., & Rosenblum, L. A. (1978). Introduction: Issues in affect development. In M. Lewis & L. Rosenblum (Eds.), *The development of affect* (pp. 1–10). New York: Plenum Press.

Levenson, R. W. (1994). Human emotion: A functional view. In P. Ekman & R. J. Davidson (Eds.), *The nature of emotion: Fundamental questions* (pp. 123–126). New York: Oxford University Press.

Levenson, R. W., Ekman, P., Heider, K., & Friesen, W. V. (1992). Emotion and autonomic nervous system activity in the Minangkabau of West Sumatra. *Journal of Personality and Social Psychology, 62,* 972–988.

Lutz, C. A. (1987). Goals, events and understanding in Ifaluk emotion theory. In N. Quinn & D. Holland (Eds.), *Cultural models in language and thought* (pp. 290–312). Cambridge, UK: Cambridge University Press.

Lutz, C. A. (1998). *Unnatural emotions: Everyday sentiments on a Micronesian atoll and their challenge to Western theory.* Chicago: University of Chicago Press.

Lutz, C. A., & Abu-Lughod, L. (Eds.). (1990). *Language and the politics of emotion.* Cambridge, UK: Cambridge University Press.

Markus, H. R., & Kitayama, S. (1991). Culture and the self: Implications for cognition, emotion, and motivation. *Psychological Review, 98,* 224–253.

Markus, H. R., & Kitayama, S. (1994). The cultural construction of self and emotion: Implications for social behavior. In S. Kitayama & M. R. Markus (Eds.), *Emotion and culture: Empirical studies of mutual influence* (pp. 89–130). Washington, DC: American Psychological Association.

Matsumoto, D., & Ekman, P. (1989). American-Japanese cultural differences in intensity ratings of facial expressions of emotion. *Motivation and Emotion, 13,* 143–157.

Mauro, R., Sato, K., & Tucker, J. (1992). The role of appraisal in human emotions: A cross-cultural study. *Journal of Personality and Social Psychology, 62,* 301–317.

Mesquita, B. (2000). *Cultural variations in emotions: A comparative study of Dutch, Surinamese and Turkish people in the Netherlands*. Manuscript in preparation.

Mesquita, B. (in press). Emotions in collectivist and individualist contexts. *Journal of Personality and Social Psychology*.

Mesquita, B., & Ellsworth, P. (in press). The role of culture in appraisal. In K. R. Scherer & A. Schorr (Eds.), *Appraisal processes in emotion: Theory, research, application*. New York: Oxford University Press.

Mesquita, B., & Frijda, N. H. (1992). Cultural variations in emotions: A review. *Psychological Bulletin, 112*, 179–204.

Mesquita, B., Frijda, N. H., & Scherer, K. R. (1997). Culture and emotion. In P. Dasen & T. S. Saraswathi (Eds.), *Handbook of cross-cultural psychology* (Vol. 2, pp. 255–297). Boston: Allyn & Bacon.

Mesquita, B., & Karasawa, M. (in press). Different emotional lives. *Cognition and Emotion*.

Mesquita, B., Karasawa, M., Haire, A., & Kobata, H. (2000). *Japanese emotion: A different model*. Unpublished manuscript.

Nisbett, R. E., & Cohen, D. (1996). *Culture of honor: The psychology of violence in the South*. Boulder, CO: Westview Press.

Oatley, K., & Johnson-Laird, P. N. (1987). Towards a cognitive theory of emotions. *Cognition and Emotion, 1*, 29–50.

Oatley, K., & Johnson-Laird, P. N. (1996). The communicative theory of emotions: Empirical tests, mental models, and implications for social interaction. In L. L. Martin & A. Tesser (Eds.), *Striving and feeling: Interactions among goals, affect and self-regulation* (pp. 363–380). Mahwah, NJ: Erlbaum.

Ortony, A., & Turner, T. (1990). What's basic about basic emotions? *Psychological Review, 97*, 315–331.

Plutchik, R. (1980). *Emotion: A psychoevolutionary synthesis*. New York: Harper & Row.

Reise, S. P., & Flannery, W. P. (1996). Assessing person-fit measures of typical performance. *Applied Measurement in Education, 9*, 9–26.

Rosaldo, M. Z. (1980). *Knowledge and passion: Ilongot notions of self and social life*. Cambridge, UK: Cambridge University Press.

Rosch, E. (1978). Principles of categorization. In E. Rosch & B. L. Lloyd (Eds.), *Cognition and categorization* (pp. 27–48). Hillsdale, NJ: Erlbaum.

Roseman, I. J. (1984). Cognitive determinants of emotion: A structural theory. In P. Shaver (Ed.), *Review of personality and social psychology* (Vol. 5, pp. 11–36). Beverly Hills, CA: Sage.

Roseman, I. J., Dhawan, N., Rettek, S. I., Naidu, R. K., & Thapa, K. (1995). Cultural differences and cross-cultural similarities in appraisals and emotional responses. *Journal of Cross-Cultural Psychology, 26*, 23–48.

Russell, J. A. (1991). Cultural variations in emotions: A review. *Psychological Bulletin, 112*(2), 179–204.

Russell, J. A. (1994). Is there universal recognition of emotion from facial expression?: A review of cross-cultural studies. *Psychological Bulletin, 115*, 102–141.

Russell, J. A., & Fernández-Dols, J. M. (1997). What does a facial expression mean? In J. A. Russell & J. M. Fernández-Dols, *The psychology of facial expression* (pp. 14–17). New York: Cambridge University Press.

Sartre, J.-P. (1934/1965). *Esquisse d'une théorie des émotions* [An essay on the theory of emotions]. Paris: Hermann.

Scherer, K. R. (1984). Emotion as a multicomponent process: A model and some cross-cultural data. In P. Shaver (Ed.), *Review of personality and social psychology* (Vol. 5, pp. 37–63). Beverly Hills, CA: Sage.

Scherer, K. R. (1997a). Patterns of emotion-antecedent appraisal across cultures. *Cognition and Emotion, 11,* 113–150.

Scherer, K. R. (1997b). The role of culture in emotion-antecedent appraisal. *Journal of Personality and Social Psychology, 73,* 902–922.

Scherer, K. R., & Schorr, A. (Eds.). (in press). *Appraisal processes in emotion: Theory, methods, research.* New York: Oxford University Press.

Scherer, K. R., & Wallbott, H. G. (1994). Evidence for universality and cultural variation of differential emotion response patterning. *Journal of Personality and Social Psychology, 66,* 310–328.

Scherer, K. R., Wallbott, H. G., Matsumoto, D., & Kudoh, T. (1988). Emotional experience in cultural context: A comparison between Europe, Japan, and the United States. In K. R. Scherer (Ed.), *Facets of emotions* (pp. 5–30). Hillsdale, NJ: Erlbaum.

Scherer, K. R., Wallbott, H. G., & Summerfield, A. B. (Eds.). (1986). *Experiencing emotion: A cross-cultural study.* Cambridge, UK: Cambridge University Press.

Shweder, R. A. (1991). Cultural psychology: What is it? In R. A. Shweder, *Thinking through cultures* (pp. 73–110). Cambridge, MA: Harvard University Press.

Shweder, R. A. (1993). The cultural psychology of the emotions. In M. Lewis & J. M. Haviland (Eds.), *Handbook of emotions* (pp. 417–431). New York: Guilford Press.

Shweder, R. A. (1999, August). *The psychology of practice and the practice of psychology.* Paper presented at the third conference of the Asian Association for Social Psychology, Taipei, Taiwan.

Smith, C. A., & Ellsworth, P. C. (1985). Patterns of cognitive appraisal in emotion. *Journal of Personality and Social Psychology, 48,* 813–838.

Stemmler, D. G. (1989). The autonomic differentiation of emotions revisited: Convergent and discriminant validation. *Psychophysiology, 26,* 617–632.

Tsai, J. L., & Levenson, R. W. (1997). Cultural influences on emotional responding: Chinese American and European American dating couples during interpersonal conflict. *Journal of Cross-Cultural Psychology, 28,* 600–625.

Tsai, J. L., Levenson, R. W., & McCoy, K. (1999). *Are Chinese Americans less emotional than European Americans?: Culture, context, and components of emotion.* Unpublished manuscript, University of Minnesota, Minneapolis.

Van Bezooijen, R. (1984). *Characteristics and recognizability of vocal expressions of emotion.* Dordrecht, Netherlands: Floris.

Van Bezooijen, R., Otto, S. A., & Heenan, T. A. (1983). Recognition of vocal expressions of emotion: A three-nation study to identify universal characteristics. *Journal of Cross-Cultural Psychology, 14,* 387–406.

Wason, P. C., & Johnson-Laird, P. N. (1972). *Psychology of reasoning.* London, UK: Batsford.

White, G. M. (1994). Affecting culture: Emotion and morality in everyday life. In S.

Kitayama & H. Markus (Eds.), *Emotion and culture* (pp. 219–239). Washington, DC: American Psychological Association.

Wierzbicka, A. (1986). Human emotions: Universal or culture-specific? *American Anthropologist, 88,* 584–594.

Wierzbicka, A. (1992). Talking about emotions: Semantics, culture, and cognition. *Cognition and Emotion, 6,* 285–319.

Zajonc, R. B., & McIntosh, D. N. (1992). Emotion research: Some promising questions and some questionable promises. *Psychological Science, 3,* 70–74.

Zammuner, V. L., & Frijda, N. H. (1994). Felt and communication emotions: Sadness and jealousy. *Cognition and Emotion, 8,* 37–53.

8

Emotion Self-Regulation

GEORGE A. BONANNO

The abundance of research on basic emotion processes over the past few decades (and documented in this book) has distinctly demonstrated the important role emotions play in many aspects of daily experience, as well as their influence on adaptation to both ongoing and acute life stressors and transitions. How emotions are best regulated has become a crucial issue for future research on emotion. Considerable debate, for example, has been devoted to the question of whether emotions are best attended to, experienced, and expressed, or suppressed, inhibited, or ignored (Baumeister, Heatherton, & Tice, 1994; Bonanno, in press; Littrell, 1998; Wortman & Silver, 1989). Emotion theorists have only recently begun to develop systemic, guiding principals from which to consider the myriad forms and consequences of emotion regulation (Bonanno & Kaltman, 1999; Gross, 1998a, 1998b). This chapter will consider emotion regulation in the broader context of psychological self-regulation. We begin by elucidating a number of general principals of psychological self-regulation, with a specific emphasis on the role of negative feedback loops, instrumental and exploratory behaviors, schematized goals, and the hierarchical organization of regulatory processes. We integrate this material by proposing three basic categories of psychological self-regulation: control regulation, anticipatory regulation, and exploratory regulation, which we view as organized and enacted in an overarching sequence of regulatory responses. We next apply this regulatory sequence as a framework from which to review and order a number of different processes and behaviors of relevance to the specific question of emotion regulation. Finally, we conclude with suggestions for future research on emotion regulation.

PSYCHOLOGICAL SELF-REGULATION

The idea of self-regulation pivots on the concept of biological and psychological homeostasis. The idea originated with 19th-century anatomist Claude Bernard's observations of the remarkable consistency with which humans maintain a stable internal state or *milieu intérieur* despite nearly constant variation in the external environment (Campbell, 1986). Bernard's nascent observations were later elaborated by Cannon (1939), who coined the term *homeostasis* to describe the encompassing organization of the human nervous system around the goal of biological equilibrium. More recent explications of these ideas have placed increasing emphasis on mechanical metaphors, feedback loops, and goal-driven control systems.

Feedforward and Feedback Loops

An *open-loop* control system involves the instigation of a particular action that simply runs to completion. Open-loop systems are also known as *feedforward* systems because the control action continues regardless of its consequences. The toaster is a classic example. If the control setting is adjusted properly, beautiful slices of toast will dutifully leap from the machine. If, however, the setting does not function properly or is not adequately matched to the particular type of bread that had been inserted, the toast will be either underdone or burnt. Human behavior can sometimes be understood in terms of open-loop control. These are typically automated behaviors that are instigated in situations that call for immediate action and provide little chance for adjustment or monitoring (Wegner & Bargh, 1998), such as a turn of the steering wheel of an automobile to avoid a collision or reaching out a hand to grab a glass that is about to tip over. In these cases, it is usually better to ensure the aversion of a potential catastrophe by instigating a quickly enacted and tightly organized behavior program than to allow for more reflective, higher-order cognitive processes, or more flexible behavioral programs that might avoid unnecessary behaviors but would fail to meet the imperative demands of the immediate situation. LeDoux (1993, 1996) has made a similar point in arguing for the existence of precortical processes that process fear-related stimuli in a rapid but relatively crude manner. Although such processing can produce the unfortunate side effect of a biological fear response in the absence of actual physical danger, from an evolutionary standpoint this disadvantage is far outweighed by the benefits early humans gained by being able to respond quickly to the many potentially fatal dangers they faced.

The vast majority of behaviors that contribute to the ongoing maintenance of homeostasis are met using a second type of regulation based on a *closed-loop* system, or *negative feedback loop*. Negative feedback loops begin with a preset *reference value* and a monitoring mechanism, or *comparator*, which assesses the consequences of a control action in terms of the reference value (Davis, 1979; Powers, 1973). For a given loop, regulatory processes are instigated when a discrepancy or mismatch is detected between the reference value and actual internal or external functioning, and terminated when the discrepancy is no longer apparent.

The functioning of negative feedback loops has typically been illustrated using mechanical metaphors, such as a thermostat or governor. A thermostat registers the fluctuations of temperature in an external environment. When the external temperature deviates from a preset optimal range, the thermostat instigates some sort of regulatory response, usually a cooling or heat-generating device, until the optimal temperature is restored. A mechanical governor monitors the internal state for a specific variable, such as pressure, and increases or decreases this variable through a valve system.

Living systems, including the human organism, are characterized by similar, albeit far more complex, self-regulating mechanisms designed to maintain a relatively constant biological balance (Langley, 1973). Like mechanical mechanisms, human feedback control systems rely heavily on *automaticity*. For instance, humans maintain a remarkably consistent internal temperature. When the demands of the external environment induce even the slightest fluctuation in body temperature, automatic regulatory mechanisms such as sweating or shivering are activated to help return body temperature to its optimal level. However, as Powers (1978) astutely pointed out, mechanical control systems were created by observing and imitating human regulatory functioning, rather than the other way around. A too-literal interpretation of human self-regulation in terms of machine metaphors underestimates the complexity of human functioning. For instance, in addition to the intrinsic homeostatic mechanisms, animals may engage in a variety of *instrumental behaviors* to modify their body temperature, such as seeking shelter or huddling together with other creatures. Humans, of course, may further regulate body temperature using any number of relatively sophisticated instrumental behaviors, such as putting on or removing clothing, turning on an air conditioner or heating unit, or building a fire. Humans may also employ psychological solutions, such as distraction or imagery as employed in biofeedback procedures designed to alter body temperature (Schwartz, 1979).

Instrumental Planning and Exploratory Behaviors

The concept of the negative feedback loop is most clearly applicable in relation to relatively automatic or intrinsic attempts to reduce or erase a state of physical deprivation. However, the alleviation of deprivation alone accounts for only a small portion of human and animal self-regulatory behaviors. Indeed, the alleviation of deprivation does not fully explain even those behaviors associated with relatively simple drive states such as hunger or thirst. For instance, Toates (1986) has noted that although hunger appears to be associated with a strong negative feedback loop, food consumption often goes beyond satiety. Laboratory animals will typically eat to satiety when presented with a single type of food. Yet, if subsequently provided with other novel types of food, the satiated animals will resume eating (Kushner & Mook, 1984). Laboratory rats have also been found to overeat to the point of gross obesity when provided with a variety of sweet and palatable foods (Wirtshafer & Davis, 1977). The same habits have been observed for thirst. Animals that have been infused with water, either intravenously or intragastrically, do not stop drinking water (Nicolaidis & Rowland, 1975).

Although these behaviors are clearly driven by an organizing principle that goes beyond the mere reduction of a state of deprivation, they may still be explained in terms of negative feedback. A critical and often misunderstood feature of the way reference values function within negative feedback control systems is that their output, that is, behavior that might be observed from an objective perspective, is irrelevant (Powers, 1978). *Feedback control systems are organized to keep their inputs matching the reference signal.* Specific behaviors are typically not the goals that drive control systems. Rather, all that is important is that the input back into the system (i.e., the feedback) eventually be brought in line with the driving reference value. As Powers (1978) noted, "behaviors exist only to control consequences that affect the organism" (p. 410). To put this another way, only the end result of behavior, as perceived by the organism in relation to its reference goal, is of relevance to the operation of the control system. This simple but crucial point explains why humans may often behave in a manner that appears to an external observer as irrational, unhealthy, or even psychotic. What may be more appropriately considered irrational or unhealthy are the reference values that drive the control system. However, from the internal perspective of a control system, behaviors are perfectly logical as long as their consequences satisfy the driving reference goal. (We return to this idea at the close of the chapter.)

Extending even further, animal self-regulation is often driven by higher-order feedback loops that encompass instrumental behaviors related to *long-term control needs and intentions.* To return to the example of body temperature regulation, many animals *anticipate* seasonal climate changes by constructing shelters or by migrating to different climate zones. Similarly, humans may *plan* for variations in weather, and hence anticipate changes in body temperature, by watching a weather forecast on television, bringing along extra clothing, purchasing an air conditioner or heater, etc. None of these behaviors can be explained in terms of an immediate automated response to a state of deprivation, yet each is indirectly related to body temperature and may be regulated through a negative feedback control loop.

Finally, self-regulation may be enhanced incidentally through *exploratory behaviors* that foster the development of new skills or the acquisition of additional resources to promote adaptation. For instance, while visiting a Scandinavian country, a person may participate in a traditional sauna and in doing so discover new ways to extend his/her capacity to endure high temperatures. Similarly, the act of reading about expeditions to the polar ice cap or the ascension of a great mountain peak may incidentally teach a person about different ways to endure extreme cold. (We elaborate on the role played by anticipatory and exploratory self-regulation in a later section of this chapter.)

Schematized Goals

To accommodate these more elaborate behaviors, control systems theorists have expanded the concept of the negative feedback to encompass *schematized goals and expectations* (Carver & Scheier, 1981, 1982; Powers, 1973; Scheier & Carver, 1988). In this case, a specific goal serves as the reference value and what is monitored is progress toward the achievement of that goal. Feedback loops may be organized around any number of possible goals. The particular goal or set of goals that may be operative at any given moment will depend to a large extent upon the schemas that have been activated. Like all forms of schematized knowledge structure, these may be activated both by deliberate conscious intention and by relatively automated processes linked to implicit perception or environmental cues (Bargh, 1989; Wegner & Bargh, 1998).

APPLYING SELF-REGULATORY PRINCIPLES TO EMOTION

In this section, we consider several features of psychological self-regulation in their specific application to the regulation of emotion.

Emotional Homeostasis

An imperative distinction to be made is between the view of emotion self-regulation we propose in this chapter and Carver and Scheier's (1990) self-regulatory perspective on the origins and functions of affect. In their view, negative affect is generated as a by-product of the organisms' perception that goal satisfaction is progressing at a slower rate than expected. By the same token, positive affect is thought to arise whenever goal satisfaction progresses at a rate higher than expected. Although we borrow heavily in this chapter from Carver and Scheier's theoretical contributions, the model we propose here does not speak directly to the generation of emotion. Rather, our model pertains to the control, anticipation, and exploration of emotional homeostasis.

But what is emotional homeostasis? As is the case for self-regulation in general, we conceive of the maintenance of emotional homeostasis in terms of schematized goals pertaining to the optimal experience and expression of emotion. This question of optimal levels of emotion is of course rendered more complex if we consider that emotion is not a unidimensional phenomenon, but rather manifests in multiple response channels including experiential or "felt" responses, behavioral or expressive responses, and physiological responses (Buck, 1988; Ekman, 1992; Izard, 1977; Lang, 1979; Levenson, 1988; Leventhal, 1984). In this view, each of these types of emotional response contributes to emotional homeostasis and is therefore subject to emotional self-regulation. Thus, *emotional homeostasis is conceptualized in terms of reference goals pertaining to ideal frequencies, intensities, or duration of experiential, expressive, or physiological channels of emotional responses.*

The specific parameters of what may be considered optimal variants of reactivity will likely vary across emotions. At the level of basic emotional self-control, the question of optimal reactivity pertains primarily to differing degrees of limitations on negative or positive emotions. Sadness, for example, may be tolerable at relatively low intensities for considerable periods of time before it disrupts homeostatic goals. In contrast, emotions associated with strong, relatively automated action tendencies, such as fear, anger, or disgust, may have a narrow range of tolerable expression. There are also instances when it is necessary to control or down-regulate positive emotions. For example, the positive emotions of interest or excitement are thought to foster the attention to and exploration of objects or ideas (Izard, 1977). When intense and focused concentration is required, however, we seek to rein in our interest in irrelevant or distracting objects or ideas. To cite another example, the emotions associated with love or affection are generally discussed in exceedingly desirable terms. Yet, during the complex negotiations and delicacies of human intimate relationships, we sometimes need to control our amorous emotions so as to maintain appropriate conduct or avoid vulnerability.

Self-regulation may also be instigated to up-regulate emotion, that is, to produce or increase it. For example, it may be necessary to stimulate anger or anxiety as a way of focusing attention and maximizing performance. Consider the prototypical pregame speech of the football coach who strives to "pump up" or even anger his team to maximize their concentration and physical endurance. The schematized goals that drive emotional self-regulation may also include regulatory processes that instigate or increase positive emotions. For instance, positive emotions have been found to promote creativity in problem solving and to increase the efficiency and thoroughness of decision making (Isen, 1993; Isen, Daubman, & Nowicki, 1987). Thus, we may attempt to induce pride, interest, or amusement in situations that require problem-solving or decision-making skills. We consider these possibilities in greater detail below when we discuss specific regulatory processes.

The Hierarchical Organization of Regulatory Processes

A crucial feature of control systems in general is their hierarchical organization. For any given situation, a number of different types of regulatory feedback loops may be operative. These loops are organized hierarchically, with *subordinate loops* embedded within *superordinate loops* (Powers, 1973). Superordinate loops tend to be linked to longer-term, abstract goals, whereas subordinate loops are associated with proximal mechanisms (Carver & Scheier, 1981, 1982). The hierarchical organization of regulatory processes suggests a number of important implications for emotional self-regulation. For instance, Baumeister and colleagues have noted that regulatory failures, such as dysregulation, may occur when lower-order mechanisms supersede higher-order mechanisms (Baumeister et al., 1994; Leith & Baumeister, 1996). In terms of emotions, this may occur when phylogenically more immediate and automated emotional processes are instigated that temporarily override more abstracted regulatory processes.

Individual and Cultural Differences

Another important implication of the hierarchical nesting of regulatory feedback loops is that there may be considerable individual and cultural variation as a function of differences in the more abstracted structures of the self, such as *idealized self-images*. In this case, an idealized self-image functions as an abstract reference value in an overriding, superordinate feedback loop (Carver & Scheier, 1990). Because abstract goals are difficult to define and hence difficult to monitor in a regulatory system, idealized self-images function primarily to provide reference values for the subordinate feedback loop at the next lowest level (Powers, 1973). This next-lowest loop, in turn, provides *principles* to guide behavior, such as honesty, generosity, or integrity. Carver and Scheier (1990) described the example of an idealized self-image centered around an image of a kind and caring person. Nested within this idealized self-image loop is a subordinate feedback loop pertaining to the guiding principle of kindness. However, since guiding principle feedback loops, such as kindness, are still relatively abstracted, they function in turn by providing reference values for even more subordinate feedback loops related to *concrete behavioral programs*. In this case, the principle of kindness will have nested within it subordinate behavioral program loops related to such acts as shoveling snow off a neighbor's walk, offering a friend a lift, or giving money to a homeless person. Finally, nested within these behavioral programs will be even more subordinate loops related to *movement sequences*. A fundamental distinction between these two levels is that behavioral programs are more likely to be evoked by conscious intention, whereas movement sequences tend to be highly practiced and thus more likely to involve automated sequences.

Extending these ideas to emotional self-regulation suggests a similar hierarchical structuring based on *ideal emotional selves*. It seems likely that these structures will be organized along basic *personality dimensions*. For instance, emotion regulation for highly agreeable or conscientious individuals may be driven by the superordinate principle of avoiding or minimizing interpersonally disruptive emotions, such as anger or disgust, and the maximization of prosocial emotions, such as amusement or affection (Keltner, Bonanno, Caspi, Kreuger, & Stouthamer-Loeber, 1996). Other individuals may have an ideal-self schema that emphasizes calmness, or the measured expression of emotion, and may employ anticipatory strategies to avoid or obviate the possibility of intense emotion. For instance, if such individuals are participating in a group discussion just as a potentially volatile argument erupts, they may attempt to placate other involved, reappraise the situation so as to distance themselves psychologically from the discussion, dismiss those participating in the argument as "hotheads," or even physically leave the discussion so as to avoid emotional contagion.

Optimal levels of emotional experience or expression will also vary as a function of *interactions between personal self-schemas and situational constraints*. For example, embarrassment is typically instigated by relatively clear situational antecedents (e.g., tripping in public or forgetting the name of a new acquaintance) and, when expressed, tends to evoke relatively consistent responses in others (e.g., amusement, sympathy, or inferences that the embarrassed individual respects the violated norm) (Keltner & Buswell, 1997). However, the extent that individuals value adherence to social norms will also mediate the frequency with which embarrassment is experienced (Miller, 1995) or displayed (Keltner & Buswell, 1997; Keltner, Moffitt, & Stouthamer-Loeber, 1995). Thus, how people construe a situation in relation to their personal goals and values will inform their emotional responses and their subsequent regulatory needs and plans (Mischel & Shoda, 1995).

Another source of variation in the organization of self-structures for emotional self-regulation is found in *cultural norms*. The broad categories of Western and non-Western cultures have been characterized, respectively, as fostering *independent* and *interdependent construals of self* (Markus & Kitayama, 1991). In Markus and Kitayama's (1991) analysis, cultures that emphasize an independent construal of the self encourage individuals to strive for uniqueness, self-expression, direct communication, and the realization of personal goals and internal attributions, whereas cultures that emphasize an interdependent construal of the self encourage individuals to strive to fit in, to occupy their proper place, to communicate indirectly and in relation to the needs of others, and to engage in socially appropriate actions that promote others' goals.

One implication of such differences is that individuals from independent-oriented cultures will attend more to and be more concerned with the regulation of emotional states than do individuals from interdependent-oriented cultures (Ross & Nisbett, 1991; Suh, Diener, Oishi, & Triandis, 1998). For example, American and Japanese students, representing independent and interdependent cultures, respectively, report experiencing approximately similar portions of different emotions, but American students report experiencing their emotions for a longer duration and are more likely to believe that emotions require coping responses, relative to Japanese students (Matsumoto, Kudoh, Scherer, & Walbott, 1988). Similarly, in a study that examined life satisfaction data from over 40 different countries, participants from independent or "individualist" cultures tended to base their life satisfaction judgments primarily on their emotional experiences, whereas participants from interdependent or "collectivist" cultures tended to base their life satisfaction judgments more broadly, using both emotions and cultural norms (Suh et al., 1998).

We might also expect interactions between cultural differences in self-structures and the regulation of specific emotions. The expression of anger, for example, should be considerably more prevalent in cultures that value the independence of the self. Expressions of anger in interdependent or collectivist cultures, on the other hand, are widely thought to impair social harmony and so would more likely be viewed as inappropriate, dysfunctional (Markus & Kitayama, 1991), or even dangerous (Rosenblatt, 1993). To cite another example, bereaved individuals in independent-oriented cultures are typically expected to express certain grief-related emotions, such as sadness, and to minimize or even completely avoid the expression of other emotions, such as amusement or joy, that would be considered inappropriate (Averill & Nunley, 1993). In contrast, people in interdependent cultures tend to deemphasize the negative emotional experiences of bereaved individuals and instead affirm their place in the larger community, often through the overt encouragement of humor, fantasy, and amusement (Bonanno, 1998).

A SEQUENTIAL MODEL OF EMOTIONAL SELF-REGULATION

In this final section of this chapter, we propose a sequential model of emotional self-regulation that incorporates the general features of psychological self-regulation reviewed in preceding sections and serves as an integrative framework from which we can review many different aspects of emotional behavior. We begin by describing a general sequence of self-regulatory activity and then apply this model to the specific question of emotional self-regulation. Finally, we consider the implications of this approach for future research directions.

The different types of self-regulatory processes described earlier suggest three general categories of self-regulatory activity: control regulation, anticipatory regulation, and exploratory regulation. Control regulation encompasses automatic processes and instrumental behaviors associated with the immediate regulation of a psychological or physical state, that is, self-control. Many applications of self-regulation theory to psychological functioning have pertained to self-control. For instance, the concept of self-control has been applied to the delay of gratification (Funder, Block, & Block, 1983), depression (Pyszczynski & Greenberg, 1987), antisocial behaviors (Gottfredson & Hirschi, 1990), and the problems people experience with various impulses and appetites, such as eating, smoking, or gambling (Baumeister et al., 1994; Herman & Polivy, 1975). The second category, anticipatory regulation, pertains to instrumental behaviors that anticipate future control needs, such as attending a support group to gain control over a behavioral problem, or avoiding a gathering of friends in order to resist the anticipated temptation of overindulgence in alcohol. The third category, exploratory regulation, pertains to behaviors that lead to the development of new skills, knowledge, or resources that incidentally enhance self-regulatory efforts. We noted earlier the ways people may inadvertently discover new capacities to regulate body temperature. A person might also engage in a new sport or hobby and by so doing learn that it can also serve as a distraction to keep his/her mind off a tempting bad habit. Likewise, people engage in sundry activities, such as visiting an art gallery or museum, viewing a film, or riding a roller-coaster, often with no specific goal other than amusement or entertainment. Yet, engaging in these activities presents myriad opportunities to observe and understand one's emotional behavior or to learn new emotion self-regulation skills.

We conceptualize these three categories of self-regulatory activity as being activated sequentially in response to the relative immediacy of homeostatic equilibrium. Control regulation is always the most basic and imperative form of self-regulation, superseding all other regulatory behavior. Self-control processes require energy and have been found to conform to a strength and depletion model such that their enactment decreases physical stamina and renders subsequent self-control efforts less efficacious (Muraven, Tice, & Baumeister, 1998). Thus, self-regulatory behaviors normally begin with the question of whether or not there is a relatively stable state of psychological homeostasis. If the answer to this question is no, then a chain of control regulation feedback loops may be instigated with the aim of restoring emotional homeostasis. If the answer is yes, that is, a relatively stable state of homeostasis is apparent or has been achieved, the next question pertains to whether or not psychological homeostasis is likely to be maintained. If the answer to this question is no, then a chain of anticipatory regulation feedback loops may be instigated whose aim is to prepare for and if possible circumvent the need for further control regulation. If the answer is yes, that is, an impending threat to homeostasis in not perceived, then exploratory behaviors are possible that may incidentally foster future self-regulatory efforts.

In the remainder of this chapter, we consider the sequence of self-regulatory processes in terms of their specific application to the question of emotional self-regulation. This sequence is outlined as a flowchart in Figure 8.1.

Control Regulation

When applied to emotion, control regulation pertains to automatic and instrumental behaviors aimed at the immediate regulation of emotional responses that have already been instigated. Gross (1998a; see also Gross & Muñoz, 1995) has described a similar class of emotion regulation processes as *response-focused* emotion regulation These include mechanisms that dampen or short-circuit emotion responses, such as emotional dissociation and suppression, and mechanisms that accentuate emotional response, such as the intensified experience and expression of emotion. The driving reference goal behind control regulation of emotion is the maintenance or restoration of emotional homeostasis within the constraints of specific emotions and their interaction with individual, cultural, and situational variations.

Emotional Dissociation

The most basic forms of control regulation involve relatively automated shifts in attention away from the experience of undesirable emotion. Although discrete emotions are generally thought to produce a coordinate set of emotional responses or response programs, it is widely accepted that different types of emotional responses may occur partially independently from one another such that emotion may sometimes be indicated at one response channel and absent, or even contradicted, at another response channel

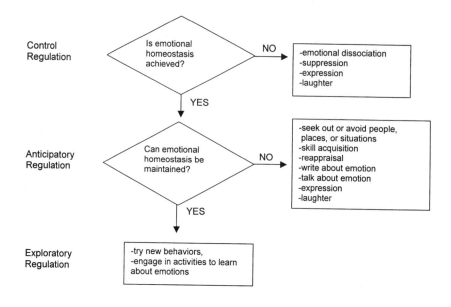

FIGURE 8.1. Self-regulation flowchart.

(Buck, 1988; Ekman, 1992; Izard, 1977, 1992; Lang, 1979; Lang, Kozak, Miller, Levin, & McLean, 1980; Levenson, 1994; Leventhal, 1984, 1991; Schwartz, Fair, Greenberg, Freedman, & Klerman, 1974; Schwartz, Fair, Salt, Mandel, & Klerman, 1976). For example, subjective emotional responses may be experienced in the absence of overt behavioral expression (Schwartz et al., 1974). By the same token, observable emotional responses or physiological changes are not necessarily always accompanied by the subjective experience of emotion (Izard, 1977; Lang, Levin, Miller, & Kozak, 1983; Leventhal, 1991; Schwartz, 1982).

When relatively little negative emotion is experienced during potentially stressful situations despite evidence of emotional responsivity at other channels, it can be assumed that emotional dissociation is operative and performs a defensive or regulatory function (Bonanno & Singer, 1990; Krohne, 1992; Lazarus, 1966; Newton & Contrada, 1992). In the context of self-regulation theory, we would conclude that emotional dissociation serves the function of shifting attention so as to short-circuit or nullify the undesired emotional response output, or to instigate a competing emotional response that might override the undesired response. Although such dissociative shifts in attention may be linked to longer-term goals and personality-based emotional habits, they manifest at a subordinate point in the regulatory hierarchy, close to the output end of the chain of control responses, and thus function in a virtually automated fashion (Bonanno, Keltner, Holen, & Horowitz, 1995).

It is important to note here the distinction between emotional dissociation and the more extreme type of dissociation often linked to psychopathology. The term "dissociation," when used in clinical nomenclature, typically refers to severe or pathological splits in consciousness and identity (Bernstein & Putnam, 1986; Hilgard, 1986; James, 1890). Emotional dissociation, in contrast, refers to a transient shift in the focus of attention away from awareness of a particular, and usually negative, emotional response. (We return to this distinction below.)

One of the most widely used measures of emotional dissociation is *affective–autonomic response dissociation*, which is observed when subjective emotional experience is minimal in comparison with the strength of the autonomic response (Newton & Contrada, 1992). Evidence for the construct validity of the affective–autonomic discrepancy scores as a measure of emotional dissociation has come from several sources. Consistent with its assumed link to personality-based emotional control habits, a number of studies have shown that affective–autonomic dissociation is particularly likely to be observed among individuals categorized as repressors (Asendorpf & Scherer, 1983; Newton & Contrada, 1992; Weinberger & Davidson, 1994; Weinberger, Schwartz, & Davidson, 1979). In related research, repressors have shown a general propensity to selectively attend away from threatening information (Fox, 1993), report more interfering thoughts while attempting to focus attention in the presence of threat (Bonanno, Davis, Singer, & Schwartz, 1991), and evidence greater task interference when the selective avoidance of threatening stimuli was not possible (Dawkins & Furnham, 1989). Furthermore, despite their consistent self-reports of low distress, repressors typically exhibit elevated physiological arousal (Asendorpf, & Scherer, 1983; Newton & Contrada, 1992; Weinberger et al., 1979) and show greater observer-rated distress (Asendorpf & Scherer, 1983; Fox, O'Boyle, Barry, & McCreary, 1989). When repressors' elevated levels of arousal are brought to their attention, they tend to doubt the accuracy of the autonomic equipment rather than revise their subjective appraisals (Weinberger & Davidson, 1994). Furthermore, consistent with its personality manifestations, affective–autonomic dissociation has shown relatively high test–retest reliability over an 8-month interval (Bonanno et al., 1995).

The shift of awareness away from distressing emotion has traditionally been viewed as a form of maladaptive denial. Shedler, Mayman, and Manis (1993) argued that this form of emotional circumvention masks an individual's true level of distress, thus creating an "illusion of mental health" and increasing the risk for subsequent deterioration in mental and physical health. However, from an the perspective of emotional self-regulation, the question is less of adaptiveness than of what relationship the behavior holds to the driving reference value (Powers, 1978). If the particular reference value guiding the system is aimed at reducing the experience of emotion, than affective–autonomic dissociation would be an effective control behavior. If, on the other hand, the driving reference value is aimed at reducing the overt expression of emotion, then affective–autonomic dissociation would probably be a relatively ineffective control choice. For instance, affective–autonomic dissociation has been found to correlate with clinical ratings of the avoidance of emotional awareness, suggesting that it may be observed by others and thus an ineffective means of masking emotion.

In terms of the longer-term consequences of emotional dissociation, it has been suggested that whether this mechanism, or any other regulatory mechanism for that matter, is salubrious or deleterious will depend on myriad factors, including the frequency of its use and the particular demands of the situations in which it may be employed (Bonanno & Siddique, 1999; Paulhus, Fridhandler, & Hayes, 1997). Consistent with this reasoning, a recent study of conjugal bereavement showed that affective–autonomic dissociation was a reasonably effective means of coping with the pain of losing a spouse. In this study, affective–autonomic dissociation was measured as bereaved individuals talked about their loss and compared with clinical ratings of grief, self-reported somatic complaints, and frequency of doctor visits across 25 months of bereavement (Bonanno et al., 1995; Bonanno, Znoj, Siddique, & Horowitz, 1999). Individuals who employed affective–autonomic dissociation at the 6-month point in bereavement were rated by the clinical interviewers as having less grief than other participants through the 25 months of the study, even when initial levels of grief were statistically controlled.

It is noteworthy, however, that affective–autonomic dissociation in this same study was also linked to concurrent increases in somatic complaints, thus indicating some cost. However, participants showing affective–autonomic dissociation returned to low levels of somatic complaints at later assessments and were not different from other participants in their frequency of doctor visits. Together, these findings suggest that the "cost" of affective–autonomic dissociation during bereavement may be relatively short lived and outweighed by the coping advantages it offers. These findings are also of particular interest in light of Taylor's (1991) mobilization–minimization hypothesis, which posits that the mobilization of coping resources is an effective short-term response to adverse events, whereas long-term adaptation is generally characterized by processes that dampen, minimize, or even erase the intensity of the negative event. The fact that affective–autonomic dissociation among bereaved individuals produced an initial health cost suggests that it may interfere with the adaptive benefits of the early mobilization response. By the same token, however, the long-term salutary effects of affective–autonomic dissociation suggests that in some situations the long-term minimization response may hold a crucial and perhaps overriding impact.

In another recent study, affective–autonomic dissociation among sexually abused adolescent girls correlated with significantly fewer trauma symptoms (Bonanno, Noll, Putnam, Lomakina, & Trickett, 1999). Importantly, this study also provided direct evidence to support the distinction between affective–autonomic dissociation as a potentially adaptive emotional regulatory mechanism and pathological dissociation as a clinically relevant split in consciousness and identity. In this study, both sexually abused adolescents and nonabused controls who showed affective–autonomic dissociation as they described their most stressful experiences scored significantly *lower* on questionnaire measures of pathological dissociation (Bonanno et al., 1999).

Emotional Suppression

The minimization of emotion response outputs may also occur at a more superordinate level of the feedback control hierarchy in the form of deliberate conscious suppression of emotional output. Gross and Levenson (1993) defined suppression as the conscious inhibition of emotional expressive behaviors while emotionally aroused. To investigate this process, they showed undergraduates a disgust-eliciting film. Students in the suppression condition were instructed to behave "in such a way that a person watching you would not know you were feeling anything" (suppression condition), while control students were simply told to view the film. This approach produced two intriguing findings. First, although participants in the suppression condition showed a complex mix of physiological responses, the suppression and no suppression conditions did not differ in self-reported emotion. From a emotional self-regulation perspective, this finding suggests that if the driving reference goal is to control or reduce the experience of emotion, then the suppression of emotional response behaviors, at least for the specific emotion of disgust, is not likely to be very effective. A second set of findings, however, showed that participants in the suppression condition did manage to show less expressive behavior indicative of disgust, had reduced facial movement, less body movement, and touched their faces less often, but blinked more often than participants in the control condition. These findings indicate that if the reference goal is to conceal emotion, then suppression is likely to be an effective control strategy. However, since eye blinks are generally correlated with arousal (Stern, Walrath, & Goldstein, 1984), it is not clear to what extent this behavior may "leak" participants true emotional state to others.

In subsequent studies, Gross (1998a) and Gross and Levenson (1997) replicated these findings, again showing that the instruction to suppress emotional expression had little impact on the subjective experience of negative emotion (in this case, disgust and sadness), but was an effective means of concealing emotion from others. However, these studies also more clearly linked the suppression of emotional expression to increased cardiovascular arousal. Although longitudinal data were not collected, it was argued that repeated attempts to suppress emotional expression may have long-term health consequences (Gross, 1997).

Emotional Expression

The evolution of facial expressive behaviors is commonly understood in terms of the increased capacity for communication they afford. However, there is increasing evidence that in addition to their communicative function facial muscle movements also play an important role in the activation and regulation of emotional experience (Darwin, 1872; Izard, 1977, 1990; Laird, 1974; Tomkins, 1962). Tomkins (1962) argued that facial expressions contribute to people's awareness of their emotional experiences. Izard and Malatesta (1987) noted that the capacity to regulate emotions is closely associated with the development of skills related to the inhibition, attenuation, or amplification of spontaneous facial expressions. Zajonc, Murphy, and Inglehart (1989) argued that facial expressions influence emotional experiences by altering the flow of blood to the brain. They provided compelling evidence in support of this idea by showing that specific facial muscle movements alone, independent of cognitive mediation, altered subsequent affective experiences. Finally, Ekman and Davidson (1993) provided striking evidence that deliberately induced smiles could produce patterns of regional brain activity similar to those observed in relation to genuine positive emotion.

From a clinical perspective, the overt expression of negative or painful emotions is widely assumed to be necessary for mental health (Shedler et al., 1993). Emotional expression has long been thought to be particularly important in the aftermath of highly stressful or traumatic events (Freud, 1917/1957; Horowitz, 1986; Littrell, 1998; Pennebaker, 1989; Raphael, 1983). However, it is generally accepted that the unrestrained expression of the emotions associated with distressing events may also impede psychological recovery from those events (van der Kolk, 1996). Furthermore, it has become clear that in some types of highly stressful situations the overt expression of negative emotions may be maladaptive (Bonanno & Siddique, 1999). For example, a recent study of facial expressions and bereavement showed that the increased facial expression of negative emotion in the early months after the death of a spouse predicted a more protracted grief course, even when initial levels of grief and the self-reported experience of emotion were statistically controlled (Bonanno & Keltner, 1997). Furthermore, the associations between facial expressions and poor outcome were particularly strong for expressions of anger, an emotion whose expression many bereavement theorists believe to be essential for recovery (see, e.g., Belitsky & Jacobs, 1986; Cerney & Buskirk, 1991). This study also showed that the facial expression of positive emotions, generally assumed to be of little consequence during bereavement, predicted reduced levels of grief at subsequent assessments.

Laughter

One of the more intriguing forms of control regulation through emotional expression is laughter. Although genuine (or Duchenne) laughter is unmistakably associated with the experience of positive emotion (Duchenne de Bologne, 1862/1990; Frank, Ekman, & Friesen, 1993), it often occurs in contexts that are not necessarily positive. Indeed, a number of investigators have noted that laughter often arises in negative contexts and accompanies shifts toward more positive states. Positive emotions in general have been conceptualized as "undoers" of negative emotion (Fredrickson & Levenson, 1998; Levenson, 1988). Laughter in particular has been associated with the adoption of a novel perspective and with the experience of gaining of insight into an undesirable, unexpected, or dangerous situation, and thus appears to accompany the shift toward more positive states (Martin & Lefcourt, 1983; Rothbart, 1973).

Several pieces of evidence in support of the "laughter-as-dissociation" hypothesis were provided in the context of bereavement (Bonanno, 1999). Traditional bereavement theory has viewed positive emotions as either infrequent, and therefore insignificant, or as indicators of maladaptive denial (see, e.g., Bowlby, 1980). However, videotapes of bereaved individuals talking about the recent death of their spouses revealed that the majority (58%) showed genuine laughter at least once (Bonanno & Keltner, 1997). Furthermore, bereaved individuals who showed genuine laughter while talking about their loss tended to do so most often when discussing angry feelings about the lost deceased (Bonanno & Keltner, 1999). Finally, the bereaved individuals who laughed while talking about their loss experienced more positive and less negative emotion than did nonlaughers, and were significantly more likely than nonlaughers to evidence affective–autonomic response dissociation (Keltner & Bonanno, 1997).

Anticipatory Regulation

When a relative state of emotional homeostasis has been achieved, the immediate needs for control regulation are minimal. At this point in the regulatory sequence the next form of evaluation pertains to goals oriented around anticipated challenges to homeostasis. Anticipatory regulation includes instrumental behaviors that anticipate future control needs, such as fixing an air conditioner to help meet anticipated temperature variations, as well as approach–avoidance behaviors, such as attending a support group to help gain control over a behavioral problem or avoiding a gathering of friends to help resist the anticipated temptation of overindulgence in alcohol. In emotional self-regulation, anticipatory regulation involves identifying and adjusting facets of the emotion control hierarchy so as to better maintain emotional homeostasis. Anticipatory regulation of emotion encompasses expressive behaviors, the avoidance of or seeking out of people, places, or situations that may alter control needs, attempts to modify the meaning of potentially emotionally charged situations through reappraisal or cognitive reschematization, attempts to acquire new regulatory skills, and attempts to influence interactions with other people through the expression of emotion.

Emotional Expression

In addition to its role in the control of emotional experience, the overt expression of emotion also plays a role in the management of situational factors associated with the anticipation of control needs. It is generally acknowledged that primates utilize a wide array of gestures and expressions as a means of indicating relative social status, averting conflict, and eliciting supportive responses from other animals (Goodall, 1986; de Waal, 1989). In a similar manner, facial expressions in humans may anticipate subsequent emotion control needs by evoking responses in others that shape the demands of the social interaction (Ekman, 1992; D. Keltner & J. Haidt, Chapter 6, this volume; Lazarus, 1991; Oatley & Jenkins, 1996). For example, an overt expression of anger may by used to increase the social distance between the self and another person. Sadness may be expressed as a means of evoking support or sympathy, or dissuading others from possible aggressive behavior. Expressions of embarrassment may be evoked as a means of correcting social transgressions and prompting forgiveness from others (Goffman, 1967; Keltner & Buswell, 1997), thus averting possible negative social encounters.

Laughter

Like emotional expression in general, laughter also appears to serve important anticipatory regulation functions. For instance, laughter tends to foster group cohesiveness (Vinton, 1989) and to evoke positive emotions in others through the phenomenon of contagion (Hatfield, Cacioppo, & Rapson,

1992: Keltner & Bonanno, 1997; Provine, 1992). Laughter has also been found to evoke more favorable judgments from others and to be associated with more satisfying interpersonal relationships (Keltner & Bonanno, 1997). Thus, laughter may anticipate control needs related to negative interpersonal emotions, such as shame, sadness, or anger, by fostering interpersonal cohesion or by assuaging potential interpersonal conflicts.

Avoiding or Seeking Out People, Places, and Situations

Encounters with people, places, or specific types of situations can evoke emotion in ways that may be plainly anticipated. For example, an awkward interpersonal exchange with a neighbor may predictably result in shame or embarrassment upon a subsequent encounter. In the simplest terms, we may avoid such an encounter as a means of obviating these disquieting emotions. Behavioral avoidance of even greater urgency is often noted as a symptom of posttraumatic stress disorder (Horowitz, 1986; van der Kolk, 1996). Traumatized individuals anticipate the intense emotion they experience in situations that remind them of their traumatic past and avoid such encounters in anticipation of the psychological disruption they tend to induce. By the same token, we are drawn toward situations that may have generated past experiences of a positive nature or toward encounters that we may anticipate as being pleasant or helpful. Thus, we may seek out positive emotion-generating experiences as a means of bolstering our control resources.

Acquisition of New Skills

Just as we may decide to purchase an air conditioner in anticipation of difficulties with excessively warm weather, we may also seek out ways to develop or improve our emotion control skills. An obvious example of this type of anticipatory regulation is participation in psychotherapy to control emotion-related difficulties such as anxiety or depression. For example, exposure treatments such as systematic desensitization or stress inoculation training have as their explicit goal helping patients gain skills to confront and manage fear (Rothbaum & Foa, 1996). People may also seek new skills for regulating emotion through popular press psychology books, workshops, or by learning tension-reducing activities such as yoga or dance.

Reappraisal

Another means by which emotion regulatory needs may be anticipated is through the reappraisal of a potentially emotion-inducing situation into one that is relatively unemotional (Gross & Muñoz, 1998a). Gross (1998a) examined the correlates of reappraisal directly by informing undergraduates that they would be shown a disgust-eliciting medical film and then instructing them to "adopt a detached and unemotional attitude . . . to think about what you are seeing objectively . . . in such a way that you don't feel anything at all" (p. 227). He compared the subjective, expressive, and physiological responses of participants receiving this instruction with those of other participants who were either instructed to suppress any overt expression of emotion or instructed simply to watch the film. Participants in the reappraisal condition showed reductions in expressive behavior approximately equal to those observed among participants in the suppression condition. Further, reappraisal resulted in the reduced experience of disgust, whereas suppression, as reported above, did not influence the subjective experience of emotion. Together, these findings suggest that reappraisal may serve as an effective means of managing both the experience and expression of emotion in situations when one can anticipate the need to control these emotions. However, whether these findings generalize beyond the specific emotion of disgust has yet to be demonstrated.

Writing about Distressing Events

A related form of anticipatory regulation is found in the act of writing about emotional or distressing events. It should be noted that writing about emotion in general may act as a form of control regulation. Writing may help a person organize confused emotions, or it may provide distance so as to allow a person to understand and gain control of emotions as they are being experienced (Macnab, Beckett, Park, & Sheckter, 1998). However, as argued below, when the empirical evidence is considered as a whole, writing about emotional events is more appropriately understood as a form of anticipatory regulation similar to reappraisal. However, whereas reappraisal manifests as the reinterpretation of a potentially emotion-inducing situation in unemotional terms, writing appears to involve more elaborate cognitive restructuring of emotional experiences so as to allow their integration with existing cognitive schematic structures and to facilitate anticipated control efforts (Sgoutas-Emch & Johnson, 1998).

There is abundant empirical evidence that writing about emotional responses in the specific context of distressing or traumatic events can exert a salutary impact on long-term health (Pennebaker, 1989, 1990). In a study typical of this approach, Pennebaker and Beall (1986) randomly assigned undergraduates students to different disclosure conditions and asked them to write about specific topics on four consecutive nights. One group wrote about their emotional reactions to a trauma, defined as "a personally upsetting experience" (p. 275), while a second group wrote only about the facts associated with a trauma; a third group wrote about both trauma-related emotions and facts; and a fourth group wrote only about trivial topics each night. The student's psychological and physiological reactions were monitored each day of the study. Self-reported health data were collected 4 months later, and records from health and counseling centers were collected for a period beginning 6 months prior to the writing of the essays and for 6 months afterward. Overall, writing about traumatic experiences was associated with short-term increases in physiological arousal and negative mood. However, over the long term, writing about trauma resulted in decreased health problems. These findings were most pronounced for the groups that wrote about their emotional reactions to the traumas.

Pennebaker and colleagues' earliest theoretical explanations for the salutary impact of written disclosure were based on the idea that disclosure makes emotional suppression or inhibition unnecessary (Pennebaker, 1989). According to this view, not disclosing, or keeping private, one's personal or emotional reactions to a traumatic event is an act of emotional control similar to inhibition or suppression. Over the long term, the repeated act of inhibition produces a cumulative stress on the body and eventual increased vulnerability to stress-related illness (Selye, 1976). In contrast, the act of writing makes it possible to experience and review one's emotional responses in a relative safe and structured context and thus reduces the need for emotional inhibition. Empirical support for this explanation has been garnered in a variety of samples, including undergraduates and medical students writing about personally distressing events (Pennebaker, Hughes, & O'Heeron, 1987; Pennebaker, Kiecolt-Glaser, & Glaser, 1988; Petrie, Booth, Pennebaker, Davison, & Thomas, 1995), undergraduates who were seropositive for Epstein–Barr syndrome (Esterling, Antoni, Fletcher, Margulies, & Schneiderman, 1994), and Holocaust survivors (Pennebaker & Barger, 1988).

Importantly, several studies have also been reported that have either failed to replicate the general salutary effect or to support the inhibition theory fully. In one study (Greenberg & Stone, 1992), undergraduates wrote over a period of 4 days about either a trauma they had never previously discussed, a trauma that they had already discussed with others, or trivial events. Although the groups did not differ in physical symptoms or visits to health professionals over time, physical symptoms were reduced across groups among students who by their own subjective estimate wrote about more severe traumas. In other words, the health benefits of writing about traumatic material appeared to be less related to that act of disclosure than to the severity of the material.

More recently, Pennebaker and colleagues have adopted a broader explanatory framework that suggests an even more straightforward link to the anticipatory regulation of emotion. In this broader view, writing helps individuals structure, and ultimately understand and control, their emotional reactions (Pennebaker, 1993). For instance, Pennebaker, Colder, and Sharp (1990) observed that students transitioning to college who wrote about their experiences had not yet had time to be influenced by the long-term negative effects of inhibition yet evidenced similar health benefits to those in prior experiments who wrote about past traumas. Thus, they concluded, "the value of writing about thoughts and feelings . . . may have simply been to assimilate their leaving home with current college experiences. Assimilation rather than reduction in inhibition may have been the key variable that promoted health" (p. 535). Pennebaker (1993) analyzed the writing samples from several previous studies and found that the descriptions provided by participants who had improved the most evidenced increasingly more frequent use of insightful, causal, and cognitive words over the course of the several days of writing.

From the perspective of emotional self-regulation, these data suggest that writing about emotional events provides an opportunity to observe and recognize how traumatic or distressing events may have interacted with one's own idealized self-images (Bonanno & Kaltman, 2000; Bonanno & Keuler, 1998). This understanding, in turn, may further reveal how such events may have triggered, or may continue to activate, a hierarchical chain of subordinate emotional control responses centered around the violation of a self-schema and its guiding principles. For instance, consider again the example of an idealized self-schema leading to the guiding principle of kindness and the subordinate behavioral programs associated with kind actions. Now consider the case in which an individual possessing such a self-schema is assaulted and comes to associate kindness with vulnerability, anger, or shame. If this occurs, the guiding principle and the emotions it generates may develop links to competing behavioral programs associated with the emotional control (i.e., suppression or emotional dissociation) of the painful emotions. By writing about such an event and the emotional responses it generates, it becomes possible to identify the associative links to such emotions, to anticipate their activation, and to develop more appropriate and presumably healthier control strategies.

Consistent with this view, King and Miner (2000) recently demonstrated that writing about the perceived benefits of a traumatic event—personal growth, meaning, etc.—induced health benefits similar to that of writing about the emotional aspects of the event. Similar to the argument advanced above, they concluded that writing about perceived benefits may "spur self-regulatory processes" by providing "an opportunity to confront, control, and structure thoughts and feelings" (p. 227) associated with the trauma.

Talking about Distressing Events

In contrast to the large body of data demonstrating the health benefits of writing about such events, the efficacy of talking about emotional events as a form of self-regulation appears to be more situationally determined. Although the vast majority of highly emotional events tend to be shared with others (Rime, Mesquita, Philippot, & Boca, 1991, 1992), the verbal disclosure of private emotional experiences has not always proved adaptive (Kelly, 1998; Kelly & McKillop, 1996; Rime et al., 1991). People who experience a difficult life event may long to share the experience with another, and they may gain from sharing in a manner similar to that described above for written disclosure. However, the social nature of verbal communication brings with it the added possibility of rejection or alienation from those who might offer support (Silver, Wortman, & Crofton, 1990). Thus, choosing whether or not to talk about emotional or distressing events is somewhat of a "cruel paradox" (Harber & Pennebaker, 1992).

There is nonetheless compelling evidence that is some contexts verbal disclosure of highly emotional secrets may prove quite adaptive. A recent study examined verbal disclosure to close friends in the context of pediatric AIDS (Sherman, Bonanno, Wiener, & Battles, 2000). In this case, disclosure was particularly complex because of the social stigma associated with AIDS and because HIV/AIDS is often acquired in children through vertical transmission (i.e., it is received from the parents). Thus, verbal disclosure may generalize the negative stigma of AIDS to their family as a whole. Despite these possible untoward consequences, Sherman et al. found that children who disclosed their HIV/AIDS status to friends during the 1-year period of the study showed greater increases in immune response (CD4%) compared to children who had disclosed their HIV/AIDS status at an earlier point in time or who had not yet disclosed it.

Exploratory Regulation

The third category, exploratory regulation, pertains to behaviors that lead to the development of new skills, knowledge, or resources that incidentally enhance self-regulatory efforts. When no immediate or pending control needs are perceived, we are free to engage in exploratory behaviors that may incidentally enhance our abilities or resources for maintaining emotional homeostasis. The goals that drive exploratory regulation are less explicit and more highly abstracted than those that drive control and anticipatory regulation. For this reason, many forms of exploratory regulation involve activities that evoke positive emotions, such as interest or joy, as a means of sustaining these activities (Fredrickson, 1998; see also B. L. Frederickson & C. Branigan, Chapter 4, this volume).

Emotional Regulation in Entertainment

Exploratory regulation can occur in the context of what we would normally consider passive entertainment: reading a novel, viewing a film, or trying out a ride at an amusement part. In addition to whatever diversion, entertainment, or pleasure these experiences may provide, they also promote emotion regulation by providing a means of trying on, experiencing, and observing various emotions in a safe context. A classic example of exploratory regulation is found in the oral tradition of the folktale. Scholars of folklore have long argued that prototypic tales from a particular region can reveal both universal and local cultural values and assumptions (Dundes, 1980; Thompson, 1946/1977). Folktales take on such meanings by virtue of the fact that they are formed as part of an oral tradition and represent the experiential reality of the listener. In other words, folktales take shape gradually, through repeated telling, augmentation, and revision until they fully capture the interest of their listeners and effectively transport them to other worlds where various moral and social dilemmas are played out (Dundes, 1980; Price & Price, 1991). Even though the characters in oral tales do not always manage to resolve the dilemmas in which they find themselves, listeners can still share in the protagonists' emotions and learn what the potential solutions may feel like (Abrahams, 1983). It has been argued that modern literature emerged from the oral tradition (Thompson, 1947/1977) and that in contemporary culture the novel serves a comparable function of transporting the reader through the emotional dilemmas of its characters.

Films provide a less systematic but perhaps even more powerful avenue for exploratory emotion regulation. For instance, a person viewing a stirring romantic film may experience intense passion or sadness without the vulnerability that comes from actual interpersonal investment and commitment. Film critics have noted that romantic films, or "tearjerkers," provide tight structural boundaries through which the characters "work out complex emotional issues" (Schoemer, 1998, p. 40), all from the relative safety of a seat in a darkened movie theater. Similarly, thrillers and horror films allow viewers to experience the visceral dread of pending physical harm without the actual physical consequences. No matter how stirring or frightening such films may be, they cease when the theater lights come on and viewers return to their normal lives. The same appears to be true of films about war. Noted filmmaker Stanley Kubrick, for instance, was quoted by a friend as having said, "I'd never go to war, but I'd like to experience it if I knew I wasn't going to get hurt" (Bogdanovich, 1999, p. 25).

A person might also explore similar exhilarating or frightening emotions on an amusement ride such as the roller-coaster. In this case, as the roller-coaster slowly rises to its apex and then plunges madly downward, he/she may experience the actual physical sensations associated with fear while at the same time holding on, literally, to the knowledge that the ride is ostensibly safe. In each of these examples, the individual enters a situation with the full knowledge that no real personal harm will be possible.

Yet, the stimulus, whether a scary movie or a roller-coaster, is sufficiently intense to generate emotions we cannot normally experience in everyday circumstances. The safety of the context combined with the strength of the stimulus provides us with the opportunity to watch ourselves, to explore, observe, and learn about intense emotional responses.

Emotional Regulation in Activity

Exploratory regulation can also take the form of engaging in activities that incidentally promote emotion self-regulation. For example, a person may develop an interest in high-risk sporting activities such as rock climbing or parachuting. The ostensible motivation may be the shear thrill these sports offer. However, the person engaging in such sports may also inadvertently develop new concentration skills, or find new ways to manage negative emotions or accentuate positive emotions. To cite another example, a person may decide the time is right to finally learn formal dancing. Here the ostensible motivation may be oriented around gaining a new social outlet. Yet, dance classes may also incidentally provide a means of practicing the regulation of interpersonal emotions.

Writing about Emotion

The paradigm of writing about emotional or traumatic events as a form of anticipatory regulation, discussed above, may also be adapted in a more incidental exploratory manner. In this case, the topic of the writing would be less closely tied to concrete personal events so as to allow the exploration of possible selves and possible solutions to emotional control needs. Diary writing has long been utilized as a simple but effective tool for therapeutic exploration, self-understanding, and self-expression (Hettich, 1990; Macnab et al., 1998; Rabinor, 1998).

A recent study by Greenberg, Wortman, and Stone (1996) provided a compelling example of how exploratory writing can prove useful even with relatively traumatic material. Greenberg and colleagues preselected a sample of undergraduates who had actual traumatic experiences and then asked the students to provide the factual details of the traumatic events. Participants in this study engaged in the usual variation of writing conditions. However, Greenberg and colleagues also added a novel condition in which some participants were provided the factual details of another person's traumatic experience, asked to imagine themselves having this experience, and then to write about their emotional reactions. At a 1-month follow-up, both participants who wrote about their own traumas and participants who wrote about their imaginary reactions to another person's trauma had fewer illness visits to doctors and fewer self-reported physical symptoms than did the control group. Greenberg and colleagues' explanation for these findings, consistent with the idea of exploratory self-regulation, was that imagining another person's trauma may "foster self-empathy by allowing participants to observe their own emotional pain in . . . [a] context uncontaminated by knowledge of failed coping efforts and associated self-derogation" (p. 599) and, in doing so, may help trauma sufferers understand and gain mastery over their reactions and thus construct more "resilient possible selves" (p. 599).

FUTURE RESEARCH DIRECTIONS

The application of control systems theory to the question of emotion regulation is still in its earliest stages. Myriad avenues for future research and theory building are possible. For example, most emotion regulation theorists focus on the control or down-regulation of unpleasant or undesirable emotions. The theoretical perspective elucidated in this chapter suggests, however, that there is more to emotion self-regulation than the simple control of unwanted emotions, that anticipatory and exploratory processes are worthy of consideration, and that in some contexts emotion regulation may also involve increasing or up-regulating certain emotions. Empirical investigation in this area would greatly enhance the field.

Perhaps the most promising direction for future empirical investigations pertains to the question of whether specific emotion self-regulation stategies and behaviors are adaptive or maladaptive. Psychology has made relatively little progress in this area. Despite decades of research, questions as to whether it is best to suppress or express emotions, or confront or avoid them, remain mired in controversy (Baumeister et al., 1994; Bonanno, 1998; Littrell, 1998; Wortman & Silver, 1989). The perspective of emotional self-regulation suggests an important point of departure for future research on these questions. In contrast to the traditional approaches, which evaluate the relative adaptation of any given behavior in terms of predetermined objective criteria for outcome, the emotional self-regulation perspective places its primary emphasis on the internal logic of the control system. In other words, as noted earlier, specific regulatory behaviors such as suppression or dissociation cannot be understood from an objective perspective but only in terms of the reference values that are currently in operation and that drive the control system. As Powers (1978) noted, "behaviors exist only to control consequences that affect the organism" (p. 419).

This is not to say that any behavior is appropriate as long as it is concordant with a driving reference goal. The internal logic of the control system may be consistent but in itself may be flawed and maladaptive. To cite once again the example of an idealized self-schema for a kind person, if this schema were too rigid and dominating, it would provide guiding principles for kind behavior that would be almost impossible to maintain and that would no doubt result in conflict (e.g., attempting to be kind in a socially inappropriate or even dangerous manner). Rather, what this view implies is that before we psychologists can clearly understand any emotion self-regulation behavior, we must investigate it in the context of the broader control system. In other words, emotion self-regulation must be investigated in the context of situation-specific, culture-specific, and personality-specific self-schemas and reference goals.

REFERENCES

Abrahams, R. D. (1983). *African folktales*. New York: Pantheon.

Asendorpf, J. B., & Scherer, K. R. (1983). The discrepant repressor: Differentiation between low anxiety, high anxiety, and repression of anxiety by autonomic–facial–verbal patterns of behavior. *Journal of Personality and Social Psychology, 45*, 1334–1346.

Averill, J. R., & Nunley, E. P. (1993). Grief as an emotion and as a disease: A social-constructionist perspective. In. M. S. Stroebe, W. Stroebe, & R. O. Hansson (Eds.), *Handbook of bereavement: Theory, research, and intervention* (pp. 367–380). Cambridge, UK: Cambridge University Press.

Bargh, J. A. (1989). Conditional automaticity: Varieties of automatic influence in social perception and cognition. In J. S. Uleman & J. A. Bargh (Eds.), *Unintended thought* (pp. 3–51). New York: Guilford Press.

Baumeister, R. F., Heatherton, T. F., & Tice, D. M. (1994). *Losing control: How and why people fail at self-regulation*. New York: Academic Press.

Belitsky, R., & Jacobs, S. (1986). Bereavement, attachment theory, and mental disorders. *Psychiatric Annals, 16*, 276–280.

Bernstein, E. M., & Putnam, F. W. (1986). Development, reliability, and validity of a dissociation scale. *Journal of Nervous and Mental Disease, 174*, 727–735.

Bogdanovich, P. (1999, July 4). What they say about Stanley Kubrick. *The New York Times Magazine*, p. 25.

Bonanno, G. A. (1998). The concept of "working through" loss: A critical evaluation of the cultural, historical, and empirical evidence. In A. Maercker, M. Schuetzwohl, & Z. Solomon (Eds.), *Posttraumatic stress disorder: Vulnerability and resilience in the life-span* (pp. 221–248). Göttingen, Germany: Hogreth & Huber.

Bonanno, G. A. (1999). Laughter during bereavement. *Bereavement Care, 18*, 19–22.

Bonanno, G. A. (in press). Grief and emotion: A social-functional perspective. In M. Stroebe, R. O. Hansson, W. Stroebe, & H. Schut (Eds.), *Handbook of bereavement research: Consequences, coping, and care*. Washington, DC: American Psychological Association.

Bonanno, G. A., Davis, P. J., Singer, J. L., & Schwartz, G. E. (1991). The repressor personality and avoidant information processing: A dichotic listening study. *Journal of Research in Personality, 25*, 386–401.

Bonanno, G. A., & Kaltman, S. (1999). Toward an integrative perspective on bereavement. *Psychological Bulletin, 125,* 760–776.

Bonanno, G. A., & Kaltman, S. (2000). The assumed necessity of working through memories of traumatic experiences. In P. R. Duberstein & J. M. Masling (Eds.), *Psychodynamic perspectives on sickness and health* (pp. 165–200). Washington, DC: American Psychological Association.

Bonanno, G. A., & Keltner, D. (1997). Facial expressions of emotion and the course of bereavement. *Journal of Abnormal Psychology, 106,* 126–137.

Bonanno, G. A., & Keltner, D. (1999). *The organization of discrete emotions: A contingency analysis of facial expressions, "on-line" verbal themes, and written self-report.* Manuscript submitted for publication.

Bonanno, G. A., Keltner, D., Holen, A., & Horowitz, M. J. (1995). When avoiding unpleasant emotion might not be such a bad thing: Verbal–autonomic response dissociation and midlife conjugal bereavement. *Journal of Personality and Social Psychology, 46,* 975–989.

Bonanno, G. A., & Keuler, D. J. (1998). Psychotherapy without repressed memory: A parsimonious alternative based on contemporary memory research. In S. J. Lynn & K. M. McConkey (Eds.), *Truth in memory* (pp. 437–463). New York: Guilford Press.

Bonanno, G. A., Noll, J. G., Putnam, F. W., Lomakina, N., & Trickett, P. (1999). *Dissociation and childhood sexual abuse: A systematic comparison of pathological and nonpathological variants.* Manuscript submitted for publication.

Bonanno, G. A., & Siddique, H. (1999). Emotional dissociation, self-deception, and psychotherapy. In J. A. Singer & P. Salovey (Eds.), *At play in the field of consciousness: Essays in honor of Jerome L. Singer* (pp. 249–270). Hillsdale, NJ: Erlbaum.

Bonanno, G. A., & Singer, J. L. (1990). Repressive personality style: Theoretical and methodological implications for health and pathology. In J. L. Singer (Ed.), *Repression and dissociation* (pp. 435–470). Chicago: University of Chicago Press.

Bonanno, G. A., Znoj, H. J., Siddique, H., & Horowitz, M. J. (1999). Verbal-autonomic response dissociation and adaptation to midlife conjugal loss: A follow-up at 25 months. *Cognitive Therapy and Research, 23,* 605–624.

Bowlby, J. (1980). *Attachment and loss. Vol. 3. Loss: Sadness and depression.* New York: Basic Books.

Buck, R. (1988). *Human motivation and emotion* (2nd ed.). New York: Wiley.

Campbell, J. (1986). *Winston Churchill's afternoon nap: A wide-awake inquiry into the human nature of time.* New York: Simon & Schuster.

Cannon, W. (1939). *The wisdom of the body.* New York: Norton.

Carver, C. S., & Scheier, M. F. (1981). *Attention and self-regulation: A control theory approach to human behavior.* New York: Springer-Verlag.

Carver, C. S., & Scheier, M. F. (1982). Control theory: A useful conceptual framework for personality-social, clinical and health psychology. *Psychological Bulletin, 92,* 111–135.

Carver, C. S., & Scheier, M. F. (1990). Origins and functions of positive and negative affect: A control-process view. *Psychological Review, 97,* 19–35.

Cerney, M. W., & Buskirk, J. R. (1991). Anger: The hidden part of grief. *Bulletin of the Menninger Clinic, 55,* 228–237.

Darwin, C. (1872). *The expression of the emotions in man and animals*. London: Murray.

Davis, J. D. (1979). Broadening the homeostatic concept. *Behavioral and Brain Sciences, 1*, 104–105.

Dawkins, K., & Furnham, A. (1989). The color naming of emotional words. *British Journal of Psychology, 80*, 383–389.

de Waal, F. (1989). *Peacemaking among primates*. Cambridge, MA: Harvard University Press.

Duchenne de Bologne, G. B. (1990). *The mechanism of human facial expression* (R. A. Cuthbertson, Trans.). New York: Cambridge University Press. (Original work published 1862)

Dundes, A. (1980). *Interpreting folklore*. Bloomington: Indiana University Press.

Ekman, P. (1992). Are there basic emotions? *Psychological Review, 99*, 550–553.

Ekman, P., & Davidson, R. J. (1993). Voluntary smiling changes regional brain activity. *Psychological Science, 4*, 342–345.

Esterling, B. A., Antoni, M. H., Fletcher, M. A., Margulies, S., & Schneiderman, N. (1994). Emotional disclosure through writing or speaking modulates latent Epstein–Barr virus antibody titers. *Journal of Consulting and Clinical Psychology, 62*, 30–140.

Fox, E. (1993). Allocation of visual attention and anxiety. *Cognition and Emotion, 7*, 207–215.

Fox, E., O'Boyle, C. A., Barry, H., & McCreary, C. (1989). Repressive coping style in stressful dental surgery. *British Journal of Medical Psychology, 62*, 371–380.

Frank, M., Ekman, P., & Friesen, W. V. (1993). Behavioral markers and recognizability of the smile of enjoyment. *Journal of Personality and Social Psychology, 64*, 83–93.

Fredrickson, B. L. (1998). What good are positive emotions? *Review of General Psychology, 2*, 300–319.

Fredrickson, B. L., & Levenson, R. W. (1998). Positive emotions speed recovery from the cardiovascular sequelae of negative emotions. *Cognition and Emotion, 12*, 191–220.

Freud, S. (1957). Mourning and melancholia. In J. Strachey (Ed. & Trans.). *The standard edition of the complete psychological works of Sigmund Freud* (Vol. 14, pp. 152–170). London: Hogarth Press. (Original work published 1917)

Funder, D. C., Block, J. H., & Block, J. (1983). Delay of gratification: Some longitudinal personality correlates. *Journal of Personality and Social Psychology, 44*, 1198–1213.

Goffman, E. (1967). *Interaction ritual: Essays on face-to-face behavior*. Garden City, NY: Anchor.

Goodall, J. (1986). *The chimpanzees of Gombe*. Cambridge, MA: Harvard University Press.

Gottfredson, M. R., & Hirschi, T. (1990). *A general theory of crime*. Stanford, CA: Stanford University Press.

Greenberg, M. A., & Stone, A. A. (1992). Emotional disclosure about traumas and its relation to health: Effects of previous disclosure and trauma severity. *Journal of Personality and Social Psychology, 63*, 75–84.

Greenberg, M. A., Wortman, C. B., & Stone, A. A. (1996). Emotional expression and physical health: Revising traumatic memories or fostering self-regulation? *Journal of Personality and Social Psychology, 71,* 588–602.

Gross, J. J. (1998a). Antecedent and response-focused emotion regulation: Divergent consequences for experience, expression, and physiology. *Journal of Personality and Social Psychology, 74,* 224—237.

Gross, J. J. (1998b). The emerging field of emotion regulation: An integrative review. *Review of General Psychology, 2,* 271–299.

Gross, J. J., & Levenson, R. W. (1993). Emotional suppression: Physiology, self-report, and expressive behavior. *Journal of Personality and Social Psychology, 64,* 970–986.

Gross, J. J., & Levenson, R. W. (1997). Hiding feelings: The acute effects of inhibiting negative and positive emotion. *Journal of Abnormal Psychology, 106,* 95–103.

Gross, J. J., & Muñoz, R. F. (1995). Emotion regulation and mental health. *Clinical Psychology: Science and Practice, 2,* 151–164.

Harber, K. D., & Pennebaker, J. (1992). Overcoming traumatic memories. In S. A. Christianson (Ed.), *The handbook of emotion and memory* (pp. 359–387). Hillsdale, NJ: Erlbaum.

Hatfield, E., Cacioppo, J. T., & Rapson, R. (1992). Primitive emotional contagion. In M. S. Clark (Ed.), *Review of personality and social psychology* (Vol. 14, pp. 151–177). Newbury Park, CA: Sage.

Herman, C. P., & Polivy, J. (1975). Anxiety, restraint, and eating behavior. *Journal of Abnormal Psychology, 84,* 633–639.

Hettich, P. (1990). Journal writing: Old fare or nouvelle cuisine? *Teaching of Psychology, 17,* 36–39.

Hilgard, E. R. (1986). *Divided consciousness: Multiple controls in human thought and action* (3rd ed.). New York: Wiley.

Horowitz, M. J. (1986). *Stress response syndromes.* Northvale, NJ: Jason Aronson.

Isen, A. M. (1993). Positive affect and decision making. In M. Lewis & J. M. Haviland (Eds.), *Handbook of emotions* (pp. 261–277). New York: Guilford Press.

Isen, A. M., Daubman, K. A., & Nowicki, G. P. (1987). Positive affect facilitates creative problem solving. *Journal of Personality and Social Psychology, 47,* 1206–1217.

Izard, C. (1977). *Human emotions.* New York: Plenum Press.

Izard, C. (1990). Facial expressions and the regulation of emotion. *Journal of Personality and Social Psychology, 58,* 487–498.

Izard, C. (1992). Basic emotions, relations among emotions, and emotion–cognition relations. *Psychological Review, 99,* 561–564.

Izard, C., & Malatesta, C. Z. (1987). Perspectives on emotional development: 1. Differential emotions theory of early emotion development. In J. D. Osofsky (Ed.), *Handbook of infant development* (2nd ed., pp. 494–545). New York: Wiley-Interscience.

James, W. (1890). *The principles of psychology* (Vol. 1). New York: Dover.

Kelly, A. E. (1998). Client's secret keeping in outpatient therapy. *Journal of Counseling Psychology, 45,* 450–465.

Kelly, A. E., & McKillop, K. J. (1996). Consequences of revealing personal secrets. *Psychological Bulletin, 120,* 450–465.

Keltner, D., & Bonanno, G. A. (1997). A study of laughter and dissociation: Distinct correlates of laughter and smiling during bereavement. *Journal of Personality and Social Psychology, 73,* 687–702.

Keltner, D., Bonanno, G. A., Caspi, A., Krueger, R., & Stouthamer-Leober, M. (1996). *Personality and facial expressions of emotion.* Unpublished manuscript, University of California, Berkeley.

Keltner, D., & Buswell, B. N. (1997). Embarrassment: Its distinct form and appeasement functions. *Psychological Bulletin, 122,* 250–270.

Keltner, D., Moffitt, T. E., & Stouthamer-Loeber, M. (1995). Facial expressions of emotion and psychopathology in adolescent boys. *Journal of Abnormal Psychology, 104,* 644–652.

King, L. A., & Miner, K. N. (2000). Writing about the perceived benefits of traumatic events. Implications for physical health. *Personality and Social Psychology Bulletin, 26,* 220–230.

Krohne, H. W. (1992). Vigilance and cognitive avoidance as concepts in coping research. In H. W. Krohne (Ed.), *Attention and avoidance strategies in coping with aversiveness* (pp. 19–50). Göttingen, Germany: Hograth & Huber.

Kushner, L. R., & Mook, D. G. (1984). Behavioral correlates of oral and postingestive satiety in the rat. *Physiology and Behavior, 33,* 713–718.

Laird, J. D. (1974). Self-attribution of emotion: The effects of expressive behavior on the quality of emotional experience. *Journal of Personality and Social Psychology, 29,* 475–486.

Lang, P. J. (1979). Language, image, and emotion. In P. Pliner, K. R. Blankstein, & J. M. Spigel (Eds.), *Perception of emotion in self and others* (Vol. 5). New York: Plenum Press.

Lang, P. J., Kozak, M. J., Miller, G. A., Levin, D. N., & McLean, A. (1980). Emotional imagery: Conceptual structure and pattern of somato-visceral response. *Psychophysiology, 17,* 179–192.

Lang, P. J., Levin, D. N., Miller, G. A., & Kozak, M. J. (1983). Fear behavior, fear imagery, and the psychophysiology of emotion: The problem of affective response integration. *Journal of Abnormal Psychology, 92,* 276–306.

Langley, L. L. (1973). *Homeostasis: Origins of the concept.* Stroudsburg, PA: Dowden, Hutchinson & Ross.

Lazarus, R. S. (1966). *Psychological stress and the coping process.* New York: Oxford University Press.

Lazarus, R. S. (1991). *Emotion and adaptation.* New York: Oxford University Press.

LeDoux, J. E. (1993). Emotional memory systems in the brain. *Behavioural Brain Research, 58,* 69–79.

LeDoux, J. E. (1996). *The emotional brain.* New York: Simon & Schuster.

Leith, K. P., & Baumeister, R. F. (1996). Why do bad moods increase self-defeating behavior?: Emotion, risk-taking, and self-regulation. *Journal of Personality and Social Psychology, 71,* 1250–1267.

Levenson, R. W. (1988). Emotion and the autonomic nervous system: A prospectus for research on autonomic specificity. In H. L. Wagner (Ed.), *Social psychophysiology and emotion: Theory and clinical applications* (pp. 17–42). London: Wiley.

Levenson, R. W. (1994). Human emotion: A functional view. In P. Ekman & R. J.

Davidson (Eds.), *The nature of emotion: Fundamental questions* (pp. 123–126). Oxford, UK: Oxford University Press.

Leventhal, H. (1984). A perceptual–moter theory of emotion. *Advances in Experimental Social Psychology, 17,* 117–182.

Leventhal, H. (1991). Emotion: Prospects for conceptual and empirical development. In R. G. Lister & H. J. Weingartner (Eds.), *Perspectives on cognitive neuroscience* (pp. 325–348). Oxford, UK: Oxford University Press.

Littrell, J. (1998). Is the reexperience of painful emotion therapeutic? *Clinical Psychology Review, 18,* 71–102.

Macnab, A. J., Beckett, L. Y., Park, C. C., & Sheckter, L. (1998). Journal writing as a social support strategy for parents of premature infants: A pilot study. *Patient Education and Counseling, 33,* 49–159.

Markus, H. R., & Kitayama, S. (1991). Culture and the self: Implications for cognition, emotion, and motivation. *Psychological Review, 98,* 224–253.

Martin, R. A., & Lefcourt, H. M. (1983). The sense of humor as a moderator of the relation between stressors and moods. *Journal of Personality and Social Psychology, 45,* 1313–1324.

Matsumoto, D., Kudoh, T., Scherer, K., & Walbott, H. (1988). Antecedents of and reactions to emotions in the United States and Japan. *Journal of Cross-Cultural Psychology, 19,* 267–286.

Miller, R. S. (1995). On the nature of embarrassability: Shyness, social-evaluation, and social skill. *Journal of Personality, 63,* 315–229.

Mischel, W., & Shoda, Y. (1995). A cognitive–affective system theory of personality: Reconceptualizing situations, dispositions, dynamics, and invariance in personality structure. *Psychological Review, 102,* 246–268.

Muraven, M., Tice, D. M., & Baumeister, R. F. (1998). Self-control as a limited resource: Regulatory depletion patterns. *Journal of Personality and Social Psychology, 74,* 774–789.

Newton, T. L., & Contrada, R. J. (1992). Repressive coping and verbal–autonomic response dissociation: The influence of social context. *Journal of Personality and Social Psychology, 62,* 159–167.

Nicolaidis, S., & Rowland, N. (1975). Systemic versus oral and gastrointestinal metering of fluid intake. In G. Peters, J. T. Fitzsimons, & L. Peters-Haefeli (Eds.), *Control mechanisms of drinking.* Berlin: Springer-Verlag.

Oatley, K., & Jenkins, J. M. (1996). *Understanding emotions.* Cambridge, MA: Blackwell.

Paulhus, D. L., Fridhandler, B., & Hayes, S. (1997). Psychological defense: Contemporary theory and research. In J. Johnson, R. Hogan, & S. R. Briggs (Eds.), *Handbook of personality psychology* (pp. 543–574). New York: Academic Press.

Pennebaker, J. W. (1989). Confession, inhibition, and disease. *Advances in Experimental Social Psychology, 22,* 211–244.

Pennebaker, J. W. (1990). *Opening up: The healing power of confiding in others.* New York: Morrow.

Pennebaker, J. W. (1993). Putting stress into words: Health, linguistic, and therapeutic implications. *Behaviour Research and Therapy, 31,* 539–548.

Pennebaker, J. W., & Barger, S. D. (1988). *Autonomic and health effects of traumatic disclosure among survivors of the Holocaust.* Unpublished manuscript, Southern Methodist University, Dallas, TX.

Pennebaker, J. W., & Beall, S. K. (1986). Confronting a traumatic event: Toward an understanding of inhibition and disease. *Journal of Abnormal Psychology, 95,* 274–281.

Pennebaker, J. W., Colder, M., & Sharp, L. K. (1990). Accelerating the coping process. *Journal of Personality and Social Psychology, 58,* 528–537.

Pennebaker, J. W., Hughes, C. F., & O'Heeron, R. C. (1987). The psychophysiology of confession: Linking inhibitory and psychosomatic processes. *Journal of Personality and Social Psychology, 52,* 781–793.

Pennebaker, J. W., Kiecolt-Glaser, J. K., & Glaser, R. (1988). Disclosure of traumas and immune function: Health implications for psychotherapy. *Journal of Consulting and Clinical Psychology, 56,* 239–245.

Petrie, K. J., Booth, R. J., Pennebaker, J. W., Davison, K. P., & Thomas, M. G. (1995). Disclosure of trauma and immune response to a hepatitis B vaccination program. *Journal of Consulting and Clinical Psychology, 63,* 787–792.

Powers, W. T. (1973). *Behavior: The control of perception.* Chicago: Aldine.

Powers, W. T. (1978). Quantitative analysis of purposive systems: Some spadework at the foundations of scientific psychology. *Psychological Review, 85,* 417–435.

Price, R., & Price, S. (1991). *Two evenings in Saramaka.* Chicago: University of Chicago Press.

Provine, R. R. (1992). Contagious laughter: Laughter is a sufficient stimulus for laughs and smiles. *Bulletin of the Psychonomic Society, 30,* 1–4.

Pyszczynski, T., & Greenberg, J. (1987). Self-regulatory perseveration and the depressive self-focusing style: A self-awareness theory of reactive depression. *Psychological Bulletin, 102,* 122–138.

Rabinor, J. R. (1998). Journal writing: A guide to the inner world. *Eating Disorders: The Journal of Treatment and Prevention, 6,* 253–266.

Raphael, B. (1983). *The anatomy of bereavement.* New York: Basic Books.

Rime, B., Mesquita, B., Philippot, P., & Boca, S. (1991). Beyond the emotional events: Six studies on the social sharing of emotion. *Cognition and Emotion, 5,* 435–465.

Rime, B., Mesquita, B., Philippot, P., & Boca, S. (1992). Long-lasting cognitive and social consequences of emotion: Social sharing and rumination. *European Review of Social Psychology, 3,* 225–258.

Rosenblatt, P. C. (1993). Grief: The social context of private feelings. In. M. S. Stroebe, W. Stroebe, & R. O. Hansson (Eds.), *Handbook of bereavement: Theory, research, and intervention* (pp. 102–111). Cambridge, UK: Cambridge University Press.

Ross, L., & Nisbett, R. E. (1991). *The person and the situation.* New York: McGraw-Hill.

Rothbart, M. L. (1973). Laughter in young children. *Psychological Bulletin, 80,* 247–256.

Rothbaum, B. O., & Foa, E. B. (1996). Cognitive–behavioral therapy for posttraumatic stress disorder. In B. A. van der Kolk, A. C. McFarlane, & L. Weisaeth (Eds.), *Traumatic stress: The effects of overwhelming experience on mind, body, and society* (pp. 491–509). New York: Guilford Press.

Scheier, M. F., & Carver, C. S. (1988). A model of behavioral self-regulation: Translating intention into action. *Advances in Experimental Social Psychology, 21*, 303–346.

Schoemer, K. (1998). Love stories: The joy of the four-hankie weeper. *Newsweek*, pp. 36–40.

Schwartz, G. E. (1979). Disregulation theory and disease: A biobehavioral framework for biofeedback and behavioral medicine. In N. Birbaumer & H. D. Kimmel (Eds.), *Biofeedback and self-regulation*. Hillsdale, NJ: Erlbaum.

Schwartz, G. E. (1982). Physiological patterning and emotion: Implications for the self-regulation of emotion. In K. R. Blankstein & J. Polivy (Eds.), *Self-control and self-modification of emotional behavior* (pp. 13–27). New York: Plenum Press.

Schwartz, G. E., Fair, P. L., Greenberg, P. S., Freedman, M., & Klerman, J. L. (1974). Facial electromyography in the assessment of emotion. *Psychophysiology, 11*, 237.

Schwartz, G. E., Fair, P. L., Salt, P., Mandel, M. R., & Klerman, J. L. (1976). Facial muscle patterning to affective imagery in depressed and nondepressed subjects. *Science, 192*, 489–491.

Selye, H. (1976). *The stress of life*. New York: McGraw-Hill.

Sgoutas-Emch, S. A., & Johnson, C. J. (1998). Is journal writing an effective method of reducing anxiety towards statistics? *Journal of Instructional Psychology, 25*, 49–57.

Shedler, J., Mayman, M., & Manis, M. (1993). The illusion of mental health. *American Psychologist, 48*, 1117–1131.

Sherman, R., Bonanno, G. A., Wiener, L., & Battles, H. B. (2000). When children tell their friends they have AIDS: Possible consequences for psychological well-being and disease progression. *Psychosomatic Medicine, 62*, 238–247.

Silver, R. L., Wortman, C. B., & Crofton, C. (1990). The role of coping in support provision: The self-presentational dilemma of victims of life crises. In B. R. Sarason, I. G. Sarason, & G. R. Piece (Eds.), *Social support: An interactional view* (pp. 397–426). New York: Wiley.

Stern, J. A., Walrath, L. C., & Goldstein, R. (1984). The endogenous eyeblink. *Psychophysiology, 21*, 22–33.

Suh, E., Diener, E., Oishi, S., & Triandis, H. C. (1998). The shifting basis of life satisfaction judgments across cultures: Emotions versus norms. *Journal of Personality and Social Psychology, 74*, 482–493.

Taylor, S. E. (1991). Asymmetrical effects of positive and negative events: The mobilization–minimization hypothesis. *Psychological Review, 110*, 67–85.

Thompson, S. (1977). *The folktale*. Berkeley: University of California Press.

Toates, F. (1986). *Motivational systems*. Cambridge, UK: Cambridge University Press.

Tomkins, S. S. (1962). *Affect, imagery, consciousness: Vol. 1. The positive affects*. New York: Springer.

Van der Kolk, B. A. (1996). The complexity of adaptation to trauma: Self-regulation, stimulus discrimination, and characterological development. In B. A. van der Kolk, A. C. McFarlane, & L. Weisaeth (Eds.), *Traumatic stress: The effects of overwhelming experience on mind, body, and society* (pp. 182–213). New York: Guilford Press.

Vinton, K. L. (1989). Humor in the work place: Is it more than telling jokes? *Small Group Behavior, 20,* 151–166.

Wegner, D. M., & Bargh, J. A. (1998). Control and automaticity in social life. In D. T. Gilbert & S. T. Fiske (Eds.), *The handbook of social psychology* (4th ed., Vol. 2, pp. 446–496). Boston: McGraw-Hill.

Weinberger, D. A., & Davidson, M. N. (1994). Styles of inhibiting emotional expression: Distinguishing repressive coping from impression management. *Journal of Personality, 62,* 587–613.

Weinberger, D. A., Schwartz, G. E., & Davidson, J. R. (1979). Low-anxious and repressive coping styles: Psychometric patterns of behavioral and physiological responses to stress. *Journal of Abnormal Psychology, 88,* 369–380.

Wirtshafter, D., & Davis, J. D. (1977). Set points, settling points and the control of body weight. *Physiology and Behavior, 19,* 75–78.

Wortman, C. B., & Silver, R. C. (1989). The myths of coping with loss. *Journal of Consulting and Clinical Psychology, 57,* 349–357.

Zajonc, R. B., Murphy, S. T., & Inglehart, M. (1989). Feeling and facial efference: Implications of the vascular theory of emotion. *Psychological Review, 96,* 395–416.

9

Emotional Intelligence
A Process Model of Emotion Representation and Regulation

LISA FELDMAN BARRETT
JAMES J. GROSS

For the better part of the 20th century, a fairly narrow view of intelligence prevailed. This view held that human intelligence consisted of a limited set of cognitive capacities. Indeed, for all intents and purposes, "intelligence" was what intelligence tests such as the Wechsler Adult Intelligence Scale—Revised (WAIS-R) or the Stanford–Binet Test measured. These tests involve the manipulation of neutral objects (words, numbers, puzzles, blocks) in contexts that are designed to hold motivational and emotional factors constant.

Cognition, characterized by flexible deployment of knowledge, clearly plays a crucial role in adaptive success. However, an exclusively cognitive view of intelligence misses the important adaptive functions served by other psychological features responsible for our success. In an attempt to broaden traditional conceptions of intelligence, a number of researchers have focused on the role played by emotion in adaptive responding to environmental demands (see, e.g., Salovey & Mayer, 1980).

Emotions such as anger, sadness, and disgust represent "best guesses" as to what an individual in a certain general class of situation should do (Tooby & Cosmides, 1990). Emotions prepare an individual to make rapid motor responses (Frijda, 1986), and help to sculpt adaptive social functioning by tailoring cognitive style (Clore, 1994) and flexibly scripting complex social behavior (Averill, 1980). Mounting neuropsychological evidence suggests that impaired emotion systems leave an individual unprepared for dealing with complex social situations (Damasio, 1994).

Importantly, however, although emotions *may* contribute to adaptive behavior, they do not *always* do so. Optimal emotional responding results when individuals shape their emotions by regulating how these emotions are experienced or expressed. Such a process involves two major elements: accurately tracking one's ongoing emotional state, and knowing when and how to intervene to shape the emotion trajectory as needed.

In this chapter, we consider the place of emotional processes in intelligent behavior, a domain now known as the study of emotional intelligence. Our goal is not to provide a general review of the emotional intelligence area, but rather to suggest a more focused treatment that is rooted in the processes associated with emotion generation and modulation. Our general thesis is that emotional intelligence requires that individuals appreciate (1) how they are responding emotionally and (2) how they can shape the emotion as it unfolds. Emotions can be generated and regulated in better or worse ways, and how individuals go about doing this shapes their adaptive success.

THE TRADITIONAL VIEW OF EMOTIONAL INTELLIGENCE

Emotional intelligence refers to an interrelated set of abilities that allow an individual to recognize, use, and regulate emotion in an efficient and productive manner, thereby allowing effective dealings with the environment. Because emotionally intelligent individuals are more socially effective, definitions of the concept in the popular press (see, e.g., Bar-On, 1997; Goleman, 1995) have included personal attributes more generally related to effective personal and social functioning (for a review, see Mayer, Salovey, & Caruso, 2000). More scientific treatments have defined emotional intelligence in terms of mental abilities rather than in terms of broad social competencies. In their groundbreaking work, Mayer, Salovey, and colleagues have defined emotional intelligence to include four major elements (Mayer & Salovey, 1997; Mayer et al., 2000; Salovey & Mayer, 1990). These elements include emotion perception, emotion assimilation, emotion understanding, and emotion regulation.

First, the emotionally intelligent person can accurately identify emotion. Such identification takes place in three domains. These include his/her own emotional experiences (i.e., differentiating between discrete emotional experiences like anger, sadness, and fear); the emotional experiences of others (i.e., discerning the experience of others by reading facial expressions or listening to language use or intonation); and the emotional signal value attributed to objects (e.g., identifying the emotional experience evoked by artwork or music).

Second, not only does the emotionally intelligent person perceive emotion correctly, he/she also uses emotion to help shape judgment and behavior. Emotion may direct attention to important information in the environment (Mandler, 1984), thereby influencing information processing (see, e.g., Christianson, 1992; Forgas, 2000; Niedenthal & Kitayama, 1994), guiding judgment about past or current events (Clore & Parrott, 1991; Schwarz, 1990; Schwarz & Clore, 1983, 1996), and facilitating decision making about future events (although work on affective forecasting indicates that people generally are not terribly accurate in predicting how they will feel in response to a future event; Gilbert & Wilson, 2000).

Third, the emotionally intelligent person has a rich emotion knowledge base. This knowledge includes the abstract cause of the experience; the meaning of the situation to the individual and his/her immediate goals, bodily sensations, and expressive modes (i.e., display rules for expression); how the emotion functions interpersonally; and sequences of action to take to enhance or reduce the experience (i.e., plans of emotion management) (Mesquita & Fridja, 1992; Shweder, 1993). Such an emotion database makes it possible for the individual to function effectively in a variety of social contexts.

Fourth, the emotionally intelligent person engages in efficient emotion regulation in both self and others. He/she is able to reflectively monitor both positive emotion (see Fredrickson, 1998, for the use of positive emotions in broadening and building) and negative emotion (see Parrot, 1993, for the functional utility of negative emotions) in both self and others. This monitoring makes it possible for the individual to strategically manage emotion in self and others to produce the desired outcome in a given situation.

As it is currently articulated, the traditional view of emotional intelligence seems to make two assumptions: First, one's own or another's emotions are seen as fixed entities about which correct and incorrect judgments can be made (Mayer, Caruso, & Salovey, 1999). Presumably, the accurate detection of an emotional response in another person can be indexed by comparing an individual's response to that which the target reports or that which is consensually agreed upon (see, e.g., Mayer et al., 1999; Mayer & Geher, 1996). Second, emotional intelligence is seen as a static set of abilities, ranging from reading emotion expressions in another person's face to altering one's own emotional responses (Mayer et al., 1999). No particular ability is privileged above the others, and emotional intelligence is treated as though it were a global trait, even though its components might seem to involve quite divergent processes.

By way of contrast, we see emotions as fluid, emergent phenomena that result from the interplay of implicit and explicit processes (see, e.g., Izard, 1993; Lane, Nadel, Allen, & Kaszniak, 2000; see also K. N. Ochsner & L. Feldman Barrett, Chapter 2, this volume). This means that there is no one target for correct or incorrect evaluation, either in self or others.[1] Rather than referring to a static, graded capacity based on a fixed set of abilities, we view emotional intelligence as a set of related processes that allow an individual to successfully deploy mental representations in the generation and regulation of the emotional response as it unfolds over time.

EMOTIONAL INTELLIGENCE: A REVISED VIEW

We begin with the premise that an emotional response is an emergent phenomenon and that the processes that produce and modify its trajectory are at the root of emotional intelligence. Based on a distillation of major points of convergence among emotion researchers (see Gross, 1998a), we view emotion as originating with the evaluation of external or internal emotion cues. Emotions arise automatically via implicit processing, such as when we recoil fearfully from a snake (LeDoux, 1996), or they may also require considerable meaning analysis, such as when we grow angry after receiving a insult (Lazarus, 1991). In either case, the evaluations can be associated with behavioral, experiential, and physiological emotional response tendencies that facilitate responding to perceived challenges and opportunities. But this is not the end of the story: individuals can modulate these response tendencies, thereby modifying the resulting emotional responses.

From this perspective, emotions can be considered modes with anticipated or probable trajectories (involving an automatic set of responses) that may be modified by an executive mode of functioning that is—at least initially—deliberate and flexible. The automatic responses to a class of objects may be due to temperamental differences or to overlearned responses involving both subcortical and cortical brain centers; this aspect of the emotional response feels reflex-like. Because there is often continuity between our automatic emotional responses and our varying life circumstances, these automatically executed responses serve us well much of the time. When a response does not match the circumstance, however, we intervene by deliberately deploying emotion knowledge with varying degrees of flexibility and efficiency to modify either our experience or our expression of emotion. Both automatic responses and deliberate control processes contribute to individual differences in the ability to optimally function in a varying social context and therefore in our view constitute central components of emotional intelligence.

A process conception of emotion suggests a number of points at which individuals might differ in terms of emotion generation and emotion regulation. We believe two of these deserve special consideration due to their central role in generating meaningful individual differences in emotional intelligence. The first has to do with how emotions are represented. If an individual is not aware of an emotional response or represents it in poorly differentiated terms, it seems unlikely that the emotion will be employed (or regulated) to full advantage. The second point at which we believe meaningful individual differences in emotional intelligence might arise has to do with how and when emotions are regulated. It is not enough to simply know which emotions one is experiencing. One also needs to be able to flexibly regulate emotions in appropriate ways so as to maximize the degree to which they are tailored to the particular situation. In the following subsections, we focus on these two critical processes, emotion differentiation and emotion regulation.

Emotion Differentiation

An emerging literature suggests that there are individual differences in emotional complexity (Carstensen, Pasupathi, & Mayr, in press; Lane, Quinlan, Schwartz, Walker, & Zeitlin, 1990; Lane & Schwartz, 1987; Lane et al., 1996; Larsen & Cutler, 1996). Although happiness, fear, sadness, hostility, guilt, surprise, and interest are considered discrete either for psychobiological (see, e.g., Ekman, 1992; Izard, 1977) or social (see, e.g., Stein & Trabasso, 1992) reasons, evidence suggests that there is great variability in the representation of emotional experiences as discrete. The tendency to generate discrete emotional responses ranges along a continuum, with those who report global mood states at one end and those who report highly differentiated responses at the other.

Emotion differentiation has most often been studied using experience-sampling methodology (Carstensen et al., in press; Feldman, 1995a; Feldman Barrett, 1998a, 1998b; Larsen & Cutler, 1996). In the experience-sampling studies to be discussed here, individuals provided ratings of their emotional experience at randomly sampled times throughout the day for some period of time. An analysis of the resulting correlation matrix provides a clue to the degree of discreteness in the individual's emotional response. Emotions should be experienced separately from one another for some proportion of the time to support the claim that they are discrete and experientially separate from one another. Such a pattern of experience would produce moderate-to-small correlations between similarly valenced emotional experiences (e.g., sadness, anxiety, and anger; relaxation, happiness, and enthusiasm), with the result that emotion labels like *happy* or *sad* are being used to represent distinct and specific emotional experiences. Large correlations between such states would indicate that the different unpleasant states or the different pleasant states are not meaningfully differentiated from one another. At any given moment different negative states such as anger, sadness, and fear are not discriminated from one another, nor are different positive states such as happiness, relaxation, and enthusiasm. The result is that emotion labels like *happy* and *sad* are being used as proxy indicators of general pleasantness or unpleasantness.

Recent evidence from several experience-sampling studies indicates that there are stable individual differences in how people go about the process of applying emotion knowledge to affective feeling, leading to differences in emotional differentiation and presumably to differences in emotional intelligence (Feldman, 1995a; Feldman Barrett, 1998a). Some individuals use discrete emotion labels to name their feelings in a distinct and specific fashion, as evidenced by smaller correlations between like-valenced states and by more distinctiveness in their use of emotion labels across time. Others use emotion labels as proxies for general affective feelings ("I feel good" or "I feel bad") rather than to denote distinct experiences, as evidenced by large positive correlations between self-reports of similarly valenced emotional states across time. Such a strong degree of co-occurence between discrete emotional states indicates that these individuals do not meaningfully separate those emotions in conscious experience and calls into question whether the subjective emotional states are indeed distinct for these individuals. These individuals seem to represent their emotional experiences in an undifferentiated fashion along a single pleasant–unpleasant dimension, because their use of discrete terms conveys no unique information about the particular state itself.

It might be argued that there is a distinction between the conscious labeling of emotional experience and the biological responses that underlie that experience. From this perspective, emotion differentiation in self-report may say little about variations in emotional responses per se because subjective experience represents only the translation of biological phenomena into consciousness. We would argue, however, that in the absence of objective criteria to reference emotional experience, studies of that experience must be based on self-reports that are, of necessity, consciously given. Studying conscious reports of experience is not distinct from studying true emotion, because the same representations of emotion knowledge are likely used in the emotion generation process whether or not the person is aware of having done so (see Ochsner & Feldman Barrett, Chapter 2, this volume). From this perspective, individual differences in how people consciously represent their affective experience using emotion language might have something to tell us more generally about how individuals experience emotion with different levels of granularity, and such differences should have important implications for their emotional lives.

Understanding the concomitants of individual differences in emotion differentiation help us to identify and understand the processes that might

be important to emotional intelligence. We identify three different processes associated with emotion generation that might influence emotion differentiation specifically, and emotional intelligence more generally: (1) the
availability of emotion knowledge, (2) the accessibility of such knowledge
or motivation to use it in the generation of discrete emotional experience,
and (3) the cognitive resources to use the knowledge in any given instance.

Availability of Emotion Knowledge

Emotion differentiation does not seem to be related to the availability of
general semantic knowledge about emotion, but rather seems to be determined by the deployment of such knowledge. Mental representations of
emotion begin with two primary dimensions stored in semantic memory:
valence and activation (Feldman Barrett & Fossum, 1999; Russell, 1980;
Russell & Feldman Barrett, 1999; Russell, Yik, & Feldman Barrett, 1999).[2]
Valence refers to the hedonic quality or pleasantness of an affective experience, and activation refers to the subjective sense of arousal associated with
an affective experience. These two semantic components are often represented a circumplex configuration with discrete emotion terms arrayed
around the circumference of a circular structure anchored by valence and
arousal dimensions (Remington, Fabrigar, & Visser, 2000; Russell, 1980).
Emotion terms are thought to array in a circumplex format because valence
and activation feelings are a component of each emotion representation
(Russell & Feldman Barrett, 1999). This mental representation is essentially nomothetic. It has been identified in participants of different ages
(Russell & Ridgeway, 1983; Russell & Bullock, 1985), from different cultures (see, e.g., Russell, 1983, 1991; Russell, Lewicka, & Niit, 1989), and
in different groups of emotion terms (see, e.g., Block, 1957; Bush, 1973;
Feldman, 1995b; Russell, 1980).

  Although individuals share the same mental representation at this general level, they are thought to differentially weigh the semantic components
to arrive at judgments of their own emotion states. This differential weight-
ing produces two psychological characteristics associated with whether or
not individuals label their own emotional experiences as distinct entities.
Valence focus is defined as the extent to which individuals incorporate
pleasantness or unpleasantness into their conscious affective experience.
Arousal focus is defined as the extent to which individuals incorporate subjective experiences of arousal into a conscious affective experience. Individuals who are predominantly valence focused, that is, who give more weight
to the pleasantness or unpleasantness of their emotional experiences, tend
to differentiate distinct emotional experiences less frequently than do those
lower in valence focus. In contrast, those who weigh valence and arousal
semantic components more equally, that is, who are moderate in valence

focus while high in arousal focus, are more likely to label discrete emotional states as distinct experiences. Affective focus is computed by empirically comparing the semantic structure of emotion language to idiographically derived *P*-correlation matrices between affect ratings over time. It is possible that emotion differentiation may be related to other types of complexity in emotion representations, but thus far the evidence suggests that fine-grained emotional experiences, and perhaps emotional intelligence more generally, are more related to how people use what they know about emotion, rather than differences in what they know per se.

Accessibility and Motivation

Affective focus, as a proxy indicator of emotion differentiation, is related to two sets of personality characteristics that are, in turn, likely related to either the accessibility of emotion knowledge or motivation to construct discrete emotional experiences.

Individuals who are disproportionately focused on the valence of their experience describe themselves as higher on personality characteristics associated with motivational relevance and situational responsivity than do those who are lower in valence focus (Feldman Barrett, 1999). Motivational relevance is determined by the extent to which a situation touches upon a personal goal or concern; that is, it reflects the self-relevance or importance of the situation to the self. Judging a stimulus as self-relevant is a necessary first step in having a valenced emotional response. The stronger the motivational relevance, the more intense the emotional experience that results (Smith & Pope, 1992). Individuals who are high in valence focus are likely to judge many situations and cues as self-relevant, with the result that they more frequently generate intense valenced responses. Consistent with this evidence, individuals who are higher in valence focus also experience most interpersonal situations as having implications for their personal wellbeing and are highly reactive to changing situational cues, especially when those cues were negative (Feldman Barrett, 1999).

Individuals who focus more on the subjective experience of activation associated with their emotional experiences when labeling those experiences, thereby communicating more differentiated emotional responses, describe themselves as more introspective and sensitive to their internal state than do those who report undifferentiated emotional responses (Feldman Barrett, 1999). The significant relationship between arousal focus and reports of internal awareness does not necessarily indicate that high arousal focus individuals are more accurate in perceiving their bodily sensations, however. Subjective feelings of arousal are not illusions, but their relationship to actual neurophysiological substrates is complex and poorly understood (for a discussion, see Blascovich, 1992). In general, people tend to be inaccurate perceivers of their own interoceptive cues (Katkin, 1985; Katkin, Blascovich, & Goldband, 1981; Pennebaker, 1982; Zillmann, 1983). If the use of arousal-based semantic knowledge to label emotional experiences is related to the accurate detection of bodily cues (called interoceptive sensitivity), then this would indicate that accurate detection of physiological information is related to discrete emotional responding. If, however, arousal focus is not related to accurate perceptions of bodily activation, then arousal focus might be related to response bias (i.e., the tendency to report somatic activity regardless of whether a bodily cue is present or not), which in turn would suggest that accurate perceptions of the body are not important to the experience of discrete emotional experiences. Pilot evidence suggests that arousal focus may indeed be related to interoceptive sensitivity (Feldman Barrett & Blascovich, 1994). The number of correct detections on a heartbeat detection task (hits plus correct rejections) displayed a curvilinear relationship to arousal focus, indicating that individuals who incorporated subjective perceptions of arousal into their emotional experience were doing so based on more accurate perceptions of at least one bodily signal.

Resource Allocation

There is some indirect evidence that emotion differentiation may be related to allocation of resources during the emotion-generative process. When mental representations associated with discrete emotion knowledge are applied in a top–down manner to construct a conscious representation of emotional experience, this cognitive work probably takes place via the executive functions of working memory (for a discussion of this topic, see Baddeley, 1986; Lane, in press; LeDoux, 2000).[3] Working memory is a multicomponential system that mediates the processing and storage of internal representations. Working memory is implicated in tasks that require the storage and manipulation of internal symbolic cues, inhibition of prepotent but contextually inappropriate responses, and utilization of information from multiple sources (Gabrieli, Singh, Stebbins, & Goetz, 1996). The executive functions of working memory are thought to have limited resources, so that when the capacity is taken up with one processing task there are fewer resources left to deal with additional input. If working memory is involved in the conscious construction of discrete emotional experiences, then it should be the case that when working memory is taxed people will show less emotional differentiation and more valence focus in their emotional experience. To test this hypothesis, 38 participants made ratings of their emotional experiences and stressful life events over a 60-day period (Feldman Barrett & Aronson, 1998). It was predicted—and found—that on days that were more stressful, individuals showed larger valence focus (and less differentiation in their emotional experiences at a given moment) than on days that were less stressful. Thus, the coping resources required to deal with contextual demands may influence the degree of emotion differentiation displayed at particular moments. Note that this decrease in differentiation occurred at exactly the times when emotional specificity would seem most important, because specificity in emotional responding should have informational value to facilitate coping.

Moreover, individual differences in working memory capacity may influence the degree to which individuals differentiate their conscious emotional experience. Individual differences in working memory capacity account for variability in a range of intellectual abilities (e.g., reasoning, Kyllonen & Christal, 1990; problem solving, Carpender, Just, & Shell, 1990; reading comprehension, Daneman & Carpenter, 1980) and may be related to individual differences in emotion differentiation specifically or emotional intelligence more broadly. Emotion generation, when it involves top–down or deliberative invocation of complex emotion representations, requires that an individual be able to multitask (that is, construct his/her subjective experience at the same time as performing other ongoing social or instrumental daily functions). Thus, individuals with greater working memory capacity may well have greater resources to generate discrete emotional experiences when under cognitive load than will individuals with smaller working memory capacity.

Summary

Together, the findings thus far suggest that one aspect of emotional intelligence, namely, the tendency to report distinct emotional experiences, may be related to a number of processes associated with the generation of discrete emotional responses. Individuals who communicate discrete emotional responses do not have a greater store of general emotion knowledge available, but they do seem to differ from those who report more global emotional states on a number of variables related to the accessibility of and motivation to use discrete emotion knowledge. Individuals with more differentiated emotional lives consider themselves moderate in motivational relevance (i.e., not every situation is goal relevant) and highly introspective, are moderately responsive to changing environmental circumstances, and may be more accurate in detecting interoceptive cues. It may also be the case that they have greater resources, in the form of working memory capacity, with which to construct discrete emotional experiences while continuing to multitask and process other aspects of an experience.

Emotion Regulation

Important as emotion differentiation is, it only takes one so far. One also must be able to skillfully employ this emotion knowledge about what one is feeling so as to effectively regulate which emotions one has and how these emotions are experienced or expressed (Gross, 1998b). Indeed, we will argue that individual differences in emotion regulation constitute a second critical ingredient in emotional intelligence. But before we can address individual differences in emotion regulation, we need to have a better grasp on what people are doing when they try to regulate their emotions.

To begin to characterize emotion regulation as it occurs in everyday life, we (Gross & Richards, 2000) asked undergraduates to describe a recent occasion on which they tried to alter their emotions. Respondents had little difficulty with this task, and all were able to describe such an episode. Two representative responses are given below:

> "On Saturday, I got some really bad news that a friend—my roommate's mother—had died. So, I was really sad about that. I was kind of depressed all day, but then that night I went to a party, and so I guess I just tried to get in a party mood. You know, instead of being depressed and everything. I guess every time I would think about something sad, I would just try my hardest to . . . get my mind off of it. I think that was what I need[ed] most, which was to try and get my mind off it—that if I was talking with people and dancing and having fun, then I'd kind of forget about what was happening. And then if I started to feel a little bit down, I would try to, I don't know, just like, get myself more into talking to friends or whatever. So mostly by distracting myself."

> "We had a paper that was given back in my class and my roommate actually is in that class also. And we got very conflicting grades. He got a very bad grade, and I got a very good grade. So he was angry. Of course actually I didn't work very hard on this paper, so I got a really good grade and I was surprised. My roommate actually did some work and didn't get a good grade, so he was very, very down about it. So I kind of had to cover my emotions. Instead of acting happy and surprised, I actually kind of lied to him when I said what I got on my paper because we did kind of similar work. So I had to kind of cover up—I was very happy inside, but at the same time, I didn't want [that] to show up [to] my roommate because he's my friend too. So I kind of put on my depressed face and you know, my academic sad face and said, 'Oh well, I didn't do well either.' I guess I was trying to [change] my expressions on my face more than anything."

As the first example suggests, emotion regulation may (and often does) involve down-regulating negative emotions. However, as the second example suggests, emotion regulation encompasses more than down-regulating negative emotions (Gross, 1999b). Individuals report that they attempt to initiate, increase, maintain, and decrease both negative and positive emotions (Parrott, 1993). It also is important to note that emotion regulation involves more than altering emotion experience (e.g., trying not to feel bad), and might also include attempts to influence expressive behavior and physiological responding. Furthermore, although our method (which consisted of asking subjects to recall episodes of emotion regulation) ensured that the examples of emotion regulation given above are conscious, it is easy to imagine emotion regulation that occurs without conscious awareness. For example, individuals might hide their disappointment at an unattractive present (Cole, 1986) or turn their attention away from potentially upsetting material (Boden & Baumeister, 1997).

Emotion Regulatory Processes

One way to organize the potentially overwhelming number of emotion regulatory processes is to use the model of emotion generation described above and to identify five major points in the emotion-generative process at which individuals might intervene to influence the course of the emotion trajectory. These five points of flexibility (described below) seem likely candidates for sources of individual differences in emotionally intelligent behavior (for a more extended discussion, see Gross, 1998b).

The first is *situation selection*, which refers to approaching or avoiding certain people, places, or objects in order to influence one's emotions. Once selected, a situation may be tailored so as to modify its emotional impact. This constitutes *situation modification*. Importantly, situations differ in terms of how much they may be modified, but few situations indeed permit no latitude for situation modification whatsoever. Situations also vary in complexity, and *attentional deployment* may be used to select which aspect of a situation a person focuses on. This scheme calls to mind external situations; however, we mean to include internal "situations" as well, in which case attentional deployment may be used to select and modify imagined situations. Even after a situation has been selected, modified, and selectively attended to, it still is possible to alter its emotional impact. *Cognitive change* refers to selecting which of the many possible meanings will be attached to a given situation. It is this meaning that gives rise to emotional response tendencies, including behavioral, experiential, and physiological tendencies. Finally, *response modulation* refers to influencing these response tendencies once they have been elicited, for example, inhibiting ongoing expressive behavior.

To illustrate these distinctions, let's take the example of a couple planning an evening out (Gross, 1999a). Before they go out, one partner, aware of her shyness, vetoes several possible ways of spending the evening (e.g., a large party and a football game) because these settings would engender negative emotions. They decide to have dinner at a restaurant that is usually quiet. They are seated near a boisterous group who have been drinking for some time. Knowing that sitting this close to a loud group would frustrate their plans for a quiet conversation, they ask to be reseated. Once reseated, they relax into dinner and conversation. Each partner chooses to attend to one thought or another and pursue one topic or another, in part due to the desire to experience certain emotions and not others. Toward the end of the evening, one partner remarks how rare it is for them to have such a nice evening out. Although this comment can be read either as a compliment or a criticism, the other partner interprets it as a compliment and responds in kind, saying how much fun it had been to have a nice evening out. The first partner makes the criticism explicit: They really haven't been going out enough. Although hurt by this comment, the recipient does not want to spoil the happy evening and does not express the hurt.

In terms of the example above, *situation selection* refers to choosing how to spend the evening so as to maximize pleasant feelings. Then, a bit later in the evening, *situation modification* refers to asking for a different table at the restaurant. *Attentional deployment* refers to how the couple actively select which avenues of discussion they will pursue and which they will drop, in part on the basis of their anticipated emotional impact. In our example above, *cognitive change* refers to how one person construes the meaning of an event, such as comment about how rarely the couple has such nice evenings out. *Response modulation* is illustrated here by one partner hiding hurt feelings toward the end of the evening.

Divergent Consequences of Different Forms of Emotion Regulation

This process analysis of emotion regulation makes it clear that *what* an individual is trying to achieve (e.g., a calm expression during a heated discussion) should not be confused with *how* an individual goes about achieving that goal. This is because that one goal may be achieved in a number of quite different ways, such as by cognitively reevaluating the situation or by simply biting one's lip. How might this distinction between the what and the how of emotion regulation matter? We believe such a process conception may help resolve the apparent tension between two broad literatures relevant to the down-regulation of negative emotion. These two literatures seem to reach diametrically opposed conclusions about the implications of emotion regulation for well-being (Gross, 1998a).

On the one hand, it seems clear that emotion regulation is necessary for psychological well-being. Indeed, clinical scientists since Freud (1926/ 1959) have emphasized that the way affective impulses are managed is of central importance to mental health. Although this traditionally has been the province of psychodynamic researchers, proponents of other theoretical persuasions also have emphasized that psychological health requires that emotional impulses be regulated properly (Barlow, 1991; Beck, Rush, Shaw, & Emery, 1979; Seligman, 1991). Gross and Muñoz (1995) integrated these perspectives, arguing that the capacity to flexibly down-regulate one's negative emotions should be considered an integral part of mental health.

On the other hand, a second literature casts emotion regulation in an altogether different light. This literature is concerned with physical health and has its roots in the psychosomatic medicine tradition. In this context, the notion that emotion regulation has deleterious consequences has become a cornerstone of the entire psychosomatic enterprise (Alexander & French, 1946). Venerable hypotheses such as those linking extreme anger expression or inhibition with hypertension and coronary heart disease are still being pursued vigorously (see, e.g., Smith, 1992). In addition, new hypotheses have emerged that suggest that emotion inhibition may exacerbate minor ailments and compromise immune functioning (Pennebaker, 1990; Pennebaker, Kiecolt-Glaser, & Glaser, 1988), and that inexpressiveness may accelerate cancer progression (Fawzy et al., 1993; Gross, 1989; Spiegel, 1992; Spiegel, Bloom, Kraemer, & Gottheil, 1989). Together, these hypotheses suggest that emotion down-regulation (at least of negative emotions) may be bad for one's physical health

If one were to confuse the what and the how of emotion regulation, one might summarize these literatures by saying that emotion down-regulation is good for one's psychological health but bad for one's physical health. While this conclusion is possible, we do not believe that this is the most useful way to relate these two literatures. Instead, we believe that the process conception of emotion regulation described above may be used to distinguish between "antecedent-focused" emotion regulation (e.g., situation selection, situation modification, attentional deployment, and cognitive change) and "response-focused" emotion regulation (response modulation). Antecedent-focused forms of emotion regulation principally concern whether or not emotion response tendencies *are triggered* (psychological health literature), whereas response-focused strategies concern how emotion response tendencies *are modulated once they have been triggered* (physical health literature). Manipulating the input to the system—antecedent-focused emotion regulation—may be good for one's long-term psychological health. By contrast, manipulating the output of the emotion system—response-focused emotion regulation—may have deleterious consequences for certain aspects of physical health.

However suggestive, these literatures on the longer-term consequences of different forms of emotion regulation cannot conclusively establish differences among antecedent- and response-focused forms of emotion regulation. In everyday life, the boundaries between antecedent- and response-focused forms of regulation, as well as the distinctions between psychological and physical health, become blurred. For example, in T. W. Smith's (1992) transactional model, certain individuals create more anger-eliciting situations, to which they then respond with larger cardiovascular responses, thereby increasing their likelihood of cardiovascular disease.

What is needed, therefore, is a more direct test of the differential effects of various forms of emotion regulation. We have focused on the acute consequences of two theoretically derived forms of emotion down-regulation. Specifically, we have contrasted one form of antecedent-focused emotion regulation, which we have termed reappraisal (construing a potentially emotion-eliciting situation in nonemotional terms), with one form of response-focused emotion regulation, which we have termed expressive suppression (inhibiting ongoing emotion-expressive behavior). These studies have provided additional evidence that different forms of emotion regulation have clearly divergent consequences, at least in the short term.

Thus, in a series of studies (Gross & Levenson, 1993, 1997), we have demonstrated that expressive suppression decreases emotion-expressive behavior, decreases positive emotion experience but has no effect on negative emotion experience, and produces a mixed pattern of physiological responses, including decreased somatic activity and heart rate but increased signs of sympathetic activation of the electrodermal and cardiovascular systems. By contrast, reappraisal decreases both behavior and negative emotion experience, and produces no increases in autonomic responding (Gross, 1998a). More recently, we have shown that suppression decreases memory for information presented during the suppression period, whereas reappraisal has no such effect, either in the laboratory or in the field (Richards & Gross, 1999, 2000).

These results clearly indicate that although these two forms of emotion regulation both may be employed in the service of down-regulating emotions, their short-term consequences diverge quite markedly. Reappraisal effectively decreases both negative emotion experience and expression, and does so without apparent physiological or cognitive cost. Suppression, by contrast, has no impact on negative emotion experience, and has both physiological and cognitive costs. Although there is much that we still don't know about emotion regulation and its consequences, we believe that the evidence suggests that different forms of emotion regulation have different consequences.

Individual Differences in Emotion Regulation

Our process analysis of emotion generation and regulation suggests two broad points at which individual differences might have a substantial bearing on emotion regulation. The first has to do with emotion representation, which provides accurate and timely information regarding which emotion is likely, or already underway, and specifies precise details concerning the nature and intensity of that emotion. The second concerns emotion regulation more directly and has to do with how a given emotion is best handled within a given context.

One of the important determinants of the intelligent management of emotions is the degree to which one has differentiated emotion experience. The wealth of specific information contained in discrete emotion concepts should make emotion regulation easier, more efficient, and more effective. As a result, individuals who use emotion labels to name their feelings in a distinct and specific fashion should possess a larger repertoire of experience- and expression-related regulation strategies, thereby producing a more flexible behavioral repertoire to deal with the emotional event or the object(s) which generated the emotion. This relationship between emotion differentiation and regulation may be particularly potent for emotional experiences that have strong informational, or "signal," value (i.e., negative or intense emotional experiences). Preliminary evidence from a recent experience-sampling study (Feldman Barrett, Gross, Conner, & Benvenuto, 2000) has provided support for the hypothesis that emotion differentiation is related to emotion regulation practices. Differentiation of negative emotional experiences is associated with a larger repertoire of emotion regulation strategies, particularly for those who experience their emotions intensely.

Whether we are considering the short-term or long-term consequences of emotion regulation, it seems clear that the costs and benefits of different forms of emotion regulation may vary markedly (at least for emotion down-regulation). This suggests that in a given context there may be more and less optimal ways of regulating emotions. That is, some forms of emotion regulation produce better results with less costs than do other forms of emotion regulation. On the basis of these findings, it seems reasonable to suggest that a second important part of emotional intelligence is knowing *how* to regulate emotions when that is necessary, and we might imagine that individuals would choose to invoke different emotion regulatory processes in order to achieve a given goal. From this perspective, emotional intelligence might refer to the match of a regulatory process to a situation, as well as the range of emotion regulatory processes at an individual's disposal and the flexibility with which he/she employs these strategies.

Summary

Emotions are often helpful, but they are not always so. Emotion regulation refers to individuals' attempts to influence which emotions they have and how they experience and express these emotions. As is the case with any regulated system, a prerequisite for effective regulation is accurate and timely knowledge about the target of regulation—in this case, emotion. Thus, one important element of successful regulation would seem to be emotion differentiation, which provides information essential to determining when emotion regulation may be necessary. Yet differentiated emotion knowledge is not all there is to intelligent emotion regulation. Different forms of emotion regulation have very different consequences, and a second major aspect of emotional intelligence seems likely to be knowing how to flexibly regulate emotions in a way that is well matched to the demands of a particular situation.

FUTURE RESEARCH ON EMOTIONAL INTELLIGENCE

Classical conceptions of intelligence have prioritized a relatively narrow set of mental capacities. In the past few decades, there have been moves in a number of quarters to expand the traditional conception of intelligence (see, e.g., Gardner, 1983). One of the most important avenues of much-needed expansion has been the effort to consider individual differences in the skill with which individuals conduct their emotional lives. Emotional intelligence, which has come to be the umbrella term for such differences, now includes a broad range of attributes, from monitoring emotions in others to appreciating cultural norms regarding the emotional meaning of shared symbols. In this chapter, we have used a process conception of emotion generation and regulation to focus on two critical aspects of emotional intelligence—emotion differentiation and emotion regulation—arguing that individual differences in each of these processes have important implications for adaptive success. Important questions remain, however. In the following subsections, we touch upon three of the more pressing issues awaiting further exploration.

Intervening versus Leaving Well Enough Alone

Under certain circumstances, applying emotion knowledge in a top–down, conscious fashion so as to elaborate an emotion into a fully differentiated experience may be taxing, particularly if working memory resources are in short supply. A person who withholds the application of discrete labeling may be able to postpone a more reflective examination of an emotional response to a time or a place in which they would be more equipped to deal with the consequences. Thus, knowing when not to employ emotion knowledge may be a critical aspect of emotionally intelligent behavior. Similarly, emotionally intelligent people should know when *not* to regulate emotions. Evolution's "best guess" as to how a taxing situation should be handled certainly can be improved upon in many situations, but there are many other circumstances in which the emotion trajectory is best left alone. For example, there may be occasions when it is more adaptive to experience or express a negative emotion than to try to regulate it away (e.g., in therapy; see Parrott, 1993). More generally, it seems likely that the very act of monitoring and regulating emotion may direct precious cognitive resources away from the environment or other pressing tasks. To this extent, there is a price to be paid whenever emotions are elaborated or regulated, and emotional intelligence may consist in large measure of knowing when to leave well enough alone and when to intervene.

Optimizing versus Satisficing

According to Mayer and Salovey (1997), emotional intelligence is a real intelligence only if there are correct emotional responses. The question of evaluating the accuracy of one's own emotional response is difficult because, unlike in simpler, nonsocial tasks, negotiating complex social contexts has no clear set of "right" answers. There certainly are better and worse responses, but there may be a range of responses that are better than worse. Indeed, it may well be that emotions are designed to "satisfice," that is, to serve as adequate (although by no means perfect) solutions to a broad class of important challenges or opportunities (Simon, 1967). Although emotions may not be the optimal ("correct") solution to a given adaptive problem, they can be produced quickly, with a modest outlay of resources, and it frequently is better to have a timely and adequate solution than a better solution that is delivered at some later point.

One way to evaluate the quality of an emotional response (in emotion generation or emotion regulation) might be determined by whether or not the emotion facilitates behavior, thereby allowing an individual to effectively meet his/her goals. This view would be silent on whether or not those goals are socially productive in the first place, however. Consider this example: A young man who prides himself on being an independent, rational person is angry at his partner for being emotionally unavailable to him. Rather than directly discuss his feeling with his partner, he ends up being late for a series of business dinners that are very important to her career. As a result, his partner yells at him. An argument ensues in which the couple exchange accusations and harsh words.

We might assume that the young man is not displaying emotionally intelligent behavior. He did not approach his partner in a open manner to discuss his concerns. Indeed, in psychodynamic terms this would be considered an example of passive–aggressive behavior (i.e., aggression toward the other is expressed indirectly and ineffectively through passivity). However, consider the young man's goals: He wants to let his partner know that he is angry, yet he does not want to violate his sense of himself as an independent person who, being rational, is not verbally aggressive toward others unless provoked. Rather than acknowledge and take responsibility for his feelings, the young man engages in a behavior that angers his partner, thereby motivating her to initiate the argument. In the end, the young man is able to regulate his emotion in such a way as to have his goals met (to express anger in a way that does not challenge his self-concept), even though his behavior does not enhance his social life. Although the young man in our example may not be demonstrating social intelligence, his response is emotionally intelligent in that it has allowed him to effectively meet his goals.

Thus, from our perspective, emotional intelligence need not imply "good" (i.e., socially sanctioned) goals. The quality of the chosen goal is related more to social competence and social intelligence than to emotional intelligence per se. One may be positively evil and yet be emotionally intelligent in the sense that one knows how to manage one's emotions so as to further one's (wicked) ends. Thus, we believe that individual differences in emotion differentiation and regulation are important even though there are no correct or absolute answers to questions as to how and when to best experience, express, and regulate emotions in order to appropriately balance short-term versus longer-term goals.

Flexibility versus Efficiency

There seems to be an inevitable trade-off between efficiency and flexibility in the processes involved with emotional intelligence. Skills related to emotional intelligence that are very routinized (e.g., the automatic deployment of emotion knowledge or antecedent emotion regulation like situation selection) may be very efficient, but they may not leave the person able to calibrate to new situational demands (i.e., you need to know and have control over *when* to deploy what you know about emotion). Indeed, one of the central tensions in successful adaptation is the tension between the need for stable patterns of behavior and the need for openness and flexibility. If an individual inhabits a world that changes little in its interpersonal emotional demands, that individual may function very well using highly conserved and routinized emotion regulation procedures. Years of experience have finely tuned ways of regulating emotions, and these stable patterns have become so overlearned that little cognitive resources are necessary. However, that apparently highly adaptive set of procedures may be very maladaptive indeed when a dramatic change in the social world occurs. Since most of us live in a world with fluctuating and competing demands, some degree of flexibility is necessary in our emotional lives to leave us well adapted to our social environment.

NOTES

1. From this perspective, the accuracy of one's own emotional response to a given situation, person, or inanimate object is more difficult, because there are no straightforward criteria for validating a subjective experience in the self. There are normative object–emotion relationships that are anchored in an individual's own learning history, but these may be somewhat idiosyncratic to the person. There are also normative relationships anchored in the cultural context, but to say that an intelligent response must conform to these sounds more prescriptive than we might like.
2. Other models for parsing affective space exist. For example, the negative activation/positive activation (NA/PA) model focuses on two dimensions that are derived from rotating the valence and arousal dimensions in factor analyses of self-reported affect (Watson & Tellegen, 1985). The NA and PA dimensions do not appear in semantic analyses of emotion words, however. Moreover, recent evidence from four experience-sampling studies suggests that variations in the valence and arousal components determine when the NA/PA configuration appears and when it does not; thus, the NA/PA model can be considered a special case of the circumplex model (Feldman Barrett, 1999).
3. There is evidence for this claim from recent cognitive neuroscience investigations of subjective emotional experience (for a discussion, see Lane, in press).

REFERENCES

Alexander, F., & French, T. M. (1946). *Psychoanalytic therapy: Principles and applications.* New York: Ronald Press.

Averill, J. R. (1980). A constructivist view of emotion. In R. Plutchik & H. Kellerman (Eds.), *Theories of emotion* (pp. 339–368). New York: Plenum Press.

Baddeley, A. D. (1986). *Working memory.* Oxford, UK: Oxford University Press.

Barlow, D. H. (1991). Disorders of emotion. *Psychological Inquiry, 2,* 58–71.

Bar-On, R. (1997). *The Bar-On Emotional Quotient Inventory: A measure of emotional intelligence.* Toronto, Ontario, Canada: Multi-Health Systems.

Beck, A. T., Rush, A. J., Shaw, B. F., & Emery, G. (1979). *Cognitive therapy of depression.* New York: Guilford Press.

Blascovich, J. (1992). A biopsychosocial approach to arousal regulation. *Journal of Social and Clinical Psychology, 11,* 213–237.

Block, J. (1957). Studies in the phenomenology of emotions. *Journal of Abnormal and Social Psychology, 54,* 358–363.

Boden, J. M., & Baumeister, R. F. (1997). Repressive coping: Distraction using pleasant thoughts and memories. *Journal of Personality and Social Psychology, 73,* 45–62.

Bush, L. E., II. (1973). Individual differences multidimensional scaling of adjectives denoting feelings. *Journal of Personality and Social Psychology, 25,* 50–57.

Carpenter, P. A., Just, M. A., & Shell, P. (1990). What one intelligence test measures: A theoretical account of the processing in the Raven Progressive Matrices Test. *Psychological Review, 97,* 404–431.

Carstensen, L. L., Pasupathi, M., & Mayr, U. (in press). Emotional experience in everyday life across the adult life span. *Journal of Personality and Social Psychology*.

Christianson, S.-Å. (Ed). (1992). *The handbook of emotion and memory: Research and theory*. Hillsdale, NJ: Erlbaum.

Clore, G. C. (1994). Why emotions are felt. In P. Ekman & R. J. Davidson (Eds.), *The nature of emotion: Fundamental questions* (pp. 103–111). New York: Oxford University Press.

Clore, G. L., & Parrott W. G. (1991). Moods and their vicissitudes: Thought and feelings as information. In J. P. Forgas (Ed.), *Emotion and social judgment* (pp. 107–123). Oxford, UK: Pergamon Press.

Cole, P. M. (1986). Children's spontaneous control of facial expression. *Child Development, 57*, 1309–1321.

Damasio, A. R. (1994). *Descartes' error: Emotion, reason, and the human brain*. New York: Putnam.

Daneman, M., & Carpenter, P. A. (1980). Individual differences in working memory and reading. *Journal of Verbal Learning and Verbal Behavior, 19*, 450–466.

Ekman, P. (1992). Are there basic emotions? *Psychological Review, 99*, 550–553.

Fawzy, F., Fawzy, N., Hyun, C., Elashoff, R., Guthrie, D., Fahey, J., & Morton, D. (1993). Malignant melanoma: Effects of an early structured psychiatric intervention, coping, and affective state on recurrence and survival six years later. *Archives of General Psychiatry, 50*, 681–689.

Feldman, L. A. (1995a). Valence focus and arousal focus: Individual differences in the structure of affective experience. *Journal of Personality and Social Psychology, 69*, 153–166.

Feldman, L. A. (1995b). Variations in the circumplex structure of emotion. *Personality and Social Psychology Bulletin, 21*, 806–817.

Feldman Barrett, L. (1998a). Discrete emotions or dimensions?: The role of valence focus and arousal focus. *Cognition and Emotion, 12*, 579–599.

Feldman Barrett, L. (1998b, October). *Discrete emotions or dimensions?: Evidence from idiographic studies of affective experience*. Paper presented at the annual meeting of the Society of Experimental Social Psychology, Lexington, KY.

Feldman Barrett, L. (1999). *Personality process and affective focus*. Unpublished manuscript, Boston College.

Feldman Barrett, L., & Aronson, K. (1998). [Emotion differentiation and stressful life events]. Unpublished raw data.

Feldman Barrett, L., & Blascovich, J. (1994). [Arousal focus and heartbeat sensitivity]. Unpublished raw data, University of California, Santa Barbara.

Feldman Barrett, L., & Fossum, T. (in press). Mental representations of affective knowledge. *Cognition and Emotion*.

Feldman Barrett, L., Gross, J., Conner, T., & Benvenuto, M. (2000). *Knowing what you're feeling and knowing what to do about it: Mapping the relation between emotion differentiation and emotion regulation*. Manuscript submitted for publication.

Forgas, J. (Ed.). (2000). *Thinking and feeling: The role of affect in social cognition*. Cambridge, UK: Cambridge University Press.

Fredrickson, B. L. (1998). What good are positive emotions? *Review of General Psychology, 2,* 300–319.

Freud, S. (1959). *Inhibitions, symptoms and anxiety* (J. Strachey, Ed. & Trans.). New York: Norton. (Original work published 1926)

Frijda, N. H. (1986). *The emotions.* Cambridge, UK: Cambridge University Press.

Gabrieli, J. D. E., Singh, J., Stebbins, G. T., & Goetz, C. G. (1996). Reduced working memory span in Parkinson's disease: Evidence for the role of frontostriatal system in working and strategic memory. *Neuropsychology, 10,* 322–332.

Gardner, H. (1983). *Frames of mind.* New York: Basic Books.

Gilbert, D. T., & Wilson, T. D. (2000). Miswanting: Some problems in the forecasting of future affective states. In J. Forgas (Ed.), *Thinking and feeling: The role of affect in social cognition* (pp. 178–197). Cambridge, UK: Cambridge University Press.

Goleman, D. (1995). *Emotional intelligence.* New York: Bantam Books.

Gross, J. J. (1989). Emotional expression in cancer onset and progression. *Social Science and Medicine, 28,* 1239–1248.

Gross, J. J. (1998a). Antecedent- and response-focused emotion regulation: Divergent consequences for experience, expression, and physiology. *Journal of Personality and Social Psychology, 74,* 224–237.

Gross, J. J. (1998b). The emerging field of emotion regulation: An integrative review. *Review of General Psychology, 2,* 271–299.

Gross, J. J. (1999a). Emotion and emotion regulation. In L. A. Pervin & O. P. John (Eds.), *Handbook of personality: Theory and research* (2nd ed., pp. 525–552). New York: Guilford Press.

Gross, J. J. (1999b). Emotion regulation: Past, present, future. *Cognition and Emotion, 13,* 551–573.

Gross, J. J., & Richards, J. M. (2000). *Emotion regulation in everyday life: Sex, ethnicity, and social context.* Manuscript in preparation.

Gross, J. J., & Levenson, R. W. (1993). Emotional suppression: Physiology, self-report, and expressive behavior. *Journal of Personality and Social Psychology, 64,* 970–986.

Gross, J. J., & Levenson, R. W. (1997). Hiding feelings: The acute effects of inhibiting positive and negative emotions. *Journal of Abnormal Psychology, 106,* 95–103.

Gross, J. J., & Muñoz, R. F. (1995). Emotion regulation and mental health. *Clinical Psychology: Science and Practice, 2,* 151–164.

Izard, C. E. (1977). *Human emotions.* New York: Plenum Press.

Izard, C. (1993). Four systems for emotion activation: Cognitive and non-cognitive processes. *Psychological Review, 100,* 68–90.

Katkin, E. S. (1985). Blood sweat and tears: Individual differences in autonomic self-perception. *Psychophysiology, 22,* 125–137.

Katkin, E. S., Blascovich, J., & Goldband, S. (1981). Empirical assessment of visceral self-perception: Individual and sex differences in the acquisition of heartbeat discrimination. *Journal of Personality and Social Psychology, 40,* 1095–1101.

Kyllonen, P. C., & Christal, R. E. (1990). Reasoning ability is (little more than) working memory capacity. *Intelligence, 14,* 389–433.

Lane, R. D. (in press). Levels of emotional awareness: Application to emotional intelligence. In J. Parker & R. Bar-On (Eds.), *Handbook of emotional intelligence*. San Francisco: Jossey-Bass.

Lane, R. D., Nadel, L., Allen, J. J. B., & Kaszniak, A. W. (2000). The study of emotion from the perspective of cognitive neuroscience. In R. D. Lane, L. Nadel, G. Ahern, J. J. B. Allen, A. W. Kaszniak, S. Rapscak, & G. E. Schwartz (Eds.), *The cognitive neuroscience of emotion* (pp. 3–11). New York: Oxford University Press.

Lane, R. D., Quinlan, D. M., Schwartz, G. E., Walker, P. A., & Zeitlin, S. B. (1990). The Levels of Emotional Awareness Scale: A cognitive-developmental measure of emotion. *Journal of Personality Assessment, 55*, 124–134.

Lane, R. D., & Schwartz, G. E. (1987). Levels of emotional awareness: A cognitive-developmental theory and its application to psychopathology. *American Journal of Psychiatry, 144*, 133–143.

Lane, R. D., Sechrest, B., Reidel, R., Weldon, V., Kaszniak, A. W., & Schwartz, G. (1996). Impaired verbal and nonverbal emotion recognition in alexithymia. *Psychosomatic Medicine, 58*, 203–210.

Larsen, R. J., & Cutler, S. E. (1996). The complexity of individual emotional lives: A within-subject analysis of affect structure. *Journal of Social and Clinical Psychology, 15*, 206–230.

Lazarus, R. S. (1991). *Emotion and adaptation*. New York: Oxford University Press.

LeDoux, J. E. (1996). *The emotional brain: The mysterious underpinnings of emotional life*. New York: Simon & Schuster.

LeDoux, J. E. (2000). Cognitive-emotional interactions: Listening to the brain. In R. Lane, L. Nadel, G. Ahern, J. Allen, A. Kaszniak, S. Rapcsak, & G. Schwartz (Eds.), *Cognitive neuroscience of emotion* (pp. 129–155). New York: Oxford University Press.

Mandler, G. (1984). *Mind and body: Psychology of emotion and stress*. New York: Norton.

Mayer, J. D., Caruso, D. R., & Salovey, P. (1999). Emotional intelligence meets traditional standards for an intelligence. *Intelligence, 27*, 267–298.

Mayer, J. D., & Geher, G. (1996). Emotional intelligence and the identification of emotion. *Intelligence, 22*, 89–113.

Mayer, J. D., & Salovey, P. (1997). What is emotional intelligence? In P. Salovey & D. Sluyter (Eds.), *Emotional development and emotional intelligence: Implications for educators* (pp. 3–31). New York: Basic Books.

Mayer, J. D., Salovey, P., & Caruso, D. (2000). Competing models of emotional intelligence. In R. J. Sternberg (Ed.), *Handbook of human intelligence* (2nd ed., pp. 396–420). New York: Cambridge University Press.

Mesquita, B., & Fridja, N. H. (1992). Cultural variations in emotion. *Psychological Bulletin, 112*, 179–204.

Niedenthal, P. M., & Kitayama, S. (Eds.). (1994). *The heart's eye: Emotional influences in perception and attention*. New York: Academic Press.

Parrott, W. G. (1993). Beyond hedonism: Motives for inhibiting good moods and for maintaining bad moods. In D. M. Wegner & J. M. Pennebaker (Eds.), *Handbook of mental control* (pp. 279–305). Englewood Cliffs, NJ: Prentice-Hall.

Pennebaker, J. W. (1982). *The psychology of physical symptoms*. New York: Springer-Verlag.

Pennebaker, J. W. (1990). *Opening up: The healing powers of confiding in others.* New York: Morrow.

Pennebaker, J. W., Kiecolt-Glaser, J. K., & Glaser, R. (1988). Disclosure of traumas and immune function: Health implications for psychotherapy. *Journal of Consulting and Clinical Psychology, 56,* 239–245.

Remington, N. A., Fabrigan, L. R., & Visser, P. S. (2000). Re-examining the circumplex model of affect. *Journal of Personality and Social Psychology, 79,* 286–300.

Richards, J., & Gross, J. J. (1999). Composure at any cost? The cognitive consequences of emotion suppression. *Personality and Social Psychology Bulletin, 25,* 1033–1044.

Richards, J., & Gross, J. J. (2000). Emotion regulation and memory: The cognitive costs of keeping one's cool. *Journal of Personality and Social Psychology, 79,* 410–424.

Russell, J. A. (1980). A circumplex model of affect. *Journal of Personality and Social Psychology, 39,* 1161–1178.

Russell, J. A. (1983). Pancultural aspects of the human conceptual organization of emotions. *Journal of Personality and Social Psychology, 45,* 1281–1288.

Russell, J. A. (1991). Culture and the categorization of emotions. *Psychological Bulletin, 110,* 426–450.

Russell, J. A., & Bullock, M. (1985). Multidimensional scaling of emotional facial expression: Similarity from preschoolers to adults. *Journal of Personality and Social Psychology, 38,* 1290–1298.

Russell, J. A., & Feldman Barrett, L. (1999). Core affect, prototypical emotional episodes, and other things called *emotion*: Dissecting the elephant. *Journal of Personality and Social Psychology, 76,* 805–819.

Russell, J. A., Lewicka, M., & Niit, T. (1989). A cross-cultural study of a circumplex model of affect. *Journal of Personality and Social Psychology, 57,* 848–856.

Russell, J. A., & Ridgeway, D. (1983). Dimensions underlying children's emotion concepts. *Developmental Psychology, 19,* 795–804.

Russell, J. A., Yik, M. S. M., & Feldman Barrett, L. (1999). Integrating four structures of current mood into a circumplex: Integration and beyond. *Journal of Personality and Social Psychology, 77,* 600–619.

Salovey, P., & Mayer, J. D. (1990). Emotional intelligence. *Imagination, Cognition, and Personality, 9,* 185–211.

Schwarz, N. (1990). Feelings as information: Informational and motivational functions of affective states. In E. T. Higgins & R. M. Sorentino (Eds.), *Handbook of motivation and cognition: Foundations of social behavior* (Vol. 2, pp. 527–561). New York: Guilford Press.

Schwarz, N., & Clore, G. L. (1983). Mood, misattribution, and judgments of well-being: Informative and directive functions of affective states. *Journal of Personality and Social Psychology, 45,* 513–523.

Schwarz, N., & Clore, G. L. (1996). Feelings and phenomenal experiences. In E. T. Higgins & A. W. Kruglanski (Eds.), *Social psychology: Handbook of basic principles* (pp. 433–465). New York: Guilford Press.

Seligman, M. (1991). *Learned optimism.* New York: Knopf.

Shweder, R. A. (1993). The cultural psychology of emotions. In M. Lewis & J. M. Haviland (Eds.), *Handbook of emotions* (pp. 417–431). New York: Guilford Press.

Simon, H. A. (1967). Motivational and emotional controls of cognition. *Psychological Review, 74*, 29–39.

Smith, C. A., & Lazarus, R. S. (1990). Emotion and adaptation. In L. A. Pervin (Ed.), *Handbook of personality: Theory and research* (pp. 609–637). New York: Guilford Press.

Smith, C. A., & Pope, L. K. (1992). Appraisal and emotion: The interactional contributions of dispositional and situational factors. *Review of Personality and Social Psychology, 14*, 32–62.

Smith, T. W. (1992). Hostility and health: Current status of a psychosomatic hypothesis. *Health Psychology, 11*, 139–150.

Spiegel, D. (1992). Effects of psychosocial support on patients with metastatic breast cancer. *Journal of Psychosocial Oncology, 10*, 113–120.

Spiegel, D., Bloom, J. R., Kraemer, H. C., & Gottheil, E. (1989, October 14). Effect of psychosocial treatment on survival of patients with metastatic breast cancer. *The Lancet, 2*, 888–891.

Stein, N., & Trabasso, T. (1992). The organization of emotional experience: Creating links among emotion, thinking, language, and intentional action. *Cognition and Emotion, 6*, 225–245.

Taylor, G. J., Bagby, R. M., & Parker, J. D. A. (1997). *Disorders of affect regulation: Alexithymia in medical and psychiatric illness.* Cambridge, UK: Cambridge University Press.

Tooby, J., & Cosmides, L. (1990). The past explains the present: Emotional adaptations and the structure of ancestral environments. *Ethology and Sociobiology, 11*, 375–424.

Watson, D., & Tellegen, A. (1985). Towards a consensual structure of mood. *Psychological Bulletin, 98*, 219–235.

Zajonc, R. B. (1998). Emotions. In D. Gilbert, S. T. Fiske, & G. Lindzey (Eds.), *Handbook of social psychology* (4th ed., Vol. 1, pp. 591–632). New York: McGraw-Hill.

Zillmann, D. (1983). Transfer of excitation in emotional behavior. In J. T. Cacioppo & R. E. Petty (Eds.), *Social psychophysiology: A sourcebook* (pp. 215–240). New York: Guilford Press.

10

Emotion and Coping

JUDITH TEDLIE MOSKOWITZ

The human response to stress, including the associated coping responses and negative emotional reactions, has long been a subject of interest for scientists (Cannon, 1932; Lazarus, Averill, & Opton, 1974; Selye, 1956). In the past 30 years, there has been a proliferation of research into how people react to stressful events, what they do in response to the events, and the extent to which the responses are effective or ineffective (see Aldwin, 1994, for a review). Much of this coping research has focused on short-term, or acute, stressful events with less attention given to ongoing, or chronic, stress (Gottlieb, 1997). Chronic stress may result from a single acute event that has lasting negative sequelae (e.g., natural disaster, death of a spouse), or it may be a function of a stressful situation that is unresolved and ongoing (e.g., providing care for an ill loved one). Living with chronic stress can result in frequent or ongoing high levels of negative emotions such as anxiety, sadness, and anger, and the chronic experience of excessive negative emotions may cause serious disruptions in physical, psychological, and social functioning (see Mayne, 1999, for a review). Despite the destructive consequences of ongoing elevated negative emotion, chronic stress is not universally detrimental. Some individuals who undergo chronic stress fare remarkably well and even manage to find some benefit in their experience. A key factor in determining how well a person adjusts to chronic stress is coping.

In this chapter I discuss coping and emotion in the context of chronic stress.[1] Specifically, I review findings regarding the co-occurrence of positive and negative emotions under conditions of chronic stress, and I focus on the possibility that positive emotions help to sustain individuals who are experiencing chronic stress. I begin by presenting an overview of Lazarus and Folkman's (1984) theory of stress and coping, the theoretical framework on which this work is based.

STRESS AND COPING THEORY

Coping is defined as efforts to deal with demands perceived as taxing or exceeding the resources of the person (Lazarus & Folkman, 1984). In other words, coping is a response to something perceived as stressful. The majority of coping research has been based on a transactional theory of stress and coping (Lazarus & Folkman, 1984) in which coping is viewed as part of a process that unfolds in response to the demands of the situation. A central tenet of the transactional theory of stress and coping is that coping needs to be assessed within the context of the stressful situation (Lazarus & Folkman, 1984). According to the theory, it is more informative to ask what someone did to cope with a particular stressful event than it is to ask what he/she did to cope in general because both the responses used and the effectiveness of those responses depend on characteristics of the situation.

There are three major components in the stress-and-coping process: appraisal, emotion, and coping. In the context of a given stressful event, appraisal produces emotion and prompts coping which, in turn, influences emotion and subsequent reappraisal of the situation. This appraisal–emotion–coping–emotion–reappraisal process continues until the situation is resolved or the appraisals are such that the event is no longer viewed as stressful. Empirically, it is difficult to capture a causal direction among appraisal, coping, and emotion because they influence each other, often in a very short period of time. There is, however, some emerging evidence that coping may be more likely to predict subsequent emotion than emotion is likely to predict subsequent coping (Carver & Scheier, 1994). The strength of the causal links is likely to depend on a variety of factors including the particular coping response, the nature of the stressful event, and the time between measurements.

Lazarus and Folkman (1984) differentiate two types of appraisal: primary and secondary. Primary appraisal is the individual's evaluation of an event in terms of his/her goals, values, and beliefs. Primary appraisal addresses the question of whether anything is at stake for the individual in the context of the event. Secondary appraisal indicates what, if anything, can be done in response to the event. It involves the assessment of available coping resources and the likelihood that those coping resources will be effective in the particular situation.

Lazarus and Folkman (1984) further differentiate five types of primary appraisal: irrelevant, benign/positive, harm/loss, threat, and challenge.

Events appraised as irrelevant are not associated with any particular emotion because the event has no bearing on the individual's values, beliefs, or goals. Events appraised as benign/positive are likely to give rise to positive emotions such as happiness or satisfaction and are unlikely to call for any type of coping response. Events appraised as harm/loss are usually associated with negative emotions such as sadness or anger, and those appraised as threat are usually associated with negative emotions such as anxiety (Lazarus, 1991). A challenge appraisal, the evaluation of a situation as having the potential for gain, is usually associated with both positive and negative emotions. Whereas an appraisal of challenge is likely to prompt feelings such as excitement and enthusiasm, there is also the potential for anxiety and fear because the outcome is uncertain (Folkman & Lazarus, 1985; Lazarus, 1991).

Harm/loss, threat, and challenge are what Lazarus and Folkman (1984) call the stress appraisals, and they, together with their associated emotions, prompt coping responses. On a theoretical level, there are two major functions of coping: Problem-focused coping involves taking steps to deal with the problem directly, whereas emotion-focused coping is aimed at ameliorating the negative emotions associated with the problem. Some examples of problem-focused coping are making a plan of action or concentrating on the next step. Some examples of emotion-focused coping are engaging in distracting activities, using alcohol or drugs, or focusing on the benefits that might come out of the stressful experience.

The theoretical distinction between problem-focused and emotion focused types of coping is useful for classifying and discussing the many types of coping, and it is used extensively in the coping literature. However, in practice, the distinction between coping aimed at addressing the problem and coping aimed at addressing the emotion isn't always clear. Problem-focused coping can also serve an emotion-focused function because by addressing the problem itself the individual is also addressing the source of his/her negative emotions. Thus, if the problem-focused efforts are successful, the negative emotions associated with the problem will also be reduced. For example, a problem-focused response to having a car that repeatedly breaks down would be to buy a new car. Buying a new car effectively eliminates the negative emotions associated with the repeated breakdowns of the old car. Thus, the problem-focused coping response has also served an emotion-focused function. There are also occasions in which emotion-focused types of coping can ultimately serve a problem-focused function. Studying in response to an upcoming exam is a form of problem-focused coping. However, high levels of anxiety may prohibit effective studying. Therefore, doing something to reduce the anxiety such as going to the gym or getting a massage may facilitate subsequent problem-focused coping. People rarely rely on just problem-focused or emotion-focused types of coping alone.

Usually, in response to a given stressful event, they employ a mix of problem-focused and emotion-focused responses (Folkman & Lazarus, 1985).

Categorization of Coping

One of the difficulties in synthesizing findings from the coping literature
comes from the wide variety of possible ways to categorize and label coping
responses. On a theoretical level, in addition to the problem-focused–
emotion-focused distinction, researchers have used approach–avoidance,
cognitive–behavioral, and engagement–disengagement coping categorizations and various combinations of these. Empirically, the number of different coping categorizations is vast and varies widely depending on the subject population, the stressful event under study, and the particular coping
measure used.

　　To simplify comparisons in the present chapter, I will group most coping responses into one of the three general categories of problem-focused
coping, social coping, or avoidant coping. *Problem-focused coping responses* include any behavioral or cognitive efforts to directly address the
source of the stress. *Social coping responses* involve turning to others for
information, advice, or support. *Avoidant coping responses* are aimed at
putting the stress out of mind, at least temporarily, and include responses
such as use of alcohol or drugs or engaging in a distracting activity to avoid
thinking about the stressor. Versions of these three factors have emerged in
a number of studies (see, e.g., Amirkhan, 1990; Aspinwall & Taylor, 1992;
Ayers, Sandler, West, & Roosa, 1996; Carver, Scheier, & Weintraub, 1989).
Although the majority of coping responses can be grouped into one of these
three categories, there are some that do not fit neatly into this structure.
For example, positive reappraisal, which involves seeing the benefit in a difficult situation, usually correlates most highly with problem-focused types
of coping (Folkman, Lazarus, Dunkel-Schetter, DeLongis, & Gruen, 1986;
Scheier, Weintraub, & Carver, 1986) even though it is aimed at reinterpret-
ing the stressor as something positive and thus is more of an emotion-
focused type of response (Carver et al., 1989; Folkman & Lazarus, 1985). I
will note these occasional exceptions below.

Coping and Emotion

Intuitively, it seems that the types of coping that are associated with high
levels of positive emotions should be associated with low levels of negative
emotions, and this is often the case. In general, problem-focused strategies
are associated with lower levels of negative emotions (see, e.g., Amirkhan,
1990; Carver et al., 1989; Endler & Parker, 1990; Folkman & Lazarus,
1988; Moskowitz, Folkman, Collette, & Vittinghoff, 1996; Revenson &

Felton, 1989) and higher levels of positive emotions (see, e.g., Blalock, DeVellis, & Giorgino, 1995; Folkman & Lazarus, 1988; Ntoumanis & Biddle, 1998; Revenson & Felton, 1989). Thus, actively addressing the source of the stress appears to result in a reduction in the stress-related negative emotions and an increase in the positive emotions that may reflect successful coping efforts. Even if problem-focused efforts are not successful in completely solving the problem causing distress (as is often the case in chronically stressful conditions), active, constructive efforts at addressing the problem (e.g., making a to-do list, formulating a plan, researching pros and cons of various options) can provide a sense of mastery and efficacy that results in greater well-being. It is likely that there is an adaptive cyclical association in which problem-focused coping leads to increased positive affect and decreased negative affect, which, in turn, promotes further problem-focused coping.

Avoidant coping strategies are usually associated with increased negative emotions (see, e.g., Amirkhan, 1990; Carver et al., 1989) and decreased positive emotions (see, e.g., Folkman & Lazarus, 1988; Revenson & Felton, 1989). One exception was reported by Stone, Kennedy-Moore, and Neale (1995) in a study of the association between daily coping and mood at the end of the day. They found that the use of distraction (a form of avoidant coping) in response to the "most bothersome event of the day" was associated with decreased negative emotions and increased positive emotions at the end of the day. It appears that in the short term, avoidant types of coping can be effective but in the longer term they are less adaptive (Suls & Fletcher, 1985).

Despite the evidence from a number of studies that positive and negative emotions are associated with coping in symmetrically opposite ways, there are several studies that indicate that positive and negative emotions are uniquely associated with different types of coping (see, e.g., Aspinwall & Taylor, 1992; Billings, Folkman, Acree, & Moskowitz, 2000; Blalock et al., 1995; Carver & Scheier, 1994; McCrae & Costa, 1986; Stanton & Snider, 1993; Zautra, et al., 1995). For example, in a longitudinal study of older adults with osteoarthritis, Blalock and colleagues (1995) found that problem-focused coping at entry into the study was associated with higher levels of positive emotions 6 months later but unrelated to negative emotions, whereas social and avoidant types of coping at entry were associated with higher levels of negative emotion at the 6-month follow-up but unrelated to positive emotions. These findings reinforce the importance of measuring both positive and negative emotions in studies of the role of coping in adjustment to stressful events. Even though there are cases in which a particular type of coping will be associated with both increased positive emotions and decreased negative emotions, there are also cases in which particular types of coping will affect only one or the other.

The exact conditions under which positive and negative emotions have different coping antecedents and consequences have yet to be fully explicated, but possibilities include differential time frames of effectiveness for different coping responses, situational factors such as controllability of the stressor, and personality characteristics that the individual brings to the stressful situation. To further investigate these possibilities, it is imperative that researchers examine positive as well as negative emotions. Fortunately, investigators have begun to heed the call for fuller assessment of adjustment to stressful events and are now more often measuring both positive and negative affective outcomes.

POSITIVE EMOTIONS IN THE CONTEXT OF STRESSFUL EVENTS

Negative emotions are to be expected in the context of chronic stress, because the environment is likely to be appraised as harmful or threatening. The experience of negative emotions in response to highly stressful conditions such as the death of a spouse, chronic work stress, or one's own or a loved one's illness is clearly the norm and, within limits, is adaptive. Negative emotions serve important attentional, motivational, and social functions in that they focus attention on the stressful situation, motivate the individual to act to change the situation, and may signal to others that help is needed (Levenson, 1994). However, as noted by B. L. Fredrickson and C. Branigan (Chapter 4, this volume) excessive negative emotions are associated with a wide array of clinical problems such as impaired immune functioning, unipolar depression, sexual dysfunction, and suicide. Thus, it isn't surprising that much of the psychological literature concerning adaptation to stress has focused on ways to lessen the severity or shorten the duration of negative emotions with comparatively little focus on the maintenance of positive emotions.

However, mounting evidence indicates that positive emotions may be an important focus of study and intervention (see Fredrickson & Branigan, Chapter 4, this volume). Positive emotions can occur with relatively high frequency, even in the most dire stressful contexts, and they can occur at the same time that depression and distress are significantly elevated. This suggests that positive emotions may play an adaptive role under chronically stressful conditions. In our study of caregiving partners of men with AIDS, the depression scores of the men in the study were in the range that would classify them as at risk for clinical depression, both during caregiving and after the death of the partner (Folkman, Chesney, Collette, Boccellari, & Cooke, 1996). However, with the exception of the time immediately surrounding the death of the partner, the participants reported experiencing positive emotions as frequently as they experienced negative emotions

(Folkman, 1997). Three years after the death of the partner, the mean depression score of the bereaved caregivers was still significantly higher than the general population mean (Moskowitz, Acree, & Folkman, 1998). Again, however, positive emotions were predominant. Beginning at 1 year postbereavement, positive emotions were reported significantly more frequently than negative emotions despite the fact that the men were still experiencing high levels of depressive mood.[2]

Researchers have reported similar findings in other populations experiencing severe or chronic stress. R. C. Silver and C. B. Wortman (1987; as reported in Wortman, 1987) assessed positive and negative emotions in a sample of people who had severe spinal cord injuries and a sample of parents who had lost a child to sudden infant death syndrome (SIDS). In both samples, despite the severity of the loss and the fairly high levels of negative emotions reported, positive emotions occurred with surprising frequency. In the sample with spinal cord injury, happiness was reported more frequently than negative emotions by the third week after injury. In a sample of parents who lost a child to SIDS, positive and negative emotions were reported with approximately the same frequency 3 weeks after the child's death, and by 3 months positive emotions were reported more frequently then negative emotions. Westbrook and Viney (1982) interviewed a sample of patients who were hospitalized with a chronic or disabling illness and a comparison group of healthy adults, regarding their "life at the moment, the good things and the bad; what it's like for you" (p. 901). As expected, when compared with the control group, patients' responses revealed significantly more anxiety, depression, anger, and helplessness. However, their responses also showed significantly *more* positive feelings than did the responses of the comparison group. The fact that the patients actually had higher levels of positive emotions than the (nonstressed) comparison group suggests that positive emotions may be playing a functional role in coping with the stress of being hospitalized with a chronic illness.

Given that positive emotions occur with surprising frequency in the face of chronically adverse circumstances, the question then becomes: What purpose do they serve?

FUNCTIONS AND CONSEQUENCES OF POSITIVE EMOTIONS IN STRESSFUL CONTEXTS

Negative emotions clearly serve important functions. They focus attention on the problem at hand and in some cases are associated with specific evolutionarily adaptive forms of action (e.g., anger prompts the urge to attack, fear prompts the urge to flee). Early emotion theories, if they addressed positive emotions at all, proposed that positive emotions served as a safety signal and were likely to lead to decreased vigilance and shallower processing of information compared to negative emotions (see Aspinwall, 1998; Fredrickson, 1998; and Fredrickson & Branigan, Chapter 4, this volume, for reviews). If this were the case, positive emotions would be detrimental in the context of chronic stress because they would counteract the adaptive attentional and motivational effects of negative emotions. There is, however, theoretical and empirical support for adaptive cognitive, social, and physiological functions of positive emotions.

Some two decades ago, Lazarus, Kanner, and Folkman (1980) considered the functional role that positive emotions serve in the context of stressful events. They hypothesized that in the context of negative emotions, positive emotions may serve as breathers, sustainers, or restorers. Under stressful conditions, when negative emotions are predominant, positive emotions may provide a psychological break or respite (breather), support continued coping efforts (sustainer), and replenish resources that have been depleted by the stress (restorer). Fredrickson (1998) proposed a complementary "broaden-and-build" model of the function of positive emotions. In contrast to the narrowing of attention and specific action tendencies associated with negative emotions, Fredrickson reviews evidence that positive emotions broaden the individual's attentional focus and behavioral repertoire and, as a consequence, build social, intellectual, and physical resources (for further discussion, see Fredrickson & Branigan, Chapter 4, this volume). Although the broaden-and-build model is not specific to chronic stress, under chronically stressful conditions the functions of positive emotions suggested by the model become especially important. The "broadening" function of positive emotions would enable the individual to see beyond the immediate stressor and possibly come up with creative alternative solutions to problems. The "building" function would help to rebuild resources (such as self-esteem and social support) depleted by enduring stressful conditions.

Despite the neglect of positive emotions in emotion research and theory, empirical evidence for the function of positive emotions has begun to accumulate. Below I review evidence that positive emotions facilitate cognitive processing, counteract physiological effects of negative emotion, and may encourage social support.

Positive Emotions Facilitate Some Cognitive Processes

Recent experimental work indicates that positive emotions may facilitate the processing of important (e.g., self-relevant) information and protect self-esteem even if that information is negative. In one set of studies (Trope & Neter, 1994; Trope & Pomerantz, 1998), people who were put in a positive mood (compared to those in a neutral or negative mood) were more interested in information regarding their personal weaknesses than in information regarding their personal strengths. Trope and colleagues suggest that positive emotions may buffer the individual from the potential negative effects of the information.

Reed and Aspinwall (1998) found that women who were given the opportunity to affirm a positive aspect of themselves oriented to information regarding their risk of a serious illness more quickly than did those not given the opportunity to affirm another aspect of the self. They also found the information more convincing and recalled more of the risk-confirming information at a 1-week follow-up session. This study provides further evidence that affirmative experiences that presumably increase positive affect directed toward the self can facilitate effective cognitive processing and self-regulation.

Isen and her colleagues have shown in a number of studies that positive affect promotes creativity and flexibility in thinking and problem solving (Estrada, Isen, & Young, 1997; Isen & Daubman, 1984; Isen, Daubman, & Nowicki, 1987; Isen & Geva, 1987; Isen, Johnson, Mertz, & Robinson, 1985). For example, Estrada and colleagues (1997) induced positive affect in a sample of physicians by giving them a small bag of candy. The researchers then asked them to "think aloud" through their decision process as they determined the diagnosis of a clinical case. Compared to a control group, participants in the positive-affect condition considered the correct diagnosis sooner but showed significantly less anchoring (insensitivity to disconfirming information).

Contrary to the traditionally held view that positive emotions hinder, or at least do not help, cognitive processing, these studies indicate that positive emotions actually facilitate attention to and processing of important information. It isn't clear, however, whether positive emotions have the same impact on cognitive processes under stressful conditions. This question awaits further research.

Positive Emotions Counteract Physiological Effects of Negative Emotions

Negative emotions may have serious physiological consequences if they are experienced for prolonged periods at excessive levels (Selye, 1956). There is experimental evidence that positive emotions may help to offset the damaging effects of negative emotions. Fredrickson and Levenson (1998) induced negative emotions in subjects by showing them a film that elicited fear. Subjects were then shown one of four films designed to elicit contentment, amusement, sadness, or no emotion (neutral condition). Measures of cardiovascular reactivity indicated that those individuals who were shown the contentment or amusement film had faster recovery to baseline than subjects shown the sad or neutral film. In a second study, Fredrickson and Levenson (1998) found that subjects who spontaneously smiled during a

sadness-eliciting film had faster recovery on measures of cardiovascular reactivity than subjects who did not smile during the film even though the
smilers and nonsmilers did not differ on their subjective experience of emotion and on most measures of cardiovascular activity during the film. Together, these studies indicate that positive emotions may "undo" some of
the negative physiological effects associated with negative emotions. Ex-
trapolated to the context of chronic stress, these findings indicate that the
experience of positive emotions may prevent the occurrence of stress-
induced illness and disease.

Positive Emotions Encourage Social Support

It is no surprise that negative emotions tend to repel social support (see,
e.g., Coyne, 1976). A study of emotional expression in the context of bereavement indicates, however, that positive emotions may facilitate social
support. Keltner and Bonanno (1997) found that those individuals who
showed genuine, or Duchenne, laughs or smiles while describing their relationship with their deceased spouse elicited more positive emotions and less
frustration in observers. In addition, untrained observers indicated that
they would be more likely to offer comfort to those individuals who
showed the Duchenne laughs or smiles. These findings suggest that positive
emotions in the context of chronic stress could serve to elicit social support,
consistent with Fredrickson's (1998) broaden-and-build model positing
that positive emotions serve to build social resources. Bereavement is
commonly thought of as a time in which the bereaved individuals are at
risk for becoming isolated and lonely. The experience and expression of
positive emotions during this stressful period may elicit social support and
strengthen social bonds.

In summary, theoretical and empirical work indicates that positive
emotions support greater creativity, more efficient cognitive processing and
decision making, elicit social support, and may provide a psychological respite from the distress associated with chronically stressful conditions. In
addition, it is hypothesized that positive emotions help to sustain coping efforts and to restore depleted resources. Whereas negative emotions motivate the individual to focus on the stressful situation itself, positive emotions may help the individual to take a step back and see the bigger picture,
perhaps allowing for a more creative or flexible solution.

HOW ARE POSITIVE EMOTIONS GENERATED IN THE CONTEXT OF CHRONIC STRESS?

I have reviewed evidence showing that positive emotions occur even in the
midst of extremely stressful circumstances and that positive emotions serve

important functions in these circumstances. The next logical question concerns *how* positive emotions are generated in the face of such high levels of negative emotions. If the information regarding the occurrence and function of positive emotions is to be useful for individuals experiencing stress or for clinicians who work with this population, we need to know the process by which positive emotions arise in the context of chronic stress (for a related discussion, see Folkman & Moskowitz, 2000). I will discuss three possibilities: (1) positive emotions are purely a physiological reaction to the negative emotions occurring in response to the stressful event; (2) positive emotions are a by-product of posttraumatic growth that often occurs in response to extreme stress; and (3) positive emotions are generated as part of the process of coping with chronic stress.

A Physiological Process

The opponent process theory of emotion (Soloman, 1980) proposes that a departure from emotional neutrality prompts an opposite emotional reaction that serves to counteract the departure and returns the individual back to an emotional steady state. So, for example, intense negative emotions such as those that occur in response to a stressful event would automatically trigger positive emotions as the opponent process and, overall, return the individual back to his/her emotional baseline. Based on opponent process theory, the co-occurrence of positive and negative emotions in the context of chronic stress would be explained as a physiological process geared toward maintaining an emotional equilibrium in the individual. The major problem with this explanation is that there is extensive empirical evidence that people monitor their emotions actively and often consciously act to change their negative affective states (Mayor & Gaschke, 1988; Mayer, Salovey, Gomberg-Kaufman, & Blainey, 1991; Thayer, Newman, & McClain, 1994). If the opponent process truly worked as hypothesized, people would not need to deliberately try to work themselves out of a bad mood—it would happen automatically as a function of the opponent process (Taylor, 1991). Therefore, although opponent process is a useful theory in some contexts, it is not sufficient to explain the positive emotions that occur in the context of chronic stress.

Posttraumatic Growth

The process of finding beneficial effects in negative experiences has been referred to as posttraumatic growth (Tedeschi, Park, & Calhoun, 1998), stress-related growth (Park, Cohen, & Murch, 1996), positive psychological changes (Yalom & Lieberman, 1991), transformational coping (Aldwin, 1994), benefit finding (Affleck & Tennen, 1996), and thriving (O'Leary &

Ickovics, 1995). Although the majority of research into the experience of stress has focused on its negative sequelae, there is evidence that stressful experiences can have beneficial effects such as improved personal relationships, changes in philosophy of life, and positive changes in aspects of the self such as increased self-reliance and perceptions of mastery (Tedeschi & Calhoun, 1995). A second possible explanation for the occurrence of positive emotions in the context of chronic stress is that they are a by-product of this process of growth in response to stressful experience. For example, Nolen-Hoeksema and Larson (1999) conducted a longitudinal study of people who had experienced the death of a loved one. When asked whether they had found anything positive in the experience, by 1 month after the loss 73% of the bereaved responded that they had found something positive. By the end of the 18-month study, more than 80% had found something positive in the death. The respondents cited reprioritization of goals, increased self-confidence and strength, and greater appreciation of family relationships, as some of the benefits that they found. Although the researchers did not measure positive emotions as an outcome, they found that finding benefit in the stressful experience of a loved one's death was associated with lower levels of distress. The respondents who found something positive in their loss were significantly less distressed at 6, 13, and 18 months after the loss than those who had not found something positive, even when initial levels of distress were statistically controlled (Davis, Nolen-Hoeksema, & Larson, 1998).

At the conclusion of our caregivers' study, we asked the men to reflect on what they had learned and how they had been changed by their caregiving and bereavement experiences. Their responses indicated that many of them perceived significant benefit as a result of these stressful experiences. Responses included "I've grown up," "I gained a lot of competence and respect about myself," "I feel I can do anything," "I'm a stronger better person," "I've never before found that kind of purity of my own intentions," "I'm stronger, than I've ever seen myself, more fortitude, more determination, more discipline," "I'm more giving and more loving" (Richards, Wrubel, & Folkman, 1998).

In an effort to quantify the benefits that the men perceived in the caregiving experience, we developed a measure of positive meaning in caregiving. We administered the scale throughout caregiving and then, retrospectively, at one assessment approximately 1 month after the death of the partner. Positive meaning in caregiving was significantly associated with positive emotions both during caregiving and after the death of the partner but was not significantly associated with negative emotions. These data indicate that the perception of positive aspects of stressful experiences may, at least partly, account for the occurrence of positive emotions in the context of chronic stress. Further research explicitly examining the association between perceptions of growth and positive emotions is needed to more definitively address this question.

Despite the empirical evidence of an association between perceptions of growth and positive emotions, it isn't likely that finding a silver lining in the midst of a stressful experience is the sole explanation for the occurrence of positive emotions under such extreme conditions. The majority of the research into posttraumatic growth focuses on what occurs *after* the traumatic event (as evidenced by the term "*post*traumatic growth"; Tedeschi et al., 1998). The question remains: How are positive emotions produced and maintained *during* the stressful event? Coping is one factor that may play a role by directly producing positive emotions as well as by prompting perceptions of benefits associated with the stress.

Coping

Recently, Folkman (1997) proposed a revision of stress and coping theory that makes the role of positive emotions in the coping process explicit and implicates several coping mechanisms in the occurrence of positive emotions in the context of a stressful event. In this revised model, Folkman discusses two main paths by which positive emotions are promoted and maintained: as a result of coping efforts concerned with the focal stressor itself, and as a result of efforts directed largely outside of the focal stressful event.

The coping responses concerned with the focal stressor that we found promote positive emotions, often independent of negative emotions, are problem-focused coping and positive reappraisal. Problem-focused coping involves behaviors such as gathering information, decision making, and planning aimed at the problem that is causing the stress. Positive reappraisal is the cognitive reframing of a situation to see it in a more positive light. In the case of providing care for a partner with AIDS, problem-focused responses may include such tasks as changing linens, refilling the partner's prescription, or simply making him comfortable. Even though the main source of stress, the partner's illness progression, continues, the successful completion of these seemingly mundane tasks can increase feelings of control during a period that is characterized by an absence of control, and can provide a sense of satisfaction that, in turn, promotes positive emotion. Similarly, following the partner's death, there are often many matters regarding memorials, insurance, and business transactions whose successful completion can help provide closure, increase feelings of self-efficacy, and signify moving on. The completion of these tasks during bereavement may be especially important in the maintenance of positive emotions in a period that is otherwise characterized by feelings of sadness, loss, and helplessness.

Positive reappraisal includes such responses as "I changed or grew as a person in a good way" and is likely to be a reflection of the process of post-traumatic growth. As noted earlier, positive reappraisal is generally considered a form of emotion-focused coping (Carver et al., 1989; Folkman & Lazarus, 1985), but is usually strongly correlated with problem-focused types of coping (Folkman et al., 1986; Scheier et al., 1986). It may be that positive reappraisal "travels with" problem-focused coping because it facilitates problem-focused efforts by providing some hope for a positive outcome, or at least for some silver lining in an otherwise gloomy situation, or because it follows in the wake of problem-focused coping that was effective.

We investigated the association between various types of coping with positive and negative moods at four time points over the course of caregiving and bereavement: 3 months and 1 month prior to the death of the partner, and 1 month and 3 months after the death of the partner (Moskowitz et al., 1996). We found that problem-focused coping was associated with increased positive mood both during caregiving and bereavement but associated with decreased negative mood only at 1 month prior to the death of the partner. Positive reappraisal was associated with positive emotions both during caregiving and bereavement and was associated with decreased negative emotions during bereavement only. Both of these findings remained significant even when emotions at the previous interview and the other types of coping were statistically controlled.

Beyond the coping responses aimed at the focal stressor, however, our data indicate that there may be other types of coping that are likely to be related to positive emotions in the context of ongoing stress (Folkman, 1997). When we started our caregivers study, we asked the participants only about the most stressful event they had experienced associated with caregiving or (after the death of their partner) bereavement. The participants told us that we also needed to ask about the positive things in their lives, the events that helped to sustain them. So we added a section to the interview in which we asked the participants to describe "something that you did, or something that happened to you that made you feel good and that was meaningful to you and helped you get through the day."

There was a total of 1,794 interviews in which this question was posed to the participants, and in 99.5% of those interviews the participants were able to report positive meaningful event. This finding is quite striking given the stress that these men were experiencing. We analyzed a subsample of these positive meaningful events (215 events reported by 36 participants; Folkman, Moskowitz, Ozer, & Park, 1997). The events often concerned something other than caregiving or bereavement (the subject of the focal stressors) and instead were associated with other roles the participants had (e.g., coworker, family member). In addition, they often concerned what on the surface appeared to be comparatively minor events (e.g., a beautiful sunset, a kind word from a friend, a good grade on a test). For example, one participant reported, "in the past week the thing I felt good about was on Sunday. I went into the backyard, weeded, cleaned up the yard, which is quite a chore, cleaned up the patio, cleaned the patio furniture, and got the backyard livable again." Another participant reported, "I started taking a tax course to help me get a part-time job because I've been out of work for two years. I got 100% on the first quiz last night. I've been out of school for so long the I'm not used to studying, especially with all the interruptions at home now with [my partner]."

These findings led us to hypothesize that under enduring stressful conditions such as caregiving or bereavement, people consciously or unconsciously seek out positive meaningful events that increase their positive emotions and, perhaps as a result, replenish their psychological resources and help to sustain their coping efforts. We were not able to test the hypothesis that positive meaningful events were associated with positive emotions because almost everyone who was asked the above question was able to report an event and thus we had little variance on reporting. Investigation of other facets of the events such as content, source of meaning, whether the event was related to the stressful event reported, whether the event was normatively positive, and whether the event was specific or global revealed few significant associations with positive or negative emotions (Moskowitz, Oorbeck, & Folkman, 1997). However, we have begun data collection in another group of caregivers, women caring for their children with HIV/AIDS, in which we will be able to more fully address this question of the role of meaningful events in the maintenance of positive emotions under stressful conditions.

In summary, although coping research has largely been concerned with the role of coping in relation to negative emotions, there are empirical data to indicate that coping may also be implicated in the occurrence and maintenance of positive emotions. At least three types of coping are associated with positive emotions even under the chronic stress of caregiving and bereavement. Problem-focused coping and positive reappraisal are two types of coping generally measured in response to a focal stressor that are consistently associated with positive emotions. Finding meaning in seemingly ordinary events is a third coping response that appeared to be associated with positive emotions in our sample of caregiving partners of men with AIDS.

FUTURE RESEARCH DIRECTIONS

Multiple studies have shown that positive emotions occur with surprising frequency even under conditions of extreme chronic stress when distress and depression are the norm. I have discussed several possible functions of positive emotions and have proposed several ways in which positive emotions may be created and supported in the midst of enduring stress. Although researchers and theorists have begun to turn their attention to positive emotions, the study of the function and maintenance of positive emotions in the context of chronic stress is still in its infancy and thus there are multiple research avenues that have particular promise. In the following subsections, I highlight a few of the measurement issues that deserve closer attention. Specifically I discuss the measurement of coping, the measurement of emotion, and the issue of chronic stress as a forum for the study of the stress and coping process.

Measurement of Coping

There has been a great deal of discussion in the field about the various approaches to the measurement and study of coping (see, e.g., Porter & Stone, 1996; Schwarzer & Schwarzer, 1996; Zautra, 1997), and each approach has its strengths and limitations. However, with respect to the occurrence and maintenance of positive emotions in the context of chronic stress, there are a few recommendations that can be made regarding the measurement of coping. As mentioned previously, coping as measured by most current coping checklists tends to be strongly associated with negative emotions. It may be that this is simply the nature of coping because it arises in response to distressing situations. However, there is more that we can do to tap into types of coping that are associated with positive emotions. Most coping questionnaires are not designed to assess strategies that promote positive emotions. A coping measure that is specifically designed to measure these "positive" coping responses is currently under development. It is called the Positive Coping Inventory (Billings & Folkman, 2000), and it is modeled on the Ways of Coping Questionnaire in that the respondent is asked to report a specific stressful event, then fill out a series of possible responses to that focal stressor. The Positive Coping Inventory consists of 13 subscales: autonomy, environmental mastery of stressor-associated activities, environmental mastery of other activities, personal growth, positive relations with others, purpose in life, self-acceptance, respite/positive distraction, energetic arousal, relaxation, religiosity, downward social comparison, and benefit reminding/capitalizing. Drawing on diverse personality and social-psychological approaches to positive emotions, including the well-being literature (see, e.g. Ryff, 1989), self complexity studies (Linville, 1985, 1987; Morgan & Janoff-Bulman, 1994), arousal and self-regulation models (Thayer, 1989), and research into the effects on emotions and health and religion/spirituality (McFadden & Levin, 1996), these 13 ways of coping were hypothesized to be strongly associated with positive emotions. Preliminary data indicate that the scales have acceptable reliability, and we are currently conducting validity analyses.

In addition to improving quantitative coping measurement, researchers should begin to include narrative assessments of stress and coping, which in our caregivers study were more sensitive to the types of coping that were related to positive emotions (e.g., positive meaningful events; Folkman et al., 1997). The richness and depth of the data that are collected through these narratives would be difficult to match in a quantitative measure,[3] and we have found that the quantitative and qualitative coping measures complement one another. For example, in a sample of HIV+ men, we compared narrative reports of coping in response to recent HIV-associated stressful events to coping with the same events as reported on the Ways of Coping Questionnaire (Moskowitz & Wrubel, 2000). Participants reported more types of coping per interview on the Ways of Coping Questionnaire than they did in the narratives, but narratives revealed coping responses that were not captured on the quantitative instrument, for example, goal choice, goal relinquishment, and contingency/flexible coping. The Ways of Coping Questionnaire taps a wider range of responses by prompting reports of thoughts and behaviors that the participant may not consider to be actions and therefore may not report in the narrative. The qualitative approach, on the other hand, provides understanding of process and content because the narratives capture the kind of situation being coped with and what's at stake for the person in the situation. By using both qualitative and quantitative approaches to the same question, we gained a fuller understanding of coping with HIV in the context of the participants' lives. Although qualitative analysis can be time and labor intensive, the insight provided by such analysis can be invaluable.

Measurement of Emotions

Based on the findings I have reviewed, the importance of measuring positive emotions as well as negative emotions should be clear. At the risk of stating the obvious, I emphasize that if positive emotions are not measured, we cannot test hypotheses regarding their occurrence and function in the context of chronic stress. In addition, although in my review I did not differentiate among positive emotions, future studies should consider the possibility of divergent effects of different positive emotions. For example, high-activation positive emotions such as excitement and elation are motivating emotions, whereas others such as satisfaction and pleasure indicate satiation and are less likely to prompt action. The different motivational properties inherent in different emotions may discriminate between those that serve to replenish psychological and social resources and those that sustain continued coping efforts. For example, pride may be associated with increases in self-esteem (a personal resource), whereas happiness is more likely to be associated with progress toward goals and thus prompt continued coping efforts (Lazarus, 1991). See Fredrickson (1998) and Fredrickson and Branigan (Chapter 4, this volume) for excellent discussions of the likely consequences of various positive emotions.

Chronic versus Acute Stresses versus Other Life Aspects

Throughout this chapter I have emphasized that the process of coping with chronic stress is different than that of coping with acute stress. However, researchers who study chronic stress (including myself) have for the most part adopted methods used in the study of acute stress by asking the participants to focus on the most recent stressful event associated with their chronic stress. It is important in future studies to consider the possibility that a different methodology may be more appropriate in the study of coping with chronic stress. Gottlieb (1997) points out that "many contexts of chronic stress do not lend themselves to an event-centered strategy of measuring coping, and much of coping with chronic stress will be missed if attention is focused only on effortful response to perceived stress on those occasions when acute events punctuate the chronic stress process" (p. 12). Methodologies that provide data on a range of coping episodes—from extremely stressful events to seemingly more minor events that might not otherwise be recalled as stressful at all—could provide a much richer picture of coping with chronic stress. Gottlieb suggests using thought-sampling techniques (Kendall & Hollon, 1981; Wegner, Schneider, Carter, & White, 1987), diaries (Eckenrode & Bolger, 1995), within-day reporting (Stone & Shiffman, 1992), and observation by trained personnel (Suls & Martin, 1993) as alternatives.

Furthermore, by having a participant report how he/she responded to a particular focal event, we tend to overlook other aspects of his/her life that may support well-being. Participants in our caregivers study wanted to tell us about other events in their lives besides the stressful events associated with caregiving or bereavement. This alerted us to the possibility that coping efforts extend beyond the focal stressor and that individuals may be sustaining their well-being through other means. Thus, future work should consider the participants' lives beyond their experience of chronic stress and be open to the possibility that other life events, roles, or aspects of the self are contributing to the maintenance of well-being. Techniques borrowed from the fields of sociology and anthropology such as participant observation and ethnography may also be useful to this end (see, e.g., Burawoy, 1991). For example, extended observation of caregivers both in the home with the care recipients and outside of the caregiving relationship could provide extremely rich data regarding the place of the caregiving role in the overall picture of the participants' experience. Triangulation of a variety of methodologies in gathering both quantitative and qualitative data is necessary in order for the field of coping to continue progress toward a fuller understanding of the factors involved in the maintenance of well-being in stressful contexts.

IMPLICATIONS FOR INTERVENTION

The data I have presented indicate that it may be useful for clinicians to focus on helping clients to increase positive emotions in addition to decreasing negative emotions. This is not a new idea in the clinical literature. For example, Lewinsohn and his colleagues recognized the importance of pleasant events (and the associated positive emotions) in the treatment of depression years ago (Lewinsohn & Amenson, 1978; Lewinsohn, Hoberman, & Clarke, 1989; Lewinsohn, Sullivan, & Grosscup, 1980). More recent work has pursued the idea that helping clients identify thoughts and beliefs that interfere with positive experiences is an important component of therapy (Fava, Rafanelli, Cazzaro, Conti, & Grandi, 1998).

One of the appealing aspects of studying the role of coping in adjustment to chronic stress (as opposed to the role of personality or genetic predisposition) is that coping immediately suggests a point of intervention. If we can identify coping strategies that are adaptive and the conditions under which they are adaptive, we can then attempt to teach people which coping strategies to use and when to use them. Based on the data presented here, interventions that include helping clients to identify and take advantage of opportunities for problem-focused coping and positive reappraisal may be useful in increasing frequency of positive emotions even under chronically stressful conditions. In addition, helping clients to identify and focus on positive meaningful events may help to increase the frequency of positive emotions. In fact, if the participants in our study are any indication, the very act of relating a positive meaningful event to someone else may help to bolster well-being.

CONCLUSIONS AND THOUGHTS ON POLLYANNA

The risk in proclaiming the importance of positive emotions in the stress and coping process is that I may appear to be minimizing the pain and serious individual and societal consequences associated with chronic stress. I am not advocating a simplistic "don't-worry—be-happy" approach. Such a Pollyannaish stance could easily degenerate into blaming the victim if he/

she does not think the positive thoughts that prevent depression in the face of enduring stress. Rather, my point is that the human response to stress is very complex and includes positive as well as negative emotional responses. Therefore, the research focus needs to expand to include the significant role that positive emotions play in the context of ongoing stress. I believe I have made the case for tolerating this additional layer of research complexity by suggesting pathways by which positive emotions arise in stressful circumstances and discussing how positive emotions then serve to maintain well-being under chronically stressful conditions.

ACKNOWLEDGMENTS

The writing of this chapter was supported by Grant Nos. MH49985, MH52517, and MH58069 from the National Institute of Mental Health. My thanks to Susan Folkman, George A. Bonanno, and Tracy J. Mayne for helpful comments on an earlier version of this chapter. I am indebted to the participants in the Coping Project of the University of California, San Francisco, who have taught us so much.

NOTES

1. For the purposes of this chapter, I do not differentiate between moods and emotions. There is discussion in the literature regarding various criteria (e.g., duration, antecedents, consequences, and relation to facial expression) for differentiating between the two, and the interested reader should consult Ekman and Davidson (1994, pp. 49–94) for a discussion of these issues. The data presented here are largely concerned with self-reports from participants in the context of stressful events. It isn't likely that asking participants to report their emotions versus their moods under these circumstances would have a large impact on what they actually report, and it isn't clear whether the lay person in this context would be able to make this distinction. Therefore, I use the term "emotion" to refer to affective states that participants report under these conditions.

2. There has been a great deal of discussion in the literature regarding the independence or bipolarity of positive and negative emotions (for reviews, see Feldman Barrett & Russell, 1998, and Russell & Carroll, 1999). As Russell and Carroll (1999) note, when all the measurement issues are considered, a bipolar model fits the data best. It should be noted that by making the assertion that both positive and negative emotions occur in chronically stressful situations, I am not implying that they are independent and that at any given *moment* high levels of negative emotions co-occur with high levels of positive emotions. Rather, my point is that over a period of time (the previous week in the case of our caregiver study) the data indicate that although participants, as expected, experience frequent negative affect, they also report fairly frequent positive affect. This finding is not in conflict with the conclusions of Russell and Carroll (1999).

3. Examples of the analysis of narrative data from our caregivers study include papers by Nolen-Hoeksema, McBride, and Larson (1997); Pennebaker, Mayne, and Francis (1997); Stein, Folkman, Trabasso, and Richards (1997); and Weiss and Richards (1997).

REFERENCES

Affleck, G., & Tennen, H. (1996). Construing benefits from adversity: Adaptational significance and dispositional underpinnings. *Journal of Personality, 64,* 899–922.

Aldwin, C. M. (1994). *Stress, coping, and development: An integrative perspective.* New York: Guilford Press.

Amirkhan, J. H. (1990). A factor analytically derived measure of coping: The coping strategy indicator. *Journal of Personality and Social Psychology, 59,* 1066–1074.

Aspinwall, L. G. (1998). Rethinking the role of positive affect in self-regulation. *Motivation and Emotion, 22,* 1–32.

Aspinwall, L. G., & Taylor, S. E. (1992). Modeling cognitive adaptation: A longitudinal investigation of the impact of individual differences and coping on college adjustment performance. *Journal of Personality and Social Psychology, 63,* 989–1003.

Ayers, T. S., Sandler, I. N., West, S. G., & Roosa, M. W. (1996). A dispositional and situational assessment of children's coping: Testing alternative models of coping. *Journal of Personality, 64,* 923–958.

Billings, D. W., & Folkman, S. (2000). *Assessing coping strategies designed to regulate positive affect during stress: The Positive Coping Inventory.* Manuscript in preparation.

Billings, D. W., Folkman, S., Acree, M., & Moskowitz, J. T. (2000). Coping and physical health during caregiving: The roles of positive and negative affect. *Journal of Personality and Social Psychology, 79,* 131–142.

Blalock, S. J., DeVellis, B. M., & Giorgino, K. B. (1995). The relationship between coping and psychological well-being among people with osteoarthritis: A problem-specific approach. *Annals of Behavioral Medicine, 17,* 107–115.

Burawoy, M. (1991). *Ethnography unbound: Power and resistance in the modern metropolis.* Berkeley: University of California Press.

Cannon, W. B. (1932). *The wisdom of the body.* New York: Norton.

Carver, C. S., & Scheier, M. F. (1994). Situational coping and coping dispositions in a stressful transaction. *Journal of Personality and Social Psychology, 66,* 184–195.

Carver, C. S., Scheier, M. F., & Weintraub, J. K. (1989). Assessing coping strategies: A theoretically based approach. *Journal of Personality and Social Psychology, 56,* 267–283.

Coyne, J. C. (1976). Depression and the response of others. *Journal of Abnormal Psychology, 85,* 186–193.

Davis, C. G., Nolen-Hoeksema, S., & Larson, J. (1998). Making sense of loss and benefiting from the experience: Two construals of meaning. *Journal of Personality and Social Psychology, 75,* 561–574.

Eckenrode, J., & Bolger, N. (1995). Daily and within day event measurement. In S. Cohen, R. C. Kessler, & L. U. Gordon (Eds.), *Measuring stress* (pp. 80–101). New York: Oxford University Press.

Ekman, P., & Davidson, R. J. (1994). *The nature of emotion: Fundamental questions.* New York: Oxford University Press.

Endler, N. S., & Parker, J. D. A. (1990). The multidimensional assessment of coping: A critical evaluation. *Journal of Personality and Social Psychology, 58,* 844–854.

Estrada, C. A., Isen, A. M., & Young, M. J. (1997). Positive affect facilitates integration of information and decreases anchoring in reasoning among physicians. *Organizational Behavior and Human Decision Processes, 72,* 117–135.

Fava, G. A., Rafanelli, C., Cazzaro, M., Conti, S., & Grandi, S. (1998). Well-being therapy: A novel psychotherapeutic approach for residual symptoms of affective disorders. *Psychological Medicine, 28,* 475–480.

Feldman Barrett, L. A., & Russell, J. A. (1998). Independence and bipolarity in the structure of current affect. *Journal of Personality and Social Psychology, 65,* 45–55.

Folkman, S. (1997). Positive psychological states and coping with severe stress. *Social Science and Medicine, 45,* 1207–1221.

Folkman, S., Chesney, M., Collette, L., Boccellari, A., & Cooke, M. (1996). Postbereavement depressive mood and its prebereavement predictors in HIV+ and HIV− gay men. *Journal of Personality and Social Psychology, 70,* 336–348.

Folkman, S., & Lazarus, R. S. (1985). If it changes it must be a process: Study of emotion and coping during three stages of a college examination. *Journal of Personality and Social Psychology, 48,* 150–170.

Folkman, S., & Lazarus, R. S. (1988). Coping as a mediator of emotion. *Journal of Personality and Social Psychology, 54,* 466–475.

Folkman, S., Lazarus, R. S., Dunkel-Schetter, C., DeLongis, A., & Gruen, R. J. (1986). Dynamics of a stressful encounter: Cognitive appraisal, coping, and encounter outcomes. *Journal of Personality and Social Psychology, 50,* 992–1003.

Folkman, S., & Moskowitz, J. T. (2000). Positive affect and the other side of coping. *American Psychologist, 55,* 647–654.

Folkman, S., Moskowitz, J. T., Ozer, E. M., & Park, C. L. (1997). Meaningful events as coping in the context of HIV/AIDS. In B. H. Gottlieb (Ed.), *Coping with chronic stress* (pp. 293–314). New York: Plenum Press.

Fredrickson, B. L. (1998). What good are positive emotions? *Review of General Psychology, 2,* 300–319.

Fredrickson, B. L., & Levenson, R. W. (1998). Positive emotions speed recovery from the cardiovascular sequelae of negative emotions. *Cognition and Emotion, 12,* 191–220.

Gottlieb, B. H. (1997). Conceptual and measurement issues in the study of coping with chronic stress. In B. H. Gottlieb (Ed.), *Coping with chronic stress* (pp. 3–40). New York: Plenum Press.

Isen, A. M., & Daubman, K. A. (1984). The influence of affect on categorization. *Journal of Personality and Social Psychology, 47,* 1206–1217.

Isen, A. M., Daubman, K. A., & Nowicki, G. P. (1987). Positive affect facilitates creative problem solving. *Journal of Personality and Social Psychology, 52,* 1122–1131.

Isen, A. M., & Geva, N. (1987). The influence of positive affect on acceptable level of risk: The person with a large canoe has a large worry. *Organizational Behavior and Human Decision Processes, 39,* 145–154.

Isen, A. M., Johnson, M. M. S., Mertz, E., & Robinson, G. F. (1985). The influence of positive affect on the unusualness of word associations. *Journal of Personality and Social Psychology, 48,* 1413–1426.

Keltner, D., & Bonanno, G. A. (1997). A study of laughter and dissociation: Distinct correlates of laughter and smiling during bereavement. *Journal of Personality and Social Psychology, 73,* 687–702.

Kendall, P. C., & Hollon, S. D. (1981). Assessing self-referent speech: Methods in the measurement of self-statements. In P. C. Kendall & S. D. Hollon (Eds.), *Assessment strategies for cognitive–behavioral intervention* (pp. 85–118). New York: Academic Press.

Lazarus, R. S. (1991). *Emotion and adaptation.* New York: Oxford University Press.

Lazarus, R. S., Averill, J. R., & Opton, E. M., Jr. (1974). The psychology of coping: Issues of research and assessment. In G. V. Coelho, D. A. Hamburg, & J. E. Adams (Eds.), *Coping and adaptation* (pp. 249–315). New York: Basic Books.

Lazarus, R. S., & Folkman, S. (1984). *Stress, appraisal, and coping.* New York: Springer.

Lazarus, R. S., Kanner, A. D., & Folkman, S. (1980). Emotions: A cognitive-phenomenological analysis. In R. Plutchik & H. Kellerman (Eds.), *Theories of emotion* (pp. 189–217). New York: Academic Press.

Levenson, R. W. (1994). Human emotions: A functional view. In P. Ekman & R. J. Davidson (Eds.), *The nature of emotion: Fundamental questions* (pp. 123–126). New York: Oxford University Press.

Lewinsohn, P. M., & Amenson, C. S. (1978). Some relations between pleasant and unpleasant mood-related events and depression. *Journal of Abnormal Psychology, 87,* 644–654.

Lewinsohn, P. M., Hoberman, H. M., & Clarke, G. N. (1989). The coping with depression course: Review and future directions. *Canadian Journal of Behavioral Science, 21,* 470–493.

Lewinsohn, P. M., Sullivan, J. M., & Grosscup, S. J. (1980). Changing reinforcing events: An approach to the treatment of depression. *Psychotherapy: Theory, Research, and Practice, 17,* 322–334.

Linville, P. W. (1985). Self complexity and the affective extremity: Don't put all of your eggs in one cognitive basket. *Social Cognition, 3,* 94–120.

Linville, P. W. (1987). Self-complexity as a cognitive buffer against stress-related illness and depression. *Journal of Personality and Social Psychology, 52,* 663–676.

Mayer, J. D., & Gaschke, Y. N. (1988). The experience and meta-experience of mood. *Journal of Personality and Social Psychology, 55,* 102–111.

Mayer, J. D., Salovey, P., Gomberg-Kaufman, S., & Blainey, K. (1991). A broader conception of mood experience. *Journal of Personality and Social Psychology, 60,* 100–111.

Mayne, T. J. (1999). Negative affect and health: The importance of being earnest. *Cognition and Emotion, 13,* 601–635.

McCrae, R. R., & Costa, P. T. (1986). Personality, coping, and coping effectiveness in an adult sample. *Journal of Personality, 54,* 385–405.

McFadden, S. H., & Levin, J. S. (1996). Religion, emotions, and health. In C. Magai & S. H. McFadden (Eds.), *Handbook of emotion, adult development, and aging* (pp. 349–365). San Diego, CA: Academic Press.

Morgan, H. J., & Janoff-Bulman, R. (1994). Positive and negative self-complexity: Patterns of adjustment following traumatic versus non-traumatic life experiences. *Journal of Social and Clinical Psychology, 13*, 63–85.

Moskowitz, J. T., Acree, M., & Folkman, S. (1998, August). *Depression in AIDS-related bereavement: A three-year follow-up.* Paper presented at the 106th annual meeting of the American Psychological Association, San Francisco.

Moskowitz, J. T., Folkman, S., Collette, L., & Vittinghoff, E. (1996). Coping and mood during AIDS-related caregiving and bereavement. *Annals of Behavioral Medicine, 18*, 49–57.

Moskowitz, J. T., Oorbeck, J., & Folkman, S. (1997). *Positive meaningful events and mood outcomes under conditions of chronic stress.* Unpublished manuscript, University of California, San Francisco.

Moskowitz, J. T., & Wrubel, J. (2000, June). *Apples and oranges: Using qualitative and quantitative approaches to coping assessment.* Paper presented at the annual meeting of the American Psychological Society, Miami Beach, FL.

Nolen-Hoeksema, S., & Larson, J. (1999). *Coping with loss.* Mahwah, NJ: Erlbaum.

Nolen-Hoeksema, S., McBride, A., & Larson, J. (1997). Rumination and psychological distress among bereaved partners. *Journal of Personality and Social Psychology, 72*, 855–862.

Ntoumanis, N., & Biddle, S. J. H. (1998). The relationship of coping and its perceived effectiveness to positive and negative affect in sport. *Personality and Individual Differences, 24*, 773–788.

O'Leary, V., & Ickovics, J. R. (1995). Resilience and thriving in response to challenge: An opportunity for a paradigm shift in women's health. *Women's Health: Research on Gender, Behavior, and Policy, 1*, 121–142.

Park, C. L., Cohen, L., & Murch, R. (1996). Assessment and prediction of stress-related growth. *Journal of Personality, 64*, 71–105.

Pennebaker, J. W., Mayne, T. J., & Francis, M. E. (1997). Linguistic predictors of adaptive bereavement. *Journal of Personality and Social Psychology, 72*, 863–871.

Porter, L. A., & Stone, A. A. (1996). An approach to assessing daily coping. In M. Zeidner & N. S. Endler (Eds.), *Handbook of coping: Theory, research, applications* (pp. 133–150). New York: Wiley.

Reed, M. B., & Aspinwall, L. G. (1998). Self-affirmation reduces biased processing of health-risk information. *Motivation and Emotion, 22*, 99—132.

Revenson, T. A., & Felton, B. J. (1989). Disability and coping as predictors of psychological adjustment to rheumatoid arthritis. *Journal of Consulting and Clinical Psychology, 57*, 344–348.

Richards, T. A., Wrubel, J., & Folkman, S. (1998, August). *Reconstructing meaning: Changed world views in recovery from grief.* Paper presented at the 106th annual conference of the American Psychological Association, San Francisco.

Russell, J. A., & Carroll, J. M. (1999). On the bipolarity of positive and negative affect. *Psychological Bulletin, 125*, 3–30.

Ryff, C. D. (1989). Happiness is everything, or is it?: Explorations on the meaning of psychological well-being. *Journal of Personality and Social Psychology, 57*, 1069–1081.

Scheier, M. F., Weintraub, J. K., & Carver, C. S. (1986). Coping with stress: Divergent strategies of optimists and pessimists. *Journal of Personality and Social Psychology, 51*, 1257–1264.

Schwarzer, R., & Schwarzer, C. (1996). A critical survey of coping instruments. In M. Zeidner & N. S. Endler (Eds.), *Handbook of coping: Theory, research, applications* (pp. 107–132). New York: Wiley.

Selye, H. (1956). *The stress of life.* New York: McGraw-Hill.

Soloman, R. L. (1980). The opponent-process theory of acquired motivation. *American Psychologist, 35*, 691–712.

Stanton, A. L., & Snider, P. R. (1993). Coping with a breast cancer diagnosis: A prospective study. *Health Psychology, 12*, 16–23.

Stein, N., Folkman, S., Trabasso, T., & Richards, T. A. (1997). Appraisal and goal processes as predictors of psychological well-being in bereaved caregivers. *Journal of Personality and Social Psychology, 72*, 872–884.

Stone, A. A., Kennedy-Moore, E., & Neale, J. M. (1995). Association between daily coping and end-of-day mood. *Health Psychology, 14*, 341–349.

Stone, A. A., & Shiffman, S. (1992). Reflections on the intensive measurement of stress, coping, and mood, with an emphasis on daily measures. *Psychology and Health, 7*, 115–129.

Suls, J., & Fletcher, B. (1985). The relative efficacy of avoidant and nonavoidant coping strategies: A meta-analysis. *Health Psychology, 4*, 249–288.

Suls, J., & Martin, R. E. (1993). Daily recording and ambulatory monitoring methodologies in behavioral medicine. *Annals of Behavioral Medicine, 15*, 3–7.

Taylor, S. E. (1991). Asymmetrical effects of positive and negative events: The mobilization–minimization hypothesis. *Psychological Bulletin, 110*, 67–85.

Tedeschi, R. G., & Calhoun, L. G. (1995). *Trauma and transformation: Growing in the aftermath of suffering.* Thousand Oaks, CA: Sage.

Tedeschi, R. G., Park, C. L., & Calhoun, L. G. (1998). *Posttraumatic growth: Positive changes in the aftermath of crisis.* Mahwah, NJ: Erlbaum.

Thayer, R. E. (1989). *The biopsychology of mood and arousal.* New York: Oxford University Press.

Thayer, R. E., Newman, R., & McClain, T. M. (1994). Self-regulation of mood: Strategies for changing a bad mood, raising energy, and reducing tension. *Journal of Personality and Social Psychology, 67*, 910–925.

Trope, Y., & Neter, E. (1994). Reconciling competeing motives in self-evaluation: The role of self-control in feedback seeking. *Journal of Personality and Social Psychology, 66*, 646–657.

Trope, Y., & Pomerantz, E. M. (1998). Resolving conflicts among self-evaluative motives: Positive experiences as a resources for overcoming defensiveness. *Motivation and Emotion, 22*, 53–72.

Wegner, D. M., Schneider, D. J., Carter, S. R., & White, T. L. (1987). Paradoxical effects of thought suppression. *Journal of Personality and Social Psychology, 53*, 5–13.

Weiss, R. S., & Richards, T. A. (1997). A scale for predicting quality of recovery following the death of a partner. *Journal of Personality and Social Psychology, 72*, 885–891.

Westbrook, M. T., & Viney, L. L. (1982). Psychological reactions to the onset of
    chronic illness. *Social Science and Medicine, 16*, 899–905.
Wortman, C. B. (1987). Coping with irrevocable loss. In G. R. VandenBos & B. K.
    Bryant (Eds.), *Cataclysms, crises, and catastrophes: Psychology in action* (pp.
    189–235). Washington, DC: American Psychological Association.
Yalom, I. D., & Lieberman, M. A. (1991). Bereavement and heightened existential
    awareness. *Psychiatry, 54*, 334–345.
Zautra, A. J. (1997, August). *Does coping need reformulation? Four examinations of
    coping theory's utility.* Symposium conducted at the 105th annual convention of
    the American Psychological Association, Chicago.
Zautra, A. J., Burleson, M. H., Smith, C. A., Blalock, S. J., Wallston, K. A., DeVellis,
    R. F., DeVellis, B. M., & Smith, T. W. (1995). Arthritis and perceptions of quality
    of life: An examination of positive and negative affect in rheumatoid arthritis pa-
    tients. *Health Psychology, 14*, 399–408.

11

Emotion and Psychopathology

ANN M. KRING

One way we can learn about human behavior is to study what happens when things go wrong. Certainly a number of things "go wrong" in psychopathological disorders, and perhaps one of the more notable signs of things gone awry is some kind of emotional disturbance. One analysis has noted that as many as 85% of psychological disorders include disturbances in emotional processing of some kind (Thoits, 1985), whether they be "excesses" in emotion, "deficits" in emotion, or the lack of coherence among emotional components. Despite the widespread involvement of emotion dysfunction in psychopathology, systematic research into the nature, causes, and consequences of these disturbances has only recently been conducted. In this chapter, I briefly review the literature on emotion disturbance in three forms of psychopathology, with a particular emphasis on positioning these disturbances within the temporal course of the disorders. After first defining what I mean by emotion, emotion function, and emotion dysfunction, I then discuss the kinds of evidence that are needed to distinguish emotional features in psychopathology as either antecedents, concomitants, or consequences. I next review the available evidence on emotion disturbances in three different disorders: schizophrenia, unipolar depression, and social phobia. Finally, I consider the potential for basic emotion research paradigms to inform the study of the causes and manifestations of emotion disturbances in psychopathology, and conclude with suggestions for a research agenda in this area.

DEFINING AND MEASURING EMOTION

Emotion has been defined a number of different ways, and debate continues as to how to best define this somewhat elusive construct. Many emotion researchers agree, however, that emotions comprise a number of components, including (but not limited to) expressive, experiential, and physiological, which are typically coordinated within the individual. Moreover, the coordination of these components, under most circumstances, serves a number of important intra- and interpersonal functions (see, e.g., Ekman, 1994; Frijda, 1986; Keltner & Kring, 1998; Lang, Bradley, & Cuthbert, 1990; Levenson, 1992). More broadly, emotions have developed through the course of human evolutionary history to prepare organisms to act in response to a number of environmental stimuli and challenges.

It is worth noting distinctions among various terms used in the emotion literature. Although the terms "affect" and "emotion" have been used interchangeably, a number of theorists and researchers have distinguished between the terms, both conceptually and empirically. Generally speaking, the term *affect* is most often used in reference to feeling states, whereas *emotions* comprise multiple components (only one of which is a feeling state) and are hypothesized to occur in response *to* some object, person, or situation, whether real or imagined (see, e.g., Feldman Barrett & Russell, 1999). Rosenberg (1998) considers affect a broad, organizing term under which emotions and moods can be subsumed. In addition, affect is hypothesized to be *trait-like,* whereas emotions and moods are (affective) *state-like,* given their transient nature. Adopting a somewhat different perspective, Russell and Feldman Barrett (1999; see also Feldman Barrett & Russell, 1999) argue that affect, or—as they put it—*core affect,* reflects feeling states that are ever present and are just one of many constituents of what they refer to as *prototypical emotion episodes.* These prototypical episodes are hypothesized to occur in response to something and comprise cognitive, behavioral, feeling, and physiological components. In their analysis, moods are core affects that endure for a longer period of time. Unfortunately, it is often difficult to make clear distinctions between affect, emotion, and mood based on the names of the measures employed in studies (Feldman Barrett & Russell, 1999). For example, although the Positive and Negative Affect Schedule (PANAS; Watson, Clark, & Tellegen, 1988) assesses experienced *affect,* presumably so does the Differential Emotions Scale (DES; Izard, 1972). Using the framework of Russell and Feldman Barrett (1999), much of the research on emotion disturbance in psychopathology has been concerned with the various components of prototypical emotional episodes, one of which is core affect, although some research has been concerned with just one component, namely, the experience of feeling states or core affects. To ease interpretation, I will refer to feeling states in response to some stimulus (e.g., film, person, situation) as experienced emotion. Feeling states that are assessed without explicit reference to an object will be referred to as affects. Of course, some measures used in various studies reviewed may not necessarily follow this rubric and thus will preclude this distinction. In those cases, however, I will note the component of emotion each measure refers to if it is not already obvious.

As my colleagues and I have argued elsewhere (Keltner & Kring, 1998; Kring & Bachorowski, 1999), the functions of emotion in persons with various psychopathological disorders are comparable to those for nondisordered individuals. In many different disorders, however, one or more components of emotional processing are impaired in some respect, thus interfering with the achievement of emotion-related functions. For example, nonverbal displays of fear and anxiety among individuals with social phobia may evoke complementary fear and anxiety in others (Dimberg & Ohman, 1996) or discourage others from interacting with them. Similarly, schizophrenia patients' absence of facial expressions may evoke negative responses from others (Krause, Steimer-Krause, & Hufnagel, 1992) and have a number of other consequences for social relationships and interactions (see, e.g., Hooley, Richters, Weintraub, & Neale, 1987).

Adopting a multicomponential and functional definition of emotion has several implications for the study of emotion and psychopathology. First, researchers interested in specifying the nature of emotion disturbances in psychopathology ought to measure more than one component of emotion. Unfortunately, much of psychopathology research has relied upon the use of clinical rating scales that typically assess only one component of emotion. For example, a commonly used rating scale in schizophrenia called the Scale for the Assessment of Negative Symptoms (SANS; Andreasen, 1983) contains a subscale to measure the symptom called flat affect. Flat affect refers to a lack of outward expression of emotion (facially, vocally, and gesturally). To make these ratings, trained clinicians interview a patient and then rate the extent to which the patient was expressive during the interview. Although informative with respect to understanding emotional expression, using just this scale does not provide information on the experiential or physiological components of emotion. As will be discussed below, a complete understanding of emotion disturbance in schizophrenia requires assessment of the other emotion components. Second, a number of laboratory-based paradigms have been developed in the basic emotion literature that explicitly include methods for measuring and analyzing multiple components of emotion. Recently, psychopathology researchers have taken advantage of the methodological advancements made by basic emotion researchers and have incorporated these measures and paradigms into the study of different psychopathological disorders. For example, reliable self-report measures of the broad dimensions of affect (i.e., feeling states) have been developed (see, e.g., PANAS; Watson, Clark, & Tellegen, 1988) in nonpatient populations and have been successfully applied to the study of depression (see, e.g., Watson, Clark, & Carey, 1988) and social anxiety (see, e.g., Wallace & Alden, 1997). Third, understanding both the intra- and interpersonal functions of emotion informs the study of emotion dis- turbance in psychopathology much the same way, for example, that under- standing brain function informs the study of the behavioral sequelae of brain damage.

ANTECEDENTS, CONCOMITANTS, AND CONSEQUENCES

In their seminal review of cognitive theories of depression, Barnett and Gotlib (1988) distinguished between the concepts of antecedents, con- comitants, and consequences. Briefly, for a variable to be considered an antecedent of a psychological disorder, it must be shown to precede the onset of the disorder. Those features that are observed during an episode of a psychological disorder may be more accurately construed as con- comitants, and those features that persist after the episode has abated might be considered consequences. Building upon Zubin and Spring's (1977) diathesis-stress model of schizophrenia, Dawson and colleagues (Dawson & Nuechterlein, 1984; Dawson, Nuechterlein, Schell, Gitlin, & Ventura, 1994; Nuechterlein & Dawson, 1984) described related con- cepts referred to as episode and vulnerability indicators. *Episode indica- tors* are those features that are present during a psychotic episode but not during remission; *stable vulnerability indicators* are features that are pres- ent both during remission and psychosis; and *mediating vulnerability fac- tors* are features that are abnormal during remission but are markedly more deficient during psychosis.

   In order to understand the status of emotional disturbances in different psychological disorders, it is necessary to review the evidence for their oc- currence in the context of the temporal course of the disorder. Specifically, is there evidence showing that emotion disturbances precede the onset of a given disorder? Such evidence would support the role of an observed emo- tion disturbance as antecedent to the disorder or as a vulnerability indica- tor. Moreover, knowing that an emotion disturbance predates the onset of a particular disorder allows for more unambiguous claims about the causal status of that disturbance. A prospective, longitudinal study is the best de- sign to determine whether or not emotional disturbances precede the onset of a disorder. Unfortunately, few such studies have been conducted. How- ever, other forms of indirect evidence can be garnered to support the role of emotional disturbances as antecedent to the disorder, including follow-back and retrospective studies. These methods are not without their limitations, however, which I discuss below.

Is there evidence that emotional disturbances are present only during an active symptomatic state? Such evidence suggests that the disturbances are better construed as concomitants or episode indicators. Indeed, most of the research on emotional disturbances in psychopathology has employed cross-sectional designs that are ideally suited to evaluate whether particular emotional features can be construed as concomitants. Finally, if the evidence indicates that emotion disturbances persist after symptomatic recovery or predate a relapse, the disturbances can be construed as consequences of the disorder. Prospective, longitudinal designs are again the best method for ascertaining whether emotional features can be considered to be a consequence of the disorder. To examine whether emotion disturbances predict relapse, it is important to distinguish between relapse and recurrence of symptoms (Hollon & Cobb, 1993), and to distinguish symptoms from broader emotional dysfunction.

EMOTION DISTURBANCES IN SPECIFIC PSYCHOLOGICAL DISORDERS

As noted at the outset of this chapter, emotional disturbances figure prominently in many different psychological disorders. Space constraints prohibits consideration of many disorders, and thus I have chosen to focus on three disorders: schizophrenia, unipolar depression, and social phobia. My reason for choosing these three also stems from the fact that there is a growing body of theory and empirical research on the nature of emotional disturbances in these disorders. Although not typically considered an "emotional" disorder, there has been more research conducted on the emotional features of schizophrenia than on emotional disturbances in the mood or anxiety disorders. Nonetheless, a number of recent findings point to the importance of additional systematic study of emotion disturbances in the more traditional "emotional" disorders, which include unipolar depression and social phobia. I will first review the evidence for emotional disturbances in each disorder and then consider whether the disturbances can be construed as an antecedent, concomitant, or consequence (or some combination of these three) to the disorder. Where possible, the review is limited to studies that have assessed multiple components of emotions. These studies include laboratory-based as well as more naturalistic studies employing measures of facial expression, vocal expression, and self-report of emotional experience. Although recent studies of schizophrenia have also incorporated physiological indices of emotional responding heart rate, and skin conductance (see, e.g., Kring & Earnst, in press; Kring & Neale, 1996), there are not yet many published studies in depression or social phobia that have included these measures. Studies of this sort are now underway and will likely further illuminate the nature of emotional disturbances in many forms of psychopathology.

Schizophrenia

Emotion Disturbances

During the 1990s, a number of empirical studies of emotion disturbance in schizophrenia have found that schizophrenia patients show fewer observable facial expressions in response to emotional stimuli (see, e.g., Berenbaum & Oltmanns, 1992; Dworkin, Clark, Amador, & Gorman, 1996; Krause et al., 1992; Kring & Earnst, 1999; Kring, Kerr, Smith, & Neale, 1993; Kring & Neale, 1996) and during social interaction (see, e.g., Borod et al., 1989; Krause, Steimer, Sanger-Alt, & Wagner, 1989; Kring, Alpert, Neale, & Harvey, 1994; Martin, Borod, Alpert, Brozgold, & Welkowitz, 1990; Mattes, Schneider, Heimann, & Birbaumer, 1995) than do nonpatients. Interestingly, however, these laboratory studies also find that schizophrenia patients report experiencing similar or even greater amounts of emotion compared with nonpatients. Thus, schizophrenia patients' outward displays of emotion are not often an accurate reflection of their experienced emotion. Stated differently, schizophrenia patients report experiencing strong emotions in response to a variety of emotionally evocative stimuli, yet they do not often display these feelings outwardly. Clinically, dampened expressive behavior most closely resembles the symptom of schizophrenia referred to as flat affect. By all outward appearances, patients with flat affect appear to experience no emotion. Yet, as demonstrated by studies that assess multiple components of emotion, the outward display belies the internal emotional experience.

A number of studies have found that schizophrenia patients' and nonpatient controls' reports of emotional experience are similar using a wide variety of self-report measures of emotion. Nonetheless, it has been suggested that schizophrenia patients cannot report how they actually feel but instead are reporting based on how they think the investigators might want them to respond (i.e., response bias). However, additional evidence of emotional responding among schizophrenia patients renders the possibility of response bias less plausible. Although patients displayed fewer observable facial expressions in response to emotionally stimuli, recent studies have shown that patients display very subtle, microexpressive displays in a manner consistent with the valence of the stimuli (Earnst et al., 1996; Kring, Kerr, & Earnst, 1999; Mattes et al., 1995). For example, in response to positive stimuli schizophrenic patients exhibit more zygomatic (cheek) muscle activity, which is typically associated with positive emotion, than corrugator (brow) muscle activity, which is typically associated with negative emotion, in response to positive stimuli. By contrast, patients exhibit more corrugator activity than zygomatic activity in response to negative stimuli (Kring & Earnst, in press; Kring, Kerr, & Earnst, 1999). Thus, these findings of more subtle facial muscle activity in response to emotional stimuli bolster the conclusion that schizophrenic patients are responding emotionally.

Despite the well-replicated pattern of diminished expression and intact emotional experience among schizophrenia patients, the findings from laboratory studies are seemingly inconsistent with other evidence demonstrating schizophrenia patients to have the symptom of anhedonia, or the diminished capacity to experience pleasure (see, e.g., Blanchard, Bellack, & Mueser, 1994). Indeed, anhedonia appears to be fairly prevalent in schizophrenia, with one study finding as many as three-fourths of patients to have at least moderate levels of anhedonia and one-fourth of patients to have severe anhedonia (Fenton & McGlashan, 1991). More recent studies have examined the relationship between anhedonia and reports of emotional experience in response to emotional stimuli. For example, Blanchard and colleagues (1994) found that schizophrenic patients' scores on a measure of anhedonia were negatively correlated with their reports of positive emotion after both positive and negative emotion-eliciting film clips. That is, the higher the patients scored on the anhedonia measure, the less positive emotion they reported feeling after viewing emotionally evocative stimuli. Unfortunately, this study did not include a nonpatient comparison group with which the patients' reports of emotional experience could be compared. However, Berenbaum and Oltmanns (1992) found that schizophrenic patients with flat affect did *not* differ from nonpatients in their reported emotional experience to emotional film clips even though they scored higher on measures of anhedonia.

An apparent discrepancy emerges in the studies reviewed thus far. With few exceptions, studies that present emotionally evocative stimuli to schizophrenic patients find that patients report experiencing the same amount of positive emotion as nonpatients. Yet, other studies find that schizophrenic patients score higher on measures of anhedonia, indicating that they experience less positive emotion, particularly pleasure, than nonpatients. How can these findings be reconciled? This pattern of findings suggests that the nature of hedonic deficit in schizophrenia may be more circumscribed. As we have suggested elsewhere (Kring, 1999; Germans & Kring, 2000), although schizophrenic patients may not report a pleasure deficit when positive stimuli are presented to them, they may manifest an impaired ability to anticipate the hedonic value of forthcoming pleasurable experiences. It has been hypothesized that hedonic experience includes both appetitive (anticipatory) and consummatory components (see, e.g., Klein, 1987). In other words, the pleasure one derives from the imagining or the expectancy of a rewarding or pleasurable experience (appetitive pleasure) leads to the pursuit and engagement in the pleasurable activity, which results in consummatory pleasure. The research described above suggests that when presented with emotional material, patients can and do experience positive emotion. However, when asked more generally about whether they find circumstances pleasurable, they are likely to report experiencing less positive emotion.

Other evidence supports this claim. For example, Myin-Germeys, Delespaul, and deVries (in press) had schizophrenic patients complete self-reports of emotional experience at random, daily time intervals over a 2-week period and found that they reported experiencing less positive emotion and more negative emotion than did nonpatient controls. Myin-Germeys and colleagues concluded that the hedonic deficit evident in these patients' self-reports might be linked to the decreased frequency with which these patients participated in pleasurable activities and social interactions, perhaps because they could not anticipate that such activities would be pleasurable. Indeed, Delespaul (1995) found that when asked to report their daily activities, schizophrenic patients described themselves as "doing nothing" (versus engaging in hobbies, sports, social activities, or watching television) five times more frequently than did nonpatient controls. Thus, on a daily basis, schizophrenic patients may not report experiencing pleasure, particularly pleasure linked with social interaction, because they are not participating in pleasurable activities. Although these findings support the notion that anhedonia is linked to a failure to engage in pleasurable activities, it is difficult to determine whether patients' diminished engagement in rewarding pastimes is a cause or a consequence of hedonic deficit.

Other research has indicated that schizophrenia patients may have deficits in emotion perception (see, e.g., Kerr & Neale, 1993; Mueser et al., 1996; Salem, Kring, & Kerr, 1996). However, it is important to note that this deficit does not appear to be specific to emotion perception. Rather, the schizophrenic patients in these studies manifested a more generalized deficit in perceiving faces and voices. Moreover, one study did not find evidence for emotion perception deficits among acutely ill schizophrenia patients (see, e.g., Bellack, Blanchard, & Mueser, 1996), and this result has led some investigators to speculate that antipsychotic medications may be better able to ameliorate perception deficits (including emotion perception) among acutely ill patients but not more chronically disturbed patients (Mueser et al., 1996).

Antecedent, Concomitant, or Consequence?

Unfortunately, few prospective studies on emotion disturbances in schizophrenia have been conducted. Nonetheless, indirect evidence suggests that at least some of the observed emotion disturbances may predate the onset of schizophrenia. More specifically, findings from several studies suggest that schizophrenia patients may display fewer facial expressions (particularly positive expressions) and report experiencing less positive emotion and more negative emotion prior to the onset of the illness. For example, Walker, Grimes, Davis, and Smith (1993) obtained home movies of adults with schizophrenia that were made before these adults developed schizophrenia. They coded facial expressions from the home movies of preschizophrenic boys and girls and found that the girls displayed fewer joy expressions and that both the boys and the girls displayed *more* negative facial expressions compared to their healthy siblings (Walker et al., 1993). It could be the case, however, that the preschizophrenic children showed different types of behaviors or engaged in different types of social interactions captured by the home movies. Thus, these differences could have resulted in different (but appropriate) facial expressions.

Follow-up studies of adults who were seen in mental health clinics as children suggest that schizophrenia patients, particularly males, were shy, withdrawn, anxious, depressed, and socially isolated as children (Fleming & Ricks, 1970; Robbins, 1966). Follow-back studies that rely on archival data have found that preschizophrenic boys were emotionally unstable, depressed, nervous, and impulsive and that preschizophrenic girls were withdrawn and passive (Watt, 1972). Using both follow-up and follow-back method, Knight and Roff (1983, 1985) found evidence that affective disturbances appeared in childhood and persisted into adulthood. Although the findings from these studies are interesting, it remains unclear whether this pattern of social and emotional behavior was actually related to the onset of schizophrenia and whether the patterns were specific to schizophrenia due to the retrospective nature of the design and the fairly limited sample (i.e., patients seen in clinics as children are not necessarily representative of all schizophrenia patients). However, findings from prospective high-risk studies have reported similar findings. High-risk studies identify a group of children at risk for developing schizophrenia (typically defined as having a biological parent with schizophrenia) and then follow them from childhood through the period of risk (Neale & Oltmanns, 1980). Teacher ratings from the Copenhagen High-Risk Study indicated that boys and girls who were later diagnosed with schizophrenia were more emotionally labile, socially withdrawn, socially anxious, and relatively unexpressive than children who did not develop schizophrenia (Olin, John, & Mednick, 1995; Olin & Mednick, 1996). Findings from the New York High-Risk Project indicated that anhedonia was significantly associated with having a biological parent with schizophrenia but not affective disorders (Erlenmeyer-Kimling et al., 1993) and that flat affect was greater among adolescents at risk for developing schizophrenia than among adolescents at risk for developing affective disorders (Dworkin et al., 1991).

Although there is suggestive evidence that at least some type of emotion disturbance in schizophrenia may predate the onset of the disorder, many of the observed emotion disturbances in schizophrenia can perhaps be most accurately construed as concomitants of the disorder. Indeed, most of the research on emotion in schizophrenia has been cross-sectional and has included patients with at least some degree of residual symptoms. This is not to say, however, that the findings from this cross-sectional research are uninformative. Indeed, findings from these studies have further elucidated the nature of emotion disturbances in schizophrenia and have set the stage for further prospective, longitudinal studies.

With respect to whether emotion disturbances in schizophrenia can be construed as consequences of the disorder, there is some evidence that emotional disturbances in schizophrenia are fairly stable. Both the symptoms of flat affect and anhedonia are chronic (Knight, Roff, Barnett, & Moss, 1979) and stable across time (Blanchard, Mueser, & Bellack, 1998; Keefe et al., 1991; Kring & Earnst, 1999; Lewine, 1991; Pfhol & Winokur, 1982). In a longitudinal study conducted by my laboratory (Kring & Earnst, 1999), diminished emotional expression was stable across 5 months. However, our study did not specifically include assessments during and following a symptomatic episode.

Unipolar Depression

Emotion Disturbances

Two of the current diagnostic criteria (DSM-IV; American Psychiatric Association, 1994) for unipolar depression reflect emotion disturbances: sad mood and loss of interest or pleasure (anhedonia). Although the specific emotion of sadness would seem to be an ideal emotion for further study in depression, most of the research into the nature of emotion disturbances in depression has focused on broader feeling states or core affects (see Russell & Feldman Barrett, 1999). More specifically, evidence indicates that depression can be broadly characterized by low levels of positive affect and heightened levels of negative affect (see, e.g., Watson, Clark, & Carey, 1988). Positive and negative affect are associated with emotional responses, cognitive styles, and personality traits, such as extraversion and neuroticism (Watson, Clark, & Tellegen, 1988). Persons with low levels of positive affect are likely to experience emotions such as sadness and to be interpersonally disengaged. By contrast, persons with high levels of negative affect frequently experience emotions such as anxiety, guilt, and anger. Related to findings of heightened negative affect among individuals with depression, comorbid anxiety is also associated with unipolar depression (see, e.g., DiNardo & Barlow, 1990). Thus, although sadness is certainly central to emotion, it is not uncommon for individuals with depression to experience a number of different negative emotions.

Davidson, Tomarken, and colleagues have found that a particular pattern of resting brain activity is related to positive and negative affect as well as with depression. More specifically, resting left frontal *hypo*activation has been observed in both currently depressed individuals (see, e.g., Allen, Iacono, Depue, & Arbisi, 1993; Henriques & Davidson, 1991) and previously depressed individuals (Henriques & Davidson, 1990), whereas greater relative left frontal *hyper*activation has been observed in individuals who report generally experiencing high levels of positive affect and low levels of negative affect (Tomarken, Davidson, Wheeler, & Doss, 1992). Tomarken and Keener (1998) have suggested that relative left frontal hypoactivation may be a marker of risk for depression that is reflected by a number of behavioral and emotional deficits, including the relative incapacity to respond to positive emotional stimuli and self-regulatory deficits in the capacity to use positive events to shift into positive emotional states.

Additional evidence from studies that assess components of emotion episodes indicates that individuals with unipolar depression may also exhibit dampened facial, vocal, and gestural expressive behavior (Berenbaum & Oltmanns, 1992; Ekman & Friesen, 1974; Gotlib & Robinson, 1982; Hargreaves, Starkweather, & Blacker, 1965; Jones & Pansa, 1979; Kaplan, Bachorowski, & Zarlengo-Strouse, 1999; Murray & Arnott, 1993; Scherer, 1986; Ulrich & Harms, 1985; Waxer, 1974). Moreover, dampened expressive behavior among individuals with depression may be specific to positive expressions. For example, Berenbaum and Oltmanns (1992) found that depressed individuals showed fewer facial expressions in response to positive stimuli (but not to negative stimuli) than did nonpatients and schizophrenic patients with flat affect. As noted in the discussion of schizophrenia, diminished expression and experience in response to positive emotional stimuli is broadly consistent with the clinical symptom of anhedonia.

In addition to disturbances in emotion expression and experience, other studies have found that individuals with depression have deficits in emotion perception and biases in the processing of emotional material. For example, Gur and colleagues (1992) found that depressed individuals demonstrated a general negative bias in an emotion discrimination task as well as an impairment in facial expression recognition. Furthermore, some studies have shown that depression is linked to memory biases for mood-congruent stimuli (Bradley, Mogg, & Williams, 1995; Mathews & MacLeod, 1994).

Antecedent, Concomitant, or Consequence?

Similar to the research on emotional features of schizophrenia, most of the studies have been designed to more fully characterize the emotional symptoms of depression. Thus, most of the evidence reviewed above suggests that the emotional disturbances associated with unipolar depression can be construed as concomitants or episode indicators. For example, with respect to emotion-related cognitive biases, the evidence suggests that memory biases dissipate upon remission (MacLeod & Mathews, 1991), indicating that such biases are state but not trait markers of depression.

Unlike the literature on cognitive aspects of depression, very few studies have examined whether these emotion disturbances predate the onset of the first episode of depression or persist after other symptoms abate. Although a number of high-risk studies have been conducted whereby children with at least one depressed parent are compared with children of nondepressed parents (and, in some instances, children of parents with other psychological disorders), few of these studies have systematically assessed emotion disturbances among these children. Rather, high-risk studies have typically sought to determine the children's risk for developing depression and possible behavioral and psychosocial risk factors that predict the onset of depression. Thus, there is evidence that children of depressed parents are more likely to experience sad mood, anxiety, fears, and anhedonia than children of nondepressed parents (see, e.g., Billings & Moos, 1983; Welner, Welner, McCrary, & Leonard, 1977), although it remains unclear whether this pattern is specific to children of depressed parents (see, e.g., Downey & Coyne, 1990; Lee & Gotlib, 1989a, 1989b). Other recent evidence suggests that some of the emotion disturbances associated with depression may predate the onset of the first episode. Recall that relative decreased activation of left frontal brain areas has been associated with depression. This same pattern of left frontal hypoactivation has been observed in infants of depressed mothers (see, e.g., Field, Fox, Pickens, & Nawrocki, 1995). In addition, greater left frontal hypoactivation has been found among adolescents at risk for developing depression (defined by having a mother who was currently or previously depressed) even though the adolescents did not differ from a comparable control group in current depressed mood (Tomarken, Simien, & Garber, 1994). Insofar as this pattern of brain activity is linked with positive affect (Tomarken et al., 1992), these findings suggest that electroencephalographic measures of frontal brain activity may be emotion-related vulnerability indicators for depression (Tomarken & Keener, 1998).

It seems somewhat paradoxical to think that emotion disturbances in depression would persist after symptomatic recovery, since the symptoms that are alleviated comprise the observed emotion disturbances (i.e., sad mood and anhedonia). However, recent evidence suggests that certain treatments for depression may be more effective in targeting both positive and negative affect. For instance, Tomarken, Elkins, Anderson, Shelton, and Hitt (2000) have found that the combined treatment of sleep deprivation and antidepressant medication was associated with an increase in positive affect and a decrease in negative affect. By contrast, patients who received only antidepressant medication experienced a decrease in negative affect but no corresponding increase in positive affect. Thus, these findings indirectly suggest that, depending upon the treatment, low positive affect may persist after the episode of depression has gone into remission. Clearly, more research is needed to understand the changes in positive and negative affect that occur both during and after treatment.

Social Phobia

Emotion Disturbances

Social phobia is characterized by anxiety, fear, and avoidance of social situations, performance, and evaluations. Indeed, individuals with social phobia do not experience such anxiety when alone, but rather experience extreme anxiety when confronted with a social situation that involves interaction or presumed evaluation (Barlow, 1988). Theories of social anxiety hold that social anxiety is an extreme manifestation of an otherwise useful response that has evolved to promote an individual's sensitivity to others' disapproval (Barlow, 1988), to facilitate integration into a social group (Baumeister & Leary, 1995; Miller & Leary, 1992), or to negotiate power and status differences (Gilbert & Trower, 1990). When trait social anxiety reaches extreme levels, social phobia may result (Leary & Kowalski, 1995).

Social phobia's most apparent emotional disturbance is the heightened experience of anxiety, fear, and other negative emotions in the context of a social situation. Recent studies have begun to assess the nature and specificity of this disturbance in the experience component of emotion. For example, Wallace and Alden (1997) assessed reports of positive and negative affect in individuals with social phobia and nonclinical controls following successful and unsuccessful social interactions. Individuals both with and without social phobia reported experiencing more negative affect following the unsuccessful social interaction than the successful one. However, only the individuals with social phobia reported significantly greater negative affect and less positive affect than controls following both kinds of interactions.

Although a handful of studies have assessed a broad array of nonverbal behaviors associated with social phobia, no study has systematically examined facial expressions of emotion. Nevertheless, there appear to be nonverbal cues that are reliably associated with social anxiety. For example, Marcus and Wilson (1996) studied social anxiety among college women during an observed speaking task. Observers' ratings of anxiety were significantly related to speakers' reports of anxiety even though speakers rated themselves as more anxious than observers rated them. These findings indirectly suggest that social anxiety is composed of relatively easily recognizable nonverbal behaviors and cues. In our laboratory, we have examined how social anxiety influences social interactions between men and women meeting for the first time. Dyads who were more socially anxious smiled and nodded less often, exhibited greater speech dysfluencies such as stuttering, leaned to the side more often, and were generally less socially engaging and inviting than dyads who were less socially anxious (Kring, Wissman, & Schmid, 1999).

Research on emotion-related cognitive processes and social phobia indicates that socially anxious individuals may have a bias in attending to negative emotional stimuli, including threat words, facial expressions, and evaluation-related nonverbal cues (Asmundson & Stein, 1994; Hope, Rapee, Heimberg, & Dombeck, 1990; Pozo, Carver, Wellens, & Scheier, 1991; Veljaca & Rapee, 1998; Winton, Clark, & Edelmann, 1995). For example, Winton and colleagues (1995) presented slides of different facial expressions of emotion to individuals scoring high and low on a measure of social anxiety. Socially anxious participants were more likely to identify neutral facial expressions as negative and rated all the expressions more negatively than did participants who were not socially anxious.

Antecedent, Concomitant, or Consequence?

Theorists have suggested that a biological and psychological propensity to experience anxiety in combination with stressful life events involving social interaction set the stage for the development of social phobia (see, e.g., Barlow, 1988). Unfortunately, measurement and definition of this predisposition to experience heightened anxiety remain to be elucidated. One recent study, however, suggests that a particular temperamental style may be uniquely linked to social phobia. Mick and Telch (1998) found that retrospective reports of behavioral inhibition, a temperamental style that involves avoidance, isolation, excessive sympathetic arousal, and withdrawal in the face of novel situations, were related to symptoms of social phobia but not generalized anxiety disorder.

Nonetheless, that social anxiety manifests itself only in the context of a social situation suggests that the emotional disturbance is perhaps best construed as a concomitant rather than as an antecedent or a consequence. This is not to say, however, that repeated exposure to anxiety provoking social interactions will not exacerbate or at least contribute to the maintenance of social phobia over time. In addition, there are likely to be a number of interpersonal consequences of the experience and display of heightened anxiety. For example, individuals with social phobia nonverbally communicate to others the inordinate risk of embarrassment in social interaction, thus precluding the desire for interacting with those individuals. In addition, it seems likely that interactions with socially phobic individuals will be more frustrating and distressing and perhaps eventually avoided (Keltner & Kring, 1998).

CONCLUSION, INTEGRATION, AND DIRECTIONS

Emotion disturbances are common among many different forms of psychopathology. Research in the past 15 years has sought to more fully characterize the nature of these emotion disturbances. Although this chapter has focused on the disturbances that characterize just three disorders, a number of other disorders include widespread emotion disturbances. For example, many of the personality disorders include problems in emotion regulation, such as borderline personality disorder (see, e.g., Farchaus-Stein, 1996; Linehan, 1987; Shearin & Linehan, 1994) and psychopathy (Arnett, Smith, & Newman, 1997; Patrick, Bradley, & Lang, 1993; Patrick, Cuthbert, & Lang, 1994). Nearly all of the anxiety disorders are characterized by heightened negative affect (see, e.g., Chorpita & Barlow, 1998; Clark & Watson, 1991; Watson et al., 1995), yet recent research has attempted to further elucidate emotional disturbances that distinguish the specific anxiety disorders (see, e.g., Mulkens, de Jong, & Merkelbach, 1996; Zinbarg & Barlow, 1996). Challenges for the next generation of research include isolating the specificity of emotion disturbances within different disorders, more clearly locating the disturbances within the temporal course of the disorder, examining both specific, discrete emotions as well as broader emotion dimensions, linking emotion disturbances with other disorder-related disturbances, and developing and implementing interventions that target emotion disturbances.

It seems that one fruitful approach to meeting these challenges is to continue to incorporate basic emotion methods and paradigms into the study of psychopathology. For instance, researchers interested in studying emotion disturbances in psychological disorders ought to include measures of multiple emotion components and frame hypotheses about emotion disturbances with an empirically validated theoretical approach to emotion (Keltner & Kring, 1998; Kring & Bachorowski, 1999; Tomarken & Keener, 1998). Moreover, a combination of both laboratory and naturalistic research will likely yield the most complete picture of emotion disturbances in psychopathology. Thus, laboratory findings of heightened negative emotional experience among schizophrenia patients has been confirmed in studies assessing patients' emotional experience in daily life. Other approaches to the study of emotion will also generate relevant information about the nature of emotion disturbances in psychopathology. For example, narrative approaches have been successfully employed in the study of agoraphobia and bereavement (Capps & Bonanno, in press; Capps & Ochs, 1995). Personal narratives are rich sources of information about current, past, and future life events (see, e.g., McAdams, 1996; Ochs & Capps, 1996). This approach can provide information about *how* individuals use language to describe their emotions and make sense of the illness experience. Combining this approach with more traditional clinical interviews will undoubtedly help to elucidate how emotion figures prominently in various forms of psychopathology.

Although there are a number of important directions for future research, I note two here in some detail. First, the specificity of emotion disturbances in psychopathology needs to be clarified. For example, although some evidence indicates that heightened negative affect in combination with lowered positive affect is specific to unipolar depression (Watson, Clark, & Carey, 1988), other studies have found the same pattern in social phobia (Wallace & Alden, 1997) and schizophrenia (Blanchard, Mueser, & Bellack, 1998). Notably, studies finding this pattern in other disorders did not include a comparison group of individuals with unipolar depression, so it is difficult to know if these patient groups demonstrate a similar pattern of reported positive and negative affect. Indeed, it is necessary to include other psychopathological comparison groups to get at the specificity of emotion disturbances. Nonetheless, these finding suggest that lowered positive affect may not be specific to unipolar depression. Is it important to identify specific emotion disturbances for different disorders? It may be the case that broad characterizations of emotion disturbances identify a number of different disorders and that specificity is the exception rather than the rule. Indeed, heightened negative affect is a prime example of a general distress factor common to many different psychological disturbances. However, some specificity may nonetheless be detected among different disorders. For example, schizophrenia patients are less expressive of both positive and negative emotions (Kring & Earnst, 1999), whereas depressed patients may only exhibit fewer positive expressions (Berenbaum & Oltmanns, 1992). Identifying a specific emotion disturbance will aid in linking that disturbance to other known biological, cognitive, and behavioral features of a particular disorder. A second direction for research is to more clearly locate emotion disturbances within the temporal course of the disorder. A major focus of this chapter has been to consider whether the observed emotion disturbances in various disorders can be considered antecedents, concomitants, or consequences. The starting place for much of the research on emotion and psychopathology has been to more fully characterize the emotional symptoms. In essence, these studies have generated construct validity evidence for emotional symptoms and have thus provided support for the role of emotional features as concomitants of different disorders. However, in some cases, this research has gone beyond validating symptoms. For example, laboratory research has confirmed that schizophrenia patients with the symptom of flat affect are less expressive across a variety of situations. Moreover, this research has shown that the emotion disturbance in schizophrenia involves not only the expressive component of emotion; rather, it is best characterized by a pattern of expressive, experiential, and psychophysiological emotion components (Kring & Neale, 1996). Continued research that seeks to fully delineate the emotional symptoms of various psychological disorders is still an important direction for research.

This research strategy that has begun with emotional symptoms or features of a particular disorder is in contrast to, for example, research on cognitive accounts of depression. In that research, the focus is not on symptoms per se, but rather on broader cognitive styles that are hypothesized to account for the symptoms. However, psychopathology researchers interested in emotion are now well equipped to further investigate questions about mechanism. The search for mechanisms leads to questions about antecedents and consequences of emotional disturbances. As reviewed above, indirect evidence supports the role of emotion disturbances in schizophrenia and unipolar depression as antecedents and consequences of the respective disorders. Further prospective studies that assess the emotional responding in the same patients across episodes are sorely needed. Moreover, new relevant findings from ongoing high-risk studies will continue to be generated as the samples pass through the period of risk. Although these studies were not necessarily designed to study emotional risk factors, they nonetheless contain a number of measures relevant to answering questions about whether emotion disturbances predict the onset and/or maintenance of different disorders.

In summary, emotional disturbances figure prominently in psychopathology. Additional research is needed, however, to illuminate the manner in which disturbed components of emotional processes contribute to the onset, maintenance, and long-term consequences of the disorders. Research that encompasses a wide variety of methods and multiple levels of analysis is the most promising approach to further our understanding and treatment of emotion dysfunction.

ACKNOWLEDGMENT

During the preparation of this chapter, Ann M. Kring was supported in part by a grant from the National Alliance for Research on Schizophrenia and Depression.

REFERENCES

Allen, J. J., Iacono, W. G., Depue, R. A., & Arbisi, P. (1993). Regional EEG asymmetries in bipolar seasonal affective disorder before and after phototherapy. *Biological Psychiatry, 33,* 642–646.

American Psychiatric Association. (1994). *Diagnostic and statistical manual of mental disorders* (4th ed.). Washington, DC: Author.

Andreasen, N. C. (1983). *The Scale for the Assessment of Negative Symptoms (SANS).* Iowa City: University of Iowa.

Arnett, P. A., Smith, S. S., & Newman, J. P. (1997). Approach and avoidance motivation in psychopathic criminal offenders during passive avoidance. *Journal of Personality and Social Psychology, 72,* 1413–1428.

Asmundson, G. J. G., & Stein, M. B. (1994). Selective attention for social threat in patients with generalized social phobia: Evaluation using a dot-probe paradigm. *Journal of Anxiety Disorders, 8,* 107–117.

Barlow, D. H. (1988). *Anxiety and its disorders: The nature and treatment of anxiety and panic.* New York: Guilford Press.

Barnett, P. A., & Gotlib, I. H. (1988). Psychosocial functioning and depression: Distinguishing among antecedents, concomitants, and consequences. *Psychological Bulletin, 104,* 97–126.

Baumeister, R. F., & Leary, M. (1995). The need to belong: Desire for interpersonal attachments as a fundamental human motivation. *Psychological Bulletin, 117,* 497–529.

Bellack, A. S., Blanchard, J. J., & Mueser, K. T. (1996). Cue availability and affect perception in schizophrenia. *Schizophrenia Bulletin, 22,* 535–544.

Berenbaum, H., & Oltmanns, T. F. (1992). Emotional experience and expression in schizophrenia and depression. *Journal of Abnormal Psychology, 101,* 37–44.

Billings, A. G., & Moos, R. H. (1983). Comparisons of children of depressed and nondepressed parents: A socio-environmental perspective. *Journal of Abnormal Child Psychology, 11,* 463–486.

Blanchard, J. J., Bellack, A. S., & Mueser, K. T. (1994). Affective and social-behavioral correlates of physical and social anhedonia in schizophrenia. *Journal of Abnormal Psychology, 103,* 719–728.

Blanchard, J. J., Mueser, K. T., & Bellack, A. S. (1998). Anhedonia, positive and negative affect, and social functioning in schizophrenia. *Schizophrenia Bulletin, 24,* 413–424.

Borod, J. C., Alpert, M., Brozgold, A., Martin, C., Welkowitz, J., Diller, L., Peselow, E., Angrist, B., & Lieberman, A. (1989). A preliminary comparison of flat affect schizophrenics and brain-damaged patients on measures of affective processing. *Journal of Communication Disorders 22,* 93–104.

Bradley, B. P., Mogg, K., & Williams, R. (1995). Implicit and explicit memory for emotion-congruent information in clinical depression and anxiety. *Behavior Research and Therapy, 33,* 755–770.

Capps, L., & Bonanno, G. (in press). Narrating bereavement: Thematic and grammatical predictors of adjustments to loss. *Discourse Processes, 30.*

Capps, L., & Ochs, E. (1995). *Constructing panic: The discourse of agoraphobia.* Cambridge, MA: Harvard University Press.

Chorpita, B. F., & Barlow, D. H. (1998). The development of anxiety: The role of control in the early environment. *Psychological Bulletin, 124*, 3–21.

Clark, L. A., & Watson, D. (1991). Tripartite model of anxiety and depression: Psychometric evidence and taxonomic implications. *Journal of Abnormal Psychology, 100*, 316–336.

Dawson, M. E., & Nuechterlein, K. H. (1984). Psychophysiological dysfunctions in the developmental course of schizophrenic disorders. *Schizophrenia Bulletin, 10*, 204–232.

Dawson, M. E., Nuechterlein, K. H., Schell, A. M., Gitlin, M., & Ventura, J. (1994). Autonomic abnormalities in schizophrenia: State or trait indicators? *Archives of General Psychiatry, 51*, 813–824.

Delespaul, P. A. E. G. (1995). *Assessing schizophrenia in daily life*. Maastricht, The Netherlands: Universitaire Pers Maastricht.

Dimberg, U., & Ohman A. (1996). Behold the wrath: Psychophysiological responses to facial stimuli. *Motivation and Emotion, 20*, 149–182.

DiNardo, P. A., & Barlow, D. H. (1990). Syndrome and symptom comorbidity in the anxiety disorders. In J. D. Maser & C. R. Cloninger (Eds.), *Comorbidity of mood and anxiety disorders* (pp. 205–230). Washington, DC: American Psychiatric Press.

Downey, G., & Coyne, J. C. (1990). Children of depressed parents: An integrative review. *Psychological Bulletin, 108*, 50–76.

Dworkin, R. H., Bernstein, G., Kaplansky, L. M., Lipsitz, J. D., Rinaldi, A., Slater, S. L., Cornblatt, B. A., & Erlenmeyer-Kimling, L. (1991). Social competence and positive and negative symptoms: A longitudinal study of children and adolescents at risk for schizophrenia and affective disorder. *American Journal of Psychiatry, 148*, 1182–1188.

Dworkin, R., Clark, S. C., Amador, X. F., & Gorman, J. M. (1996). Does affective blunting in schizophrenia reflect affective deficit or neuromotor dysfunction? *Schizophrenia Research, 20*, 301–306.

Earnst, K. S., Kring, A. M., Kadar, M. A., Salem, J. E., Shepard, D. A., & Loosen, P. T. (1996). Facial expression in schizophrenia. *Biological Psychiatry, 40*, 556–558.

Ekman, P. (1994). All emotions are basic. In P. Ekman & R. J. Davidson (Eds.), *The nature of emotion: Fundamental questions* (pp. 15–19). New York: Oxford University Press.

Ekman, P., & Friesen, W. V. (1974). Nonverbal behavior and psychopathology. In R. J. Friedman & M. M. Katz (Eds.), *The psychology of depression: Contemporary theory and research* (pp. 203–232). Washington, DC: Wiley.

Erlenmeyer-Kimling, L., Cornblatt, B. A., Rock, D., Roberts, S., Bell, M., & West, A. (1993). The New York High-Risk Project: Anhedonia, attentional deviance, and psychopathology. *Schizophrenia Bulletin, 19*, 141–153.

Farchaus-Stein, K. (1996). Affect instability in adults with a borderline personality disorder. *Archives of Psychiatric Nursing, 10*, 32–40.

Feldman Barrett, L., & Russell, J. A. (1999). The structure of current affect: Controversies and emerging consensus. *Current Directions in Psychological Science, 8*, 10–14.

Fenton, W. S., & McGlashan, T. H. (1991). Natural history of schizophrenia subtypes: II. Positive and negative symptoms and long-term course. *Archives of General Psychiatry, 48,* 978–986.

Field, T., Fox, N. A., Pickens, J., & Nawrocki, T. (1995). Relative right frontal EEG activation in 3- to 6-month-old infants of "depressed" mothers. *Developmental Psychology, 3,* 358–363.

Fleming, P., & Ricks, D. F. (1970). Emotions of children before schizophrenia and before character disorder. In M. Roff & D. Ricks (Eds.), *Life history research in psychopathology* (pp. 240–264). Minneapolis: University of Minnesota Press.

Frijda, N. (1986). *The emotions.* Cambridge, UK: Cambridge University Press.

Germans, M. K., & Kring, A. M. (2000). Hedonic deficit in anhedonia: Support for the role of approach motivation. *Personality and Individual Differences, 28,* 659–672.

Gilbert, P., & Trower, P. (1990). The evolution and manifestation of social anxiety. In W. R. Crozier (Ed.), *Shyness and embarrassment* (pp. 144–177). New York: Cambridge University Press.

Gotlib, I. H., & Robinson, L. A. (1982). Responses to depressed individuals: Discrepancies between self-report and observer-rated behavior. *Journal of Abnormal Psychology, 91,* 231–240.

Gur, R. C., Erwin, R. J., Gur, R. E., Zwil, A. S., Heimberg, C., & Kraemer, H. C. (1992). Facial emotion discrimination: II. Behavioral findings in depression. *Psychiatry Research, 42,* 241–251.

Hargreaves, W., Starkweather, J., & Blacker, K. (1965). Voice quality in depression. *Journal of Abnormal Psychology, 70,* 218–229.

Henriques, J. B., & Davidson, R. J. (1990). Regional brain electrical asymmetries discriminate between previously depressed subjects and healthy controls. *Journal of Abnormal Psychology, 99,* 22–31.

Henriques, J. B., & Davidson, R. J. (1991). Left frontal hypoactivation in depression. *Journal of Abnormal Psychology, 100,* 535–545.

Hollon, S. D., & Cobb, R. (1993). Relapse and recurrence in psychopathological disorders. In C. G. Costello (Ed.), *Basic issues in psychopathology* (pp. 377–402). New York: Guilford Press.

Hooley, J. M., Richters, J. E., Weintraub, S., & Neale, J. M. (1987). Psychopathology and marital distress: The positive side of positive symptoms. *Journal of Abnormal Psychology, 96,* 27–33.

Hope, D. A., Rapee, R. M., Heimberg, R. G., & Dombeck M. J. (1990). Representations of the self in social phobia. *Journal of Anxiety Disorders, 6,* 63–77.

Izard, C. E. (1972). *Patterns of emotion: A new analysis of anxiety and depression.* San Diego, CA: Academic Press.

Jones, I. H., & Pansa, M. (1979). Some nonverbal aspects of depression and schizophrenia occurring during the interview. *Journal of Nervous and Mental Disease, 167,* 402–409.

Kaplan, P. S., Bachorowski, J.-A., & Zarlengo-Strouse, P. (1999). Infant directed speech produced by mothers with symptoms of depression fails to promote associated learning in four-month old infants. *Child Development, 70,* 560–570.

Keefe, R. S. E., Lobel, D. S., Mohs, R. C., Silverman, J. M., Harvey, P. D., Davidson, M., Losonczy, M. F., & Davis, K. L. (1991). Diagnostic issues in chronic schizophrenia: Kraepelinian schizophrenia, undifferentiated schizophrenia, and state-independent negative symptoms. *Schizophrenia Research, 4,* 71–79.

Keltner, D., & Kring, A. M. (1998). Emotion, social function, and psychopathology. *Review of General Psychology, 2,* 320–342.

Kerr, S. L., & Neale, J. M. (1993). Emotion perception in schizophrenia: Specific deficit or further evidence of generalized poor performance? *Journal of Abnormal Psychology, 102,* 312–318.

Klein, D. (1987). Depression and anhedonia. In D. C. Clark & J. Fawcett (Eds.), *Anhedonia and affect deficit states* (pp. 1–14). New York: PMA Publishing.

Knight, R. A., & Roff, J. D. (1983). Childhood and young adult predictors of schizophrenic outcome. In D. F. Ricks & B. S. Dohrenwend (Eds.), *Origins of psychopathology: Problems in research and public policy* (pp. 129–153). Cambridge, UK: Cambridge University Press.

Knight, R. A., & Roff, J. D. (1985). Affectivity in schizophrenia. In M. Alpert (Ed.), *Controversies in schizophrenia* (pp. 280–316). New York: Guilford Press.

Knight, R. A., Roff, J. D., Barnett, J., & Moss, J. L. (1979). Concurrent and predictive validity of thought disorder and affectivity: A 22-year follow-up of acute schizophrenics. *Journal of Abnormal Psychology, 88,* 1–12.

Krause, R., Steimer, E., Sanger-Alt, C., & Wagner, G. (1989). Facial expressions of schizophrenic patients and their interaction partners. *Psychiatry, 52,* 1–12.

Krause, R., Steimer-Krause, E., & Hufnagel, H. (1992). Expression and experience of affects in paranoid schizophrenia. *Revue Européenne de Psychologie Appliquée, 42,* 131–138.

Kring, A. M. (1999). Emotion in schizophrenia: Old mystery, new understanding. *Current Directions in Psychological Science, 8,* 160–163.

Kring, A. M., Alpert, M., Neale, J. M., & Harvey, P. D. (1994). A multichannel, multimethod assessment of affective flattening in schizophrenia. *Psychiatry Research, 54,* 211–222.

Kring, A. M., & Bachorowski, J.-.A. (1999). Emotion and psychopathology. *Cognition and Emotion, 13,* 575–599.

Kring, A. M., & Earnst, K. S. (in press). Nonverbal behavior in schizophrenia. In P. Philippot, E. Coats, & R. S. Feldman (Eds.), *Nonverbal behavior in clinical settings.* New York: Oxford University Press.

Kring, A. M., & Earnst, K. S. (1999). Stability of emotional responding in schizophrenia. *Behavior Therapy, 30,* 373–388.

Kring, A. M., Kerr, S. L., & Earnst, K. S. (1999). Schizophrenic patients show facial reactions to emotional facial expressions. *Psychophysiology, 36,* 186–192.

Kring, A. M., Kerr, S. L., Smith, D. A., & Neale, J. M. (1993). Flat affect in schizophrenia does not reflect diminished subjective experience of emotion. *Journal of Abnormal Psychology, 102,* 507–517.

Kring, A. M., & Neale, J. M. (1996). Do schizophrenics show a disjunctive relationship among expressive, experiential, and psychophysiological components of emotion? *Journal of Abnormal Psychology, 105,* 249–257.

Kring, A. M., Wissman, A. H., & Schmid, S. P. (1999, November). *Nonverbal clues to social anxiety.* Paper presented at the annual meeting of the Society for Research in Psychopathology, Montreal, Quebec, Canada.

Lang, P. J., Bradley, M. M., & Cuthbert, B. N. (1990). Emotion, attention, and the startle reflex. *Psychological Review, 97*, 377–395.

Leary, M., & Kowalski, R. M. (1995). *Social anxiety.* New York: Guilford Press.

Lee, C. M., & Gotlib, I. H. (1989a). Clinical status and emotional adjustment of children of depressed mothers. *American Journal of Psychiatry, 146*, 478–483.

Lee, C. M., & Gotlib, I. H. (1989b). Maternal depression and child adjustment: A longitudinal analysis. *Journal of Abnormal Psychology, 98*, 78–85.

Levenson, R. W. (1992). Autonomic nervous system differences among emotions. *Psychological Science, 3*, 23–27.

Lewine, R. R. J. (1991). Anhedonia and the amotivational state of schizophrenia. In A. Marneros, N. C. Andreasen, & M. T. Tsuang (Eds.), *Negative versus positive schizophrenia* (pp. 79–95). Berlin: Springer-Verlag.

Linehan, M. M. (1987). Dialectical behavior therapy for borderline personality disorder. *Bulletin of the Menninger Clinic, 51*, 261–276.

MacLeod, C., & Mathews, A. (1991). Cognitive-experimental approaches to the emotional disorders. In P. Martin (Ed.), *Handbook of behavior therapy and psychological science: An integrative approach* (pp. 116–150). New York: Pergamon Press.

Marcus, D. K., & Wilson, J. R. (1996). Interpersonal perception of social anxiety: A social relations analysis. *Journal of Social and Clinical Psychology, 15*, 471–487.

Martin, C. C., Borod, J. C., Alpert, M., Brozgold, A., & Welkowitz, J. (1990). Spontaneous expression of facial emotion in schizophrenic and right brain-damaged patients. *Journal of Communication Disorders 23*, 287–301.

Mathews, A. M., & MacLeod, C. (1994). Cognitive approaches to emotion and the emotional disorders. *Annual Review of Psychology, 45*, 25–50.

Mattes, R. M., Schneider, F., Heimann, H., & Birbaumer, N. (1995). Reduced emotional response of schizophrenic patients in remission during social interaction. *Schizophrenia Research, 17*, 249–255.

McAdams, D. (1996). Personality, modernity, and the storied self. *Psychological Inquiry, 7*, 295–321.

Mick, M. A., & Telch, M. J. (1998). Social anxiety and history of behavioral inhibition in young adults. *Journal of Anxiety Disorders, 12*, 1–20.

Miller, R. S., & Leary, M. R. (1992). Social sources and interactive functions of emotion: The case of embarrassment. In M. Clark (Ed.), *Emotion and social behavior* (pp. 202–221). Beverly Hills, CA: Sage.

Mueser, K. T., Doonan, R., Penn, D. L., Blanchard, J. J., Bellack, A. S., Nishith, P., & DeLeon, J. (1996). Emotion recognition and social competence in chronic schizophrenia. *Journal of Abnormal Psychology, 105*, 271–275.

Mulkens, S. A. N., de Jong, P. J., & Merkelbach, H. A. (1996). Disgust and spider phobia. *Journal of Abnormal Psychology, 105*, 464–468.

Murray, I. R., & Arnott, J. L. (1993). Toward the simulation of emotion in synthetic speech: A review of the literature on human vocal emotion. *Journal of the Acoustical Society of America, 93*, 1097–1108.

Myin-Germeys, I., Delespaul, P. A. E. G., & deVries, M. (in press). Flat affect: Blunted expression or experience in the daily life of schizophrenic patients? *Schizophrernia Bulletin.*

Neale, J. M., & Oltmanns, T. F. (1980). *Schizophrenia.* New York: Wiley.

Nuechterlein, K. H., & Dawson, M. E. (1984). A heuristic vulnerability/stress model of schizophrenic episodes. *Schizophrenia Bulletin, 10,* 300–312.

Ochs, E., & Capps, L. (1996). Narrating the self. *Annual Review of Anthropology, 25,* 19–43.

Olin, S. S., John, R. S., & Mednick, S. A. (1995). Assessing the predictive value of teacher reports in a high risk sample for schizophrenia: An ROC analysis. *Schizophrenia Research, 16,* 53–66.

Olin, S. S., & Mednick, S. A. (1996). Risk factors of psychosis: Identifying vulnerable populations premorbidly. *Schizophrenia Bulletin, 22,* 223–240.

Patrick, C. J., Bradley, M. M., & Lang, P. J. (1993). Emotion in the criminal psychopath: Startle reflex modulation. *Journal of Abnormal Psychology, 102,* 82–92.

Patrick, C. J., Cuthbert, B. N., & Lang, P. J. (1994). Emotion in the criminal psychopath: Fear image processing. *Journal of Abnormal Psychology, 103,* 523–534.

Pfhol, B., & Winokur, G. (1982). The evolution of symptoms in institutionalized hebephrenic/catatonic schizophrenics. *British Journal of Psychiatry, 141,* 567–572.

Pozo, C., Carver, C. S., Wellens, A. R., & Scheier, M. F. (1991). Social anxiety and social perception: Construing others' reactions to the self. *Personality and Social Psychology Bulletin, 17,* 355–362.

Robbins, L. (1966). *Deviant children grown up.* Baltimore: Williams & Wilkins.

Rosenberg, E. L. (1998). Levels of analysis and the organization of affect. *Review of General Psychology, 2,* 247–270.

Russell, J. A., & Feldman Barrett, L. (1999). Core affect, prototypical emotion episodes, and other things called *emotion*: Dissecting the elephant. *Journal of Personality and Social Psychology, 76,* 805–819.

Salem, J. E., Kring, A. M., & Kerr, S. L. (1996). More evidence for generalized poor performance in facial emotion perception in schizophrenia. *Journal of Abnormal Psychology, 105,* 480–483.

Scherer, K. R. (1986). Vocal affect expression: A review and model for future research. *Psychological Bulletin, 99,* 143–165.

Shearin, E. N., & Linehan, M. M. (1994). Dialectical behavior therapy for borderline personality disorder: Theoretical and empirical foundations. *Acta Psychiatrica Scandinavica, Supplementum, 379,* 61–68.

Thoits, P. A. (1985). Self-labeling processes in mental illness: The role of emotional deviance. *American Journal of Sociology, 92,* 221–249.

Tomarken, A. J., Davidson, R. J., Wheeler, R. E., & Doss, R. C. (1992). Individual differences in anterior brain asymmetry and fundamental dimensions of emotion. *Journal of Personality and Social Psychology, 62,* 676–687.

Tomarken, A. J., Elkins, L. E., Anderson, T., Shelton, R. E., & Hitt, S. (2000). *Sleep deprivation selectively potentiates positive affect during antidepressant treatment.* Manuscript in preparation.

Tomarken, A. J., & Keener, A. D. (1998). Frontal brain asymmetry and depression: A self-regulatory perspective. *Cognition and Emotion, 12,* 387–420.

Tomarken, A. J., Simien, C., & Garber, J. (1994). Resting frontal brain asymmetry discriminates adolescent children of depressed mothers from low-risk controls. *Psychophysiology, 31,* S97–S98.

Ulrich, G., & Harms, K. (1985). A video analysis of the nonverbal behavior of depressed patients and their relation to anxiety and depressive disorders. *Journal of Affective Disorders, 9,* 63–67.

Veljaca, K., & Rapee, R. M. (1998). Detection of negative and positive audience behaviours by socially anxious subjects. *Behaviour Research and Therapy, 36,* 311–321.

Walker, E. F., Grimes, K. E., Davis, D. M., & Smith, A. J. (1993). Childhood precursors of schizophrenia: Facial expressions of emotion. *American Journal of Psychiatry, 150,* 1654–1660.

Wallace, S. T., & Alden, L. E. (1997). Social phobia and positive social events: The price of success. *Journal of Abnormal Psychology, 106,* 416–424.

Watson, D., Clark, L. A., & Carey, G. (1988). Positive and negative affectivity and their relation to anxiety and depressive disorders. *Journal of Abnormal Psychology, 97,* 346–353.

Watson, D., Clark, L. A., & Tellegen, A. (1988). Development and validation of brief measures of positive and negative affect: The PANAS scales. *Journal of Personality and Social Psychology, 54,* 1063–1070.

Watson, D., Clark, L. A., Weber, K., Assenheimer, J. S., Strauss, M. E., & McCormick, R. A. (1995). Testing a tripartite model: II. Exploring the symptom structure of anxiety and depression in student, adult, and patient samples. *Journal of Abnormal Psychology, 104,* 15–25.

Watt, N. F. (1972). Longitudinal changes in the social behavior of children hospitalized for schizophrenia as adults. *Journal of Nervous and Mental Disease, 155,* 42–54.

Waxer, P. H. (1974). Nonverbal cues for depression. *Journal of Abnormal Psychology, 83,* 319–322.

Welner, Z., Welner, A., McCrary, D., & Leonard, M. A. (1977). Psychopathology in inpatients with depression: A controlled study. *Journal of Nervous and Mental Disease, 164,* 408–413.

Winton, W. C., Clark, D. M., & Edelmann, R. J. (1995). Social anxiety, fear of negative evaluation, and the detection of negative emotion in others. *Behaviour Research and Therapy, 33,* 193–196.

Zinbarg, R. E., & Barlow, D. H. (1996). Structure of anxiety and the anxiety disorders: A hierarchical model. *Journal of Abnormal Psychology, 105,* 181–193.

Zubin, J., & Spring, B. (1977). Vulnerability: A new view of schizophrenia. *Journal of Abnormal Psychology, 86,* 103–126.

12

Emotions and Health

TRACY J. MAYNE

At the turn of the century, there continues to be healthy and heated debate concerning basic issues of emotion: Are emotions dimensional or discrete? What are the necessary and sufficient components of emotion? Is the basic function of emotion physiological or social? Despite what appear to be some fundamental differences among affect scientists, they share one central tenet: Emotions are adaptive. Physiological researchers posit that emotions prepare an organism to quickly respond to threats in the environment (Cannon, 1911; Levenson, 1994). Social researchers postulate that emotions are central to human attachment, interaction, and social function (Lutz & White, 1986). Cognitive researchers propose that emotion is essential to memory formation and retrieval (Arnold, 1970; Bower, 1981). Taken together, research on emotion indicates that emotions are integral to many realms of healthy human functioning.

When it comes to emotion and physical health, however, a review of the literature could easily lead one to conclude that emotions may be adaptive in most areas but are detrimental to physical well-being. More specifically, negative emotions (anger, fear, distress) have been associated with morbidity and mortality from nearly every chronic illness, from cancer (Penninx et al., 1998) to AIDS (Mayne, Vittinghoff, Chesney, Barrett, & Coates, 1996) to asthma (Lehrer, Isenberg, & Hochron, 1993) to cardiovascular disease (Smith, 1992). Indeed, studies on negative emotions and health outnumber studies of positive emotions and health by a factor of 11 to 1, with the majority of studies focusing on the role of emotion in disease initiation, progression, and mortality (Mayne, 2000). This seems paradoxical for an essentially adaptive process.

This chapter looks to reconcile this apparent contradiction by proposing that emotions, including anger and fear and distress, are *health promoting*. The model I propose is in essence a systems model: Emotions play an important regulatory role in health, and when operating within a certain range, they promote overall functioning. When they operate outside of this range, they lead to disregulation and disease. The key is to know—

- What are the parameters that define healthy emotional function?
- How does each parameter affect different aspects of health?
- What is the healthy range of functioning for each parameter?

By way of analogy: A proper diet is essential to good overall health. Some of the parameters of a healthy diet include intake of calories, different proteins, vitamins and minerals, etc. One parameter, caloric intake, exists along a range from zero to tens of thousands of calories per day. Consuming too many calories results in obesity and can cause high blood pressure, arteriosclerosis, diabetes, and so on. Consuming too few calories can result in myriad health problems, from amenoria to heart failure. Within that distribution is a range of healthy caloric intake. Another parameter, vitamin C, has its own range (in milligrams) with its own health consequences: Consuming insufficient vitamin C leads to rickets, whereas too much causes kidney damage. I seek to address the following questions in this chapter: What are the parameters of health-promoting emotional functioning? How does each parameter influence health? How much of each parameter is "just right" for physical well-being and health?

THE STRUCTURE OF EMOTION: PATHWAYS TO HEALTH

In research on emotion and health, there is a key point that sometimes gets lost in the correlation between affect and various health outcomes: In order for emotion to influence health, it must affect the *physical* body. There are a number of ways for emotion to influence the body, both directly and indirectly. The bottom line, however, is that *there must be a physical impact* of an emotion in order for it to alter physical health. With that in mind, I will first explore some of these pathways that link affect to health and disease.

Direct Pathways: Physiological Activation

A great deal has been written about emotion and physiological arousal. Ekman includes physiological arousal as a central component of affect (Ekman, 1992) and has found that several negative emotions have unique patterns of activation (Ekman, Levenson, & Friesen, 1983). Evolutionary psychologists have posited that these patterns of emotion-associated arousal evolved specifically as an innate response that prepares an organism to re-act to specific classes of events in the environment (Tooby & Cosmodies, 1990). In other words, emotions produce physiological arousal patterns that support specific actions in response to environmental threats—or, in the case of positive affect, environmental opportunities (see B. L. Frederick-son & C. Branigan, Chapter 4, this volume). In this framework, anger and fear are associated with the motivation to fight and flee, and bring about sympathetic arousal that abets these behaviors: increased cardiovascular activation, greater oxygen exchange, increased glucose availability, etc. Dis-tress emotions (helplessness, depression, sadness, grief) are associated with the motivation to withdraw and to elicit help (Panksepp, 1988). Distress emotions induce activation of the hypothalamic–pituitary–adrenal cortex network, increasing blood levels of corticosteriods, which conserve energy and direct resources to vital systems, and endogenous opiates, which soothe and mediate pain (Asnis et al., 1987; Panksepp, 1988). Positive emotions are associated with increases in dopamine and seratonin, which are impli-cated in pleasure, affiliative bonding, and pain reduction (Ashby, Isen, & Turken, 1999; Jung, Staiger, & Sullivan, 1997; Knutson et al., 1998; Mor-gan & Franklin, 1991; Paalzow, 1992). Though emotions may be associ-ated with arousal in other neurohormonal systems (e.g., parasympathetic activation causing blushing during embarrassment), the majority of re-search has focused on arousal of the sympathetic adrenal–medulla system (SAM) and hypothalamic–pituitary–adrenal cortex system (HPAC). A brief summary of these systems and their effect on other physiological systems is outlined in Table 12.1.

In the Darwinian tradition, emotion-associated motivation and arousal are seen as adaptive. In this scheme, emotions function as "short-lived psychological–physiological phenomena that represent efficient modes of adaptation to changing environmental demands" (Levenson, 1994, p. 123). As shown by the work of Joseph LeDoux (1998), and reviewed by K. N. Ochsner and L. Feldman Barrett in Chapter 2 and P. Philippot and A. Schaefer in Chapter 3 of this volume, the cognitive processing that initiates emotional activation from immediate cues in the environment is primitive and automatic. In other words, a rabbit does not need to have an elabo-rated concept of a "bear" in order to flee when it hears a loud growl from behind. The evolutionary advantage of such a system is self-evident.

The physiological activation of emotion can directly influence health through its impact on the heart, lungs, immune system, etc. (see Table 12.1). Such activation was clearly adaptive to animals and has been evolutionarily conserved in humans. However, some researchers have ques-tioned whether this component of emotion is still healthy in modern hu-mans. Paul A. Obrist, a cardiologist, hypothesized that emotion-associated

TABLE 12.1. Physiological Effects of HPAC and SAM

HPAC	SAM
Glucose storage	Glucose mobilization
Decrease glucose uptake in peripheral tissues	Increased glucose uptake in peripheral tissues
Fatty acid and protein mobilization	
Immune cells centralized into lymphoid organs	Immune cells decentralized into peripheral blood
General immunosuppression	Some immunoactivation
Increased appetite and intestinal permeability	Decreased appetite and gastrointestinal activity
Decreased inflammation (including pulmonary)	Broncodilation
Cardiovascular homeostasis	Cardiovascular activation

arousal can be damaging to biological systems—especially the cardiovascular system (Obrist, 1981). Because modern humans are no longer faced with the kinds of physical threats once abundant in the environment (e.g., saber-toothed tigers), emotion-associated physiological arousal is in excess of current need. In effect, the fear of being fired from a job does not require one to run from the office as far and as quickly as possible, and yet fear-associated arousal is appropriate to this behavior. Frankenhauser (1980) suggested that such excess arousal causes "wear and tear" on the body, leading to disease (p. 58). In this framework, emotion-associated arousal *was* adaptive in primitive hominids, but is vestigial in modern humans, and like the appendix can be a source of illness and even death. This has been labeled the *psychophysiological model* (for a review, see Smith, 1992).

As cited in the opening paragraph of this chapter, there is a great deal of evidence supporting the psychophysiological model, showing that emotion can lead to initiation and progression of heart disease, cancer, AIDS, asthma, and other acute and chronic—and often fatal—illnesses. However, there is an important caveat to this literature that can easily be overlooked but is crucial to understanding and interpreting its findings. Research that falls under the rubric of the psychophysiological model examines *pathological* levels of emotion and arousal. In other words, the psychophysiological model is not a model of emotion and health but a model of emotional and physical pathology. Let me use an example to help clarify this point: the Type A coronary-prone personality.

The original Type A construct grew from cardiologists' observations that patients with heart disease shared common emotional, cognitive, and behavioral patterns—excessive anger and hostility, cynicism, a sense of time pressure, and so on (Jenkins, 1971a, 1971b). Later research confirmed that Type A individuals respond to an array of stimuli, but especially social stimuli, with "cynical hostility" and exaggerated cardiovascular arousal (Christensen & Smith, 1993; Shapiro, Goldstein, & Jamner, 1996). This excessive cardiovascular arousal bruises artery walls, leading to plaque formation, arteriosclerosis, and cardiovascular disease (Manuck, Marsland, Kaplan, & Williams, 1995; Obrist, 1981). Thus, responding to the world with cynical hostility damages the cardiovascular system through frequent and intense cardiovascular arousal.

By definition, Type A is exaggerated hostility and anger, and by definition it is unhealthy. Type A does not define what *healthy* anger and hostility might be, and one cannot infer that eliminating these is any healthier than exaggerating them. What Type A and the psychophysiological model do, however, is specify two parameters of unhealthy emotion: high *frequency* and high *intensity* of physiological activation. Thus, frequency and intensity (also known as reactivity) are two parameters that define unhealthy affect, and by induction may also define healthy affect.

The research supporting the hypothesis that frequent, intense negative affect can directly damage the body is overwhelming (for a review, see Mayne, 2000). However, in a series of studies on physiological activation and *behavioral performance*, Johansson, Frankenhaeuser, and colleagues made an interesting discovery: Greater sympathetic arousal is associated with better behavioral performance in many arenas (Ellertsen, Johnsen, & Ursin, 1978; Johansson, Frankenhaeuser, & Magnusson, 1973; Rauste–von Wright, von Wright, & Frankenhaeuser, 1981; Ursin, Baade, & Levine, 1978). Across tasks as diverse as written examinations and skydiving, individuals who excrete more catecholamines during a behavior performed better than those who showed lower levels of SAM arousal. In this case, intensity of emotion has behavioral advantages. In further analyzing their data, however, Johansson and Frankenhaeuser (1973) discovered that subjects who *recovered* more slowly from sympathetic arousal performed worse than those who recovered rapidly. Johansson and Frankenhaeuser began to develop a model in which good adjustment included a high intensity of emotion-associated physiological arousal *if* the duration of the arousal was short, that is, if there was rapid recovery. This research suggests that in addition to frequency and intensity, the third parameter that defines healthy affect versus unhealthy affect is the duration of arousal or recovery.

In summary, one component of emotion is physiological arousal. The parameters of arousal that are associated with healthy and unhealthy functioning are frequency, intensity, and duration. The psychophysiological model posits that emotions that are frequent, intense, and last for long periods cause wear and tear on the body and lead to illness. This model has focused almost exclusively on negative emotions, though the theory should hold true for positive emotions as well. What the model does not explain is whether there is some optimal level of emotional arousal associated with healthy functioning. Johansson and Frankenhaeuser (1973) suggest that intensity and frequency of arousal may not be problematic (at least for behavioral performance) as long as recovery is rapid.

Indirect Pathways: Behavior and Cognition

Physiological change, whether it is caused by emotion or exercise or some other source, is an actual component of health. Therefore, physiological arousal is considered a direct pathway by which emotions influence health. However, as we discussed in Chapter 1 of this volume, there are at least two other widely recognized components of emotion: behavior and cognition. Because behavior and cognition are *not* components of physiological function, their impact on physiological functioning and health are said to be "indirect." In effect, behavior and cognition must first influence physiology in order to affect health. Let us examine behavior first.

Behavior and Health

One function of emotion is to prime or motivate behavioral responses to threats and opportunities in the environment. For example, when faced with an insurmountable threat, a person responds with fear, which includes the motivation to flee or escape as well as the physiological arousal that supports this behavior (SAM activation). Some of the behaviors motivated by emotion can have immediate and/or long-term affects on physiology and health—suicide and substance abuse are two such examples. Conversely, some behaviors that individuals engage in to regulate health can influence emotion. For example, having your doctor examine a suspicious lump and diagnose it as a cyst can greatly alleviate breast cancer anxiety. Thus, I divide emotion-associated health behaviors into two broad categories: emotion-regulating behaviors that affect health, and health-regulating behaviors that affect emotion. Let us begin with emotion-regulating behaviors.

Emotion-Regulating Behaviors That Affect Health. Individuals differ in their ability to tolerate different emotions. Some people experience even small levels of an emotion as unpleasant, undesirable, or toxic and go to great lengths to avoid those feelings. Other individuals not only tolerate but even enjoy intense levels of affect in themselves and others. In other words, individuals are not just passive emotional responders to events in their environment, but actively seek situations and engage in behaviors that will regulate emotions up or down. This is known as the *transactional model* (Bolger & Schilling, 1991; Smith, 1992). For example, skydivers jump from planes in order to enjoy the exhilaration of fear. Severely acrophobic individuals engage in elaborate behaviors to *avoid* any of the fear associated with the potential of falling. Between these two extremes are the majority of people, who go to see Alfred Hitchcock's *Vertigo* or ride a roller-coaster to experience the fear of falling, or practice relaxation techniques to diminish those feelings when their plane hits turbulence (emotion regulation is discussed in greater detail by G. A. Bonanno in Chapter 8 and L. Feldman Barrett & J. J. Gross in Chapter 9, this volume).

Though emotion up-regulation may be quite common, some individuals fall more than a standard deviation above the mean in up-regulating behaviors. These individuals have been labeled "sensation seekers." Sensation seekers are drawn to the thrill of emotion-associated physical sensations and report enjoying the "rush" they experience in high-intensity situations (Zuckerman, Bone, Neary, Mangelsdorff, & Brustman, 1972). However, these situations often involve some degree of danger. Even skydivers who carefully prepare their equipment run the risk of a parachute failing to open and plunging to their death. Individuals who engage in sexual intercourse with many partners risk contracting a sexually transmitted disease (STD) even if they consistently use a condom (as condoms break and some STDs can be spread casually). Thus, deliberately seeking intense emotional experiences can come with a price tag: the risk of potential health damage. The more frequent, intense, and prolonged the states of emotional activation (and the behaviors that induce activation), the greater the possibility of health damage.

Other individuals up-regulate an emotion not as an end in and of itself but as a means of decreasing another competing emotion. Fredrickson and Levenson (1998) have shown that the induction of positive emotions hastens physiological recovery from negative emotions. In essence, up-regulating positive affect can down-regulate negative affect. Indeed, the increase of some neurotransmitters associated with positive affect (dopamine and seratonin) can decrease negative feelings and increase tolerance to pain, quite literally making negative emotions "feel less bad" (Knutson et al., 1998; Morgan & Franklin, 1991; Paalzow, 1992). Therefore, individuals may engage in behaviors to increase positive affect as an end unto itself (sensation seeking) or may increase positive affect as a means of "undoing" negative emotions.[1] Across emotions, there seem to be three health-affecting behaviors that reliably up-regulate positive emotion and down-regulate negative emotion: eating, substance use, and sex.

Evolutionary theorists have long suggested that foods that are high in fat and carbohydrates are pleasing for humans to eat because these foods were essential to energy storage that would later guard against starvation (Groop & Tumoi, 1997). In other words, fats and carbohydrates taste good because it is evolutionarily adaptive to have energy stored in the form of fat, motivating us to eat these foods when they are available. In parts of the world where there is no longer the large-scale threat of starvation, what was once an evolutionary advantage may now be health damaging. High-fat and carbohydrate-rich "comfort foods" continue to produce positive feelings, and in support of the "undoing" hypothesis, research has shown that high anger, anxiety, and depression are all linked to overeating (Arnow, Kennedy, & Agras, 1995). Here again, the psychophysiological model is relevant: If an individual up-regulates positive emotion and down-regulates negative emotion through caloric intake in excess of what is needed by the body, the resulting weight increase leads to disregulation and damage to many biological systems (see Green, 1997). Unanswered by the application of the psychophysiological model to eating is this question: Can the occasional use of high-fat and carbohydrate-rich foods to regulate emotion be healthy?

Psychoactive drugs induce emotional states by activating neural–hormonal systems associated with positive emotions. Cocaine is sympatho-mimetic and induces euphoria and sometimes anxiety. MDMA (3,4-methylenedioxymethamphetamine, or "Ecstasy") increases seratonin and feelings of closeness and attachment. Heroin is similar to endogenous opiates, inducing euphoria and decreasing sensations of pain. Research has shown that sensation seeking leads certain individuals to use drugs to induce intense emotional states (Scourfield, Stevens, & Merikangas, 1996). The consequences of frequent, intense, prolonged activation of these emotion-associated systems is the physiological wear and tear associated with addiction: drug tolerance, withdrawal, and overdose. In addition to up-regulating positive affect, most psychoactive drugs also (temporarily) undo the effects of negative emotions. For example, Hall and colleagues have collected convincing evidence that many smokers begin smoking and have difficulty quitting, because nicotine down-regulates depression (Hall, Muñoz, Reus, & Sees, 1993). In fact, treating individuals who are quitting tobacco with an antidepressant has been shown to increase abstinence (Hitsman et al., 1999). And across negative affects, greater intensity and frequency of emotion has been causally linked to increased alcohol and other substance use (Cox, Norton, Dorward, & Fergusson, 1989; Dielman, Leech, Miller, & Moss, 1991; Houston & Vavak, 1991; Merikangas & Angst, 1995; Mills, Berry, Dimsdale, Nelesen, & Ziegler, 1993), while substance use has also been linked to attempts to regulate affect (Cooper, Frone, Russell, & Mudar, 1995)

Like food and drugs, some sensation seekers up-regulate positive affect through sex. In recent research, sensation seekers have been shown to engage in high levels of unprotected sex and sex with multiple partners, increasing their risk of contracting HIV and other STDs (Kalichman et al., 1994). However, sensation seekers are not alone in using sex to regulate affect—it is actually a relatively common form of coping (Folkman & Lazarus, 1980). The emotions up-regulated by sex include hedonic pleasure as well as closeness and intimacy. Where early motivation theorists classified sex as a drive much like thirst and hunger, more recent affect theorists have suggested that these sexual feelings represent primitive emotions (Mayne & Buck, 1997) and may share the ability of positive emotions to "undo" negative affects. In support of this, research has found that emotions like anxiety can directly induce sexual arousal (Barlow, Sakhaira, & Beck, 1983), and that anxious and depressed individuals are more likely to engage in risky sexual practices (Coleman, 1992; Kelly et al., 1993). Though there may be evolutionary advantages to bonding and propagating after anxiety-producing natural disasters, and sexual release may be a good way of down-regulating negative emotions, the advent of HIV/AIDS also makes such behavior a health risk.

In summary, people engage in a number of different behaviors to regulate affect. Some individuals actively up-regulate feelings, both positive and negative, because they enjoy the intensity and "rush" of arousal. Others up-regulate one feeling as a means of down-regulating or "undoing" another. Though the psychophysiological model was conceptualized as a way of understanding how emotional arousal affects health, it can also be applied to behavior. Emotion regulating behaviors (but most especially eating, drinking, and drug use) can cause physical damage when they become frequent, intense, and of long duration. However, in the case of substance use or unprotected sex, even one episode can result in a fatal overdose or serious infection. And, as is the case with direct pathways between emotion and health, applying the psychophysiological model to health behaviors does not address the question of whether and at what level these behaviors may be health promoting.

Health Behaviors That Regulate Emotion. While certain behaviors used to regulate emotions can influence health, certain behaviors used to regulate health can also influence emotion. The earliest health behavior model was the *fear drive model,* which posited that inducing fear of disease can motivate individuals to stop unhealthy and initiate healthier behaviors (Higbee, 1969; Janis, 1967). In essence, people will engage in health behaviors, such as cancer screening, to down-regulate the fear of disease. In fact, if individuals believe that engaging in a health behavior will lessen the chance or severity of disease and believe that they are capable of performing this behavior, then fear does motivate that health behavior (Leventhal, Safer, & Panagis, 1983). Therefore, health behaviors can regulate emotion. This effect is not limited to negative emotions. Positive affect motivates individuals to build resources, including social resources. Several studies have shown that in couples, relationship satisfaction is associated with increased preventive and decreased risky health behaviors (Buunk & Bakkov, 1997;

Coyne & Delongis, 1986). The correlational nature of these findings do not allow causal inference: The positive feelings in the relationship may motivate healthier behavior, or healthier behavior may increase feelings of love and security. In either case, emotion-associated motivation can have a positive influence on health behavior.

One behavior stands out as particularly important in promoting and maintaining health in modern humans: health care seeking. Only in the last century and a half has medicine been able to effectively treat serious physical illness (McKinley & McKinley, 1986). Before that, bloodletting, leeches, and herbal elixirs were still the treatments of choice for most diseases. But in the last 150 years, medical treatment has flourished, and there are drugs and procedures that effectively treat (if not always cure) most chronic illnesses. In the 21st century, seeking a physician's care can prevent disease—detecting cervical dysplasia before it progresses to cancer with yearly PAP smears—as well as slow or stop progression (surgery and follow-up chemotherapy).

Given the efficacy of modern medicine, one would think that most adults would have regular physical exams, and see a physician at the first sign of illness. Unfortunately, there is strong evidence that most individuals readily accommodate their symptoms, seeking treatment only when that accommodation fails and symptoms interfere with their daily activities (Safer, Thamps, Jackson, & Leventhal, 1979). All too often this results in delays that diminish treatment efficacy. There are two emotions, however, that motivate individuals to engage in preventive behaviors and to seek treatment for their ills. These are fear/anxiety and distress/depression.

Obviously fear and distress did not evolve for the purpose of increasing medical care seeking. They developed as responses to environmental threats that are overwhelming: In the case of fear, the threat is escapable; in the case of distress, the threat is inescapable. However, fear and distress may function adaptively in ways not selected for evolutionarily. And since the elicitors of fear and distress share common characteristics, it is not surprising that they also engender some common motivations. A fearful/distressed individual does not believe that he/she has the resources to overcome the threat alone, so both emotions induce a motivation to seek help. In addition to motivating help seeking, the expression of distress and fear also motivates others to provide help (Clark, Ouelette, Powell, & Milberg, 1987; Hoffman, 1978; Stiff, Dillard, Somera, Kim, & Sleight, 1988). In fact, Tomkins (1963) hypothesized that distress is "designed" to elicit support from others. So, though distress and fear did not evolve to motivate medical care seeking, both are currently related to seeking and receiving such care (Betrus, Elmore, & Hamilton, 1995; Callahan, Hui, Nienaber, & Musick, 1994; Karlsson, Lehtinen, & Joukamaa, 1995). When care is

sought preventively or early in the course of disease, it can often be cura-
tive, thus alleviating anticipatory fear and distress around illness.

In summary, health behaviors can regulate emotions. Ceasing to smoke
can alleviate the fear of premature death from cancer or cardiovascular disease. Seeking medical help can decrease fears associated with symptoms of
an unknown illness. As in the previous subsection, the question here is how
much of these emotion-motivated behaviors is healthy.

Cognition and Health

Emotions affect health directly through emotion-associated physiological
arousal. Emotions affect health indirectly by motivating behaviors that impact the physical body. Emotions can also impact health indirectly through
cognitions, which must first influence either physiological arousal or
behavior in order to affect the body. Readers should not assume that cognition is any less powerful a predictor of health than physiological arousal or
behavior. The depressive belief that one is in an inescapably punitive, hope-
less, and helpless situation can motivate a suicide attempt—the ultimate
health-damaging behavior.

Cognitions concerning health tend to fall into three main categories:
symptom perception, illness representation/beliefs, and behavioral response/
coping. These areas have been defined within the *health beliefs model*
(Rosenstock, 1974), the *reasoned action model* (Fishbein & Ajzen, 1975),
and the *dual process model* (Leventhal, Safer, & Panagis, 1983). As will be
clear, emotion influences cognitions in each area.

Symptom Perception. In order to seek help for an illness, a person
has to be aware that he/she is sick. This begins by perceiving a symptom
or sign of illness: a fever, a lump in the breast, an irregular heart beat,
etc. And yet research has shown that, in general, people do not accurately perceive the symptoms and signs of illness (Pennebaker, 1982). One
might argue that learning requires feedback and that a generally healthy
population might not be good perceivers of a fever due to lack of feedback regarding their actual body temperature. But even in diseases where
monitoring and feedback are an essential part of treatment (asthma, diabetes mellitus, and heart disease) symptom perception is highly inaccurate
in the direction of underreporting (Barsky, Cleary, Barnett, Christiansen,
& Ruskin, 1994; Barsky, Cleary, Brener, & Ruskin, 1993; Boulet,
Turcotte, & Brochu, 1994; Rietveld, Prins, & Kolk, 1996; Schandry,
Leopold, & Vogt, 1996; Weinger, Jacobson, Draelos, Finkelstein, &
Simonson, 1995). Research on negative emotions has clearly shown that
they often increase symptom reporting and the accuracy of symptom reporting (Cohen et al., 1995; Salovey, 1992; Salovey & Birnbaum, 1989;

Wood, Saltzberg, & Goldsamt, 1990). The mechanism is unclear, though it has been suggested that depression (specifically) focuses attention inward, making bodily sensations more salient. Thus, negative emotions may be integral to overcoming a positivistic bias against recognizing symptoms of disease. The role of positive emotions in symptom perception is largely unknown, though cognitive dissonance theory (Festinger, 1957) would suggest that people experiencing positive affect should interpret illness sensation in a positivistic, affect-congruent direction.

Illness Representation, Beliefs, and Attributions. Being aware of a sign of illness is a necessary but not sufficient cognition to influence health behaviors. For example, one may perceive a fever but attribute it to being out in the sun without a hat. Until a symptom is represented as or attributed to illness, it is unlikely to generate responsive health behaviors.

Unfortunately, there are attributional biases that work against accurately representing signs of illness. In general, people represent themselves and the world as more positive than they truly are. They see the world as more controllable, the future as brighter, and themselves as more desirable than they are in reality (Taylor & Brown, 1988). This bias extends to health as well: People consistently underestimate their risk of disease (Weinstein, 1984, 1987; Weinstein & Klein, 1995). As with symptom perception, depression appears to correct this positivistic bias: Depressed individuals see the world more accurately, and depressed individuals who are sick report their illness-related symptoms more accurately (Cohen et al., 1995; Lewinsohn, Mischel, Chaplin, & Barton, 1980). Perhaps more importantly, depressed and anxious people are more likely to utilize medical care (Betrus et al., 1995; Callahan et al., 1994; Karlsson et al., 1995). For sick individuals, this may mean receiving an appropriate level of care as opposed to underutilizing medical services (Mayne, 2000).

In addition to perceiving signs of illness and attributing them to disease, several other cognitions/attributions are important in determining how people respond to an illness. These include beliefs about the consequences of the illness. The belief that a disease is severe (but not too severe), that an individual is personally vulnerable to these effects, and that the effects will be lasting all promote taking action to cope with an illness (Leventhal, Safer, & Panagis, 1983). In each of these cases a normal positivistic bias is likely to produce a minimization of illness, and in each case negative emotions (especially depression and anxiety) are likely to increase a sense of illness severity and personal vulnerability.

Behavioral Response and Coping. Once someone has identified an illness of sufficient severity, there are several cognitions that determine whether and what actions they will take to cope with the illness:

- Is there anything that can be done to improve the outcome of this disease?
- Do I have the ability to perform those behaviors?
- What are the costs and benefits (outcomes) of performing those behaviors?
- Do others engage in these behaviors?
- Do I intend to engage in these behaviors?

In each of these areas, positive and negative emotions have the ability to influence cognition, and through cognition actual behavior. Depressive affect is associated with feelings of helplessness and hopelessness, which decrease the belief that one can engage in proactive behavior and that those behaviors will lead to positive outcomes (Beck, Rush, Shaw, & Emery, 1979). A good example is adherence: Depressed individuals both believe that they are and in fact truly are less likely to adhere to medical regimens (Carney, Freedland, Eisen, Rich, & Jaffe, 1995; Carney, Freedland, Rich, & Jaffe, 1995). Paradoxically, depression is positively associated with an important health behavior—seeking health care. Anger, or what has been labeled a "fighting spirit" (the belief that action is possible and that one can control the outcome of an illness through action), has been associated with improved cancer outcomes (Greer, Morris, & Pettingale, 1979), though recent research has failed to replicate these findings (Watson, Haviland, Greer, Davidson, & Bliss, 1999). Finally, guilt, or the anticipation of "feeling bad" if one doesn't engage in healthy behaviors, has been associated with greater adherence to health behaviors (Bybee, Leckman, Mersica, & Miller, 1997). And, though specific cognitions have not been explored, there is likely to be some cognitive involvement that at least partially mediates the association between feelings of attachment and love and better health behaviors.

In a similar vein, emotion is likely to color the assessment of whether the action taken to cope with the illness has worked or not. In accordance with the positivistic attributional bias, it is likely that people who are depressed will view their efforts at coping with illness to be less effective, whereas positive affect may result in an overestimation of the efficacy of coping.

In summary, human cognition does not always result in an accurate perception of the world. In general, people show a positivistic attributional bias, seeing themselves and the world in a better light than reality would dictate. This extends to perceptions and beliefs about health as well. As such, most individuals underreport symptoms and signs of illness, often do not attribute symptoms and signs *to* illness, and often delay seeking treatment until symptoms significantly interfere with daily functioning. Negative emotions in general, and depression and fear in particular, appear to correct this bias and increase the accuracy with which people perceive symptoms, attribute them to illness, and seek help. Several negative affects, like anger and guilt, have been associated with positive health behaviors in response to disease and are associated with cognitions that support the belief that individuals can successfully take action against illness. Other emotions, like depression, may increase help seeking but decrease perceived efficacy and actual ability to engage in health-promoting behaviors (e.g., adherence to medication). Clearly, cognition is a driving force behind many health behaviors, and emotion is a powerful determinant of those cognitions.

Cognition can also influence health through its effect on emotion-associated physiological arousal. As discussed by K. N. Ochsner and L. Feldman Barrett in Chapter 2, this volume, higher level cortical processing can activate, deactivate, and up- or down-regulate an emotion. Anxiety researchers have clearly demonstrated that panic disorders hinge upon cognitive processes that amplify fear through attention to anxiety-associated physiological arousal, control attributions, etc. (Barlow, 1988). Depression researchers have shown that internal/global/stable negative attributions can cause and exacerbate depression (Beck et al., 1979). As Ochsner and Feldman Barrrett point out, emotion is under the control of more than one cortical system and at times is under more or less conscious control. It is apparent that individuals can induce emotion purely by thought. And, as the anxiety and depression literatures have shown, this can lead to intense, prolonged, frequent physiological arousal, with serious consequences to health. Once again, these parameters are consistent with those of the psychophysiological model.

Overall Summary

Emotions influence health in a number of ways. Emotion-associated physiological arousal is a component of health and directly affects health outcomes. Emotion-associated behaviors used to up-regulate or down-regulate emotions can also influence health. In both cases, in accordance with the psychophysiological model, the more frequent, intense, and prolonged the arousal/behavior, the more likely it is to damage health through wear and tear on the body. The major limitation of this model is that it does not address whether or what is a healthy level of arousal/behavior. Emotions also influence cognition, which in turn influences physiological arousal and health behavior. Negative emotions can potentiate thoughts that lead to healthy behavior by correcting the normative positivistic attributional bias and by supporting the motivation to enact an action plan (perhaps most importantly, health care seeking). But some emotions, like depression, may also undermine personal efficacy, coping, and evaluation of coping outcomes. Finally, emotion-associated cognitions can generate, intensify, and prolong physiological arousal, causing physical wear and tear and leading to disease.

What should be clear at this point is that there is no simplistic formula indicating

POSITIVE EMOTION = GOOD HEALTH
NEGATIVE EMOTION = POOR HEALTH

The next section explores the question of when and how much of which emotions is good for health, and for whom.

HEALTHY EMOTIONAL FUNCTIONING

Knowing how much of an emotion is the "right amount" is a little like the story of the three bears. When it comes to physiological arousal and emotion-regulating behaviors, the psychophysiological model makes clear that emotion can sometimes be "too hot." As reviewed in the previous sections, physiological arousal and regulating behaviors (such as eating, drinking, and sex) can be too frequent, too intense, and too long, leading to negative health outcomes that range from drug overdose to cardiovascular disease to HIV. Can emotions also be "too cold"—too infrequent, too weak, and too short? Could this negatively affect health as well? The answer is yes, but the explication is complex.

When it comes to perceiving symptoms, attributing them to illness, and seeking health care, negative emotions appear to play an important and proactive role in health. In one study, individuals living with HIV who had the lowest depression scores were the most likely to underreport symptoms of HIV later detected via medical exam and had the fewest health care visits—below the minimum recommended level (Mayne, 2000). Thus, there is some evidence that too little negative affect may provide insufficient motivation for seeking care. Another valid interpretation, however, is that individuals may be denying, repressing, or actively suppressing both emotions and the perception of symptoms and signs of illness.

What happens when individuals try to actively suppress the expression of an emotion? Gross and Levenson (1993) have found that such suppression actually results in greater emotion-specific physiological arousal. Research in the tradition of the psychophysiological model has found that emotional suppression (specifically anger suppression) is associated with decreased immune function (Petrie, Booth, & Pennebaker, 1998) and increased cardiovascular disease (Faber & Burns, 1996). Thus, if someone tries to actively suppress a feeling, physiological arousal is paradoxically heightened, which can lead to "wear and tear" and illness. Individuals can also engage in active denial by physically and/or mentally avoiding a stress-ful situation (Lazarus & Folkman, 1984). Compared to more active forms of coping such as problem solving, avoidance appears to be less effective and has been linked to poorer health behavior (Sherbourne, Hays, Ordway, DiMatteo, & Kravitz, 1992). It is important to note that intense emotions like fear can exceed an individual's affect tolerance, leading him/her to en-gage in avoidance coping or denial. This results in decrements in health care seeking and preventive behavior (Leventhal, 1970).

Conscious suppression and denial/avoidance of negative emotions is linked to heightened arousal and to decrements in health promoting behav-ior. These processes, however, are not always conscious. The research liter-ature indicates that unconscious defense mechanisms like repression (also referred to as "repressive coping") produce the same outcomes as conscious suppression. When faced with an anxiety-provoking situation, repressive copers report less anxiety but show greater physiological arousal (Newton & Contrada, 1992). Some researchers have proposed that heightened acti-vation associated with repressive coping may lead to cardiovascular disease (King, Taylor, Albright, & Haskell, 1990; Melamed, Kushnir, Strauss, & Vigiser, 1997). Others have linked repressive coping to cancer morbidity (McKenna, Zevon, Corn, & Rounds, 1999).

In summary, negative emotions that are "too cold"—short, infrequent, and weak—can undermine symptom perception and result in insufficient motivation to seek care. Whether low levels of emotion-associated physio-logical arousal have more direct effects on health (the opposite of "wear and tear") is discussed in the following subsection. Emotional suppression/denial/avoidance/repression all seem to have a negative impact on health. They appear to be associated with a paradoxical *increase* in physiological arousal and with decreases in health-promoting behaviors.

Overall, there seems to be a case for the argument that emotions that are "too hot" and "too cold" may be bad for health. The ultimate two questions for this chapter are these: How much emotion is "just right"? And is there a model for health-promoting emotion?

Psychological Toughness

Richard A. Dienstbier (1989, 1991) developed a physiological model for healthy emotional function labeled *psychological toughness*. Dienstbier's model focuses on arousal in two systems (SAM and HPAC) and three pa-rameters—intensity, recovery, and frequency. The model is summarized as follows:

- Resting levels of sympathetic and corticosteroid arousal are low.
- When faced with a new challenge, there is strong sympathetic acti-vation.

- When the challenge is over, sympathetic activation quickly returns to low levels.
- When faced with the same or similar challenges again, sympathetic activation is high but recovery becomes progressively more rapid.
- Sympathetic activation does not generalize to unrelated situations.
- When faced with continuous challenges, sympathetic activation is maintained and corticosteroid activation postponed as long as possible.
- When corticosteroid activation does occur, recovery is rapid and activation does not generalize to other situations.

In more affective terms, this model could be interpreted thus: When there are no immediate threats or challenges in the environment, baseline levels of fear, anger, and distress (and their accompanying arousal) are low. When faced with a threat or challenge, an individual reacts with strong fear or anger (action-oriented emotions) but recovers rapidly once the situation is resolved. Fear and anger do not generalize to unrelated situations, but if the same situation occurs again the fear/anger response remains intense, though recovery becomes progressively more rapid with each exposure. Individuals remain relatively resistant to distress, but if distress does occur recovery is rapid as well.

There are a number of studies indicating that the toughness pattern produces optimal behavioral responses to many challenging situations (Ader, 1970; Fride, Hilaviki, & Arora, 1990; Weiss, Glazer, Pohorecky, Brink, & Miller, 1975) and protects animals against norepinephrine depletion during episodes of stress later in life. Though toughness seems to be optimal in terms of behavioral performance, is it also optimal for health?

Toughness and Health

Though the evidence is not overwhelming and must be culled from both animal and human research, the answer to the previous question is a qualified yes. In one paradigm, animals are exposed to one of two stressors: One stressor is inescapable shock, and in time the animal responds to the stressor with distress, helplessness, and increased HPAC activation. The other stressor is escapable shock, and over time the animal learns to respond to it with fear, increased SAM activation, and active coping (jumping). In this paradigm, animals are injected with tumor cells, then exposed to one of the two stressors on an ongoing basis. The outcome variable is tumor growth. Results show that the controllable stressor and ensuing fear/SAM response are associated with greater resistance to tumors, while the uncontrollable stressor and ensuing distress/HPAC response are associated with increase tumor growth (Sklar & Anisman, 1981). In fact, the more days that animals experience their respective stressor, the greater the difference in tumor growth. Similar results have been reported elsewhere (Nieburgs et al., 1979; Sklar & Anisman, 1979; Tejwani et al., 1991). Hilaviki-Clark, Rowland, Clark, and Lipman (1993) perhaps summarized the findings best: "chronic, predictable stress may biologically help the animal to adjust towards another stressor, such as carcinogen-induced tumors" (p. 157).

What is especially interesting and supportive of the health benefits of psychological toughness is the observation that some animals exposed to the uncontrollable stressor responded by fighting with other animals as opposed to distress/helplessness. These animals do *not* show increased tumor growth in response to uncontrollable stress (Sklar & Anisman, 1981). An association between spontaneous fighting and tumor resistance has been noted elsewhere (Amkraut & Solomon, 1972).

It is risky, at best, to equate behavior and arousal in animals with emotions in humans. However, these data suggest that angry/fearful responding and the associated SAM activation protect against neoplastic disease, whereas distress/HPAC responding is associated with increase susceptibility to tumor growth. The physiological mechanism mediating this effect is cellular immunity. Within the immune system, natural killer (NK) cells seek and destroy cells that are cancerous or infected with viruses. Epinephrine (released during SAM activation) induces NK cells to seek out and kill more cancer and virally infected cells (Hellstrand, Hermodsson, & Strannegard, 1985; Targan, Britvan, & Dorey, 1981; Tonnesen, Christensen, & Brinklov, 1987; Tonnessen, Tonnessen, & Christensen, 1984). In contrast, cortisol decreases NK cell function (Tonnesen et al., 1987). Thus, periodic anger and fear, with the accompanying SAM activation, may promote health by increasing the immune system's ability to detect and kill cancerous and virally infected cells.

There are some studies in humans that also suggest that psychological toughness is associated with greater immunocompetence and resistance to neoplastic and viral disease. In one study, distressed couples engaged in marital conflict in a laboratory setting (Mayne, O'Leary, McCrady, Contrada, & Labouvie, 1997). Both the men and women reported increased anger, anxiety, and depression during the conflict and showed signs of greater SAM activation. However, the men experienced significantly faster emotional and physiological recovery than the women, and the men increased in immune function while the women showed slight decreases. In accordance with the toughness model, strong SAM responding followed by rapid recovery resulted in improved immunocompetence. Another study measured cortisol and immune function in people who had snake phobia and who were undergoing behavioral exposure treatment for their phobia (Wiedenfeld et al., 1990). As the participants succeeded in their therapy (i.e., were able to approach the snake), they decreased in HPAC activation, and immune function improved significantly. These results have been partially replicated elsewhere (Kirshbaum et al., 1995).

These studies show significant changes in immune function that indicate the toughness pattern of responding may result in increased immunocompetence in humans. However, the changes in immune function, though statistically significant, are well within the normal range of human functioning. Does the toughness pattern and the ensuing increase in immune function make any difference in morbidity and mortality? Again, the answer is a qualified yes.

Toughness not only appears to enhance immune function but also may have measurable health benefits. In one study, men living with HIV who showed more emotion-associated SAM reactivity in the laboratory also had significantly higher NK function during SAM activation and survived significantly longer than other subjects (O'Leary, Temoshok, Sweet, & Jenkins, 1989; Solomon, Temoshok, O'Leary, & Zich, 1989; Temoshok, O'Leary, & Jenkins, 1990). In another study, young children were measured for cardiac and immune reactivity in the laboratory (Boyce et al., 1995). The children who were more reactive had fewer respiratory illness. But when an uncontrollable stressor was introduced (starting school), the reactive children had more respiratory illnesses. Unfortunately, the study did not include a controllable stress condition. In such a condition, the psychological toughness model would predict that the reactive children would manifest fewer respiratory infections than the unreactive children. A recent review suggests that these small but consistent changes in immune function do, in fact, have measurable impact on immune-related health and illness (Kiecolt-Glaser & Glaser, 1999).

Research in other paradigms has also found that SAM-associated emotional arousal, followed by rapid recovery, is associated with general health benefits. Pennebaker and colleagues have induced emotional activation in and outside of the laboratory by asking participants to talk or write about upsetting and traumatic experiences. When compared to control subjects who write about mundane topics (e.g., their bedroom), participants in the trauma group show better immune function (Esterling et al., 1994; Pennebaker, Kiecolt-Glaser, & Glaser, 1988; Petrie, Booth, Pennebaker, Davison, & Thomas, 1995) and are less likely to visit a physician because of illness over the next several months (Pennebaker, Colder, & Sharp, 1990; Pennebaker et al., 1988; Richards, Pennebaker, & Beall, 1995). Using psychophysiological recording instruments, Pennebaker, Hughes, and O'Heeron (1987) found a toughness pattern of activation during disclosure: cardiovascular arousal increased during disclosure but afterward decreased below baseline levels. In accordance with the emotional suppression findings of Gross and Levenson (1993), Pennebaker and Susman (1988) suggest that inhibiting negative emotion actually results in greater physiological arousal,

whereas emotional expression temporarily increases arousal but then produces a long-term decrease. In fact, other researchers have found that expressing anger can actually hasten autonomic recovery from anger-associ-
ated SAM arousal (Hokanson & Burgess, 1962a, 1962b; Hokanson,
Burgess, & Cohen, 1963; Huber, Hauke, & Gramer, 1988).

Admittedly, the number of studies supporting the health benefits of
psychological toughness is small, some are in nonhumans, and most were
not conducted with the psychological toughness model specifically in mind.
Furthermore, the evidence supporting the premise that emotion-associated
SAM activation is good for health mostly examines immune function and
immune-related illnesses. Whether there is some healthy level of anger/fear-
associated arousal in terms of cardiovascular, pulmonary, and other health
is unknown. Still, this research indicates that periodic fear and anger, and
the associated SAM arousal, can be health promoting within the realm of
immune-related disease.

A Model

At this point, the reader may feel that the relationship between emotion
and health forms a rather muddy picture. Figure 12.1 outlines a model of
emotion and health whose components are correlated but nonlinear. In the
center of the diagram is emotion, a system that emerges when physiology,
cognition, and behavior synchronize around a precipitating event. As a system, each of its components has an effect on the other: cognition can up- or
down-regulate physiological arousal and behavior; behavior can up- or
down-regulate cognition and physiological arousal; and so on.

Emotion-associated physiological arousal manifests directly in many
of the body's individual systems (cardiovascular, gastrointestinal, etc.).
However, emotion also organizes function *between* systems. In other
words, sympathetic activation increases heart rate *and* opens the airways of
the lungs *and* increases blood glucose, etc. Therefore, emotion-associated
physiological arousal is likely to have global effects on health by influencing multiple interacting organ systems, though its health-promoting/
disease-promoting impact may not be equivalent across these systems.

Emotion-motivated behavior influences health through its effects on
physiological systems. As with physiology, behavior also forms systems.
For example, someone who drinks to down-regulate fear may also avoid
the doctor when he/she notices an irregular mole on his/her skin and may
be nonadherent with medications to avoid thinking about illness. Therefore, behavior influences multiple physiological and behavioral systems at
various levels. Finally, cognition affects health through its impact on behavior, or by up- or down-regulating emotion-associated physiological arousal.
Here, too, individual cognitions are important, but emotion influences

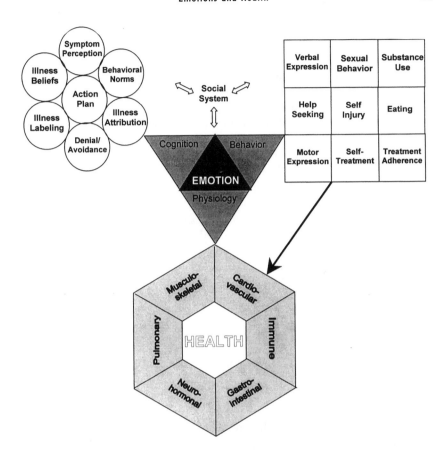

FIGURE 12.1. A dynamic model of emotion and health.

many health-relevant cognitions, often in a congruent direction. Thus, depression increases symptom perception, as well as illness attribution, illness beliefs, and so on.

  Whereas previous models of emotion and health have tended to be linear (e.g., health beliefs and reasoned action), or recursive only in part (dual process), this model suggests that emotion influences its component systems simultaneously and reciprocally. Anxiety initiates a cascade of cognitions, SAM activation, and behaviors. Central nervous system (CNS) norepinephrine increases, augmenting alertness resulting in increased symptom perception, which itself feeds back into anxiety. Simultaneously, a number of cognitions regarding illness are primed, and behaviors to escape and seek help are motivated. These thoughts and behaviors interact, and feed back on anxiety, and the relationships between components of the emotion/health system are strengthened. Over time, up- or down-regulation will occur: Health care seeking and treatment will diminish symptoms and physiological damage, illness cognitions will be quieted, and the connections between components of this system will dissipate. Alternately, an individual will attempt to down-regulate anxiety by trying not to think about the symptom. Anxiety is likely to become more chronic and to spread to other systems.

Inasmuch as emotion is the synchrony of cognition, behavior, and physiological arousal, and health is the interaction of multiple organ systems, is it possible to say how much of an emotion is good for health? The answer to this question comes in two parts: The relationships between emotion-associated cognition/behavior/physiology and physical functioning can be examined on a population level, and probably form reliable probability distributions that can be represented graphically. However, there will also be individual differences that reliably predict variance within these population distributions. The following subsections explore these two concepts in detail.

Population Norms

As humans, we have a predisposition to organizing stimuli into consistent patterns, whether or not such patterns actually exist (see Nisbett & Ross, 1980, for a discussion). When it comes to understanding the relationship between emotion and health, those impulses must be resisted. Figure 12.2 presents a hypothetical model for the relationship between fear and health. This figure includes three components of fear: arousal (SAM), health-relevant cognitions, and health behaviors. Each graph in Figure 12.2 depicts increasing emotion (and thus increasing arousal, cognition, and behavior) from left to right. For simplicity's sake, we will assume that increasing emotion implies greater frequency, duration and intensity.

In the top graph of Figure 12.2, emotion-associated SAM arousal activates the immune system, so that moderate-to-high levels of arousal have a positive impact on immune function and health. At extremely high levels, the arousal reduces immunocompetence and health. For cardiovascular function, the pattern is different. Low and moderately low levels of fear-associated SAM arousal are good for cardiovascular function and health, but moderate-to-high levels are damaging. The gastrointestinal system shows yet another pattern: Low-to-moderate levels of emotion arousal are neutral in terms of gastrointestinal health, and only at high levels does arousal begin to damage the gastrointestinal system. So, what level of fear-associated SAM arousal is best for health? It differs by organ system, and the optimal level overall is suboptimal for immune function (too low),

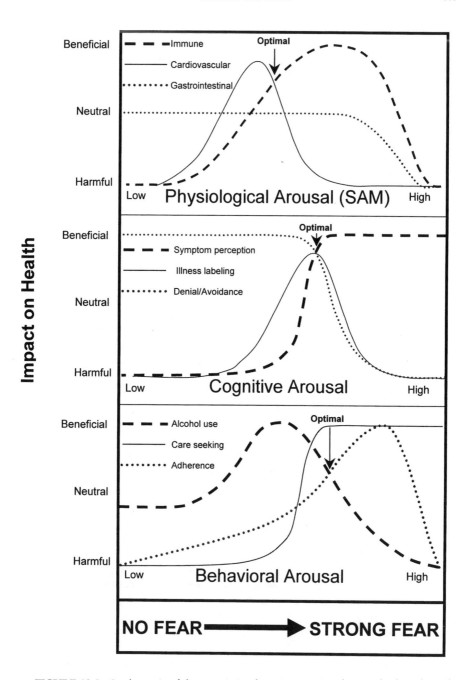

FIGURE 12.2. A schematic of the association between emotional arousal (physiological, cognitive, and behavioral) and health.

suboptimal for cardiovascular function (too high), and just right for gastro-intestinal (where optimal is defined as having a neutral effect on the system). There is no reason to force a consistent pattern on these relationships, no reason why these curves should be normal, and no reason to assume that one level of arousal is optimal for all systems.

In the middle graph of Figure 12.2, a different pattern of relationships emerges. Symptom perception is highest and most healthful at the highest levels of fear. The positive effects of illness attribution on health peak at moderate-to-high levels of fear but then decrease at extreme levels. Avoidance is lowest (and healthiest) at low levels of fear but becomes unhealthy only at high levels. In this case, the optimal level of fear-associated cognitions nearly coincides for these three cognitions. But the optimal level of health cognitions occurs at a higher level of fear than the optimal level for physiological arousal. Once again, there is no reason to assume that optimal levels will coincide across the physiological and cognitive systems.

In the bottom graph of Figure 12.2, we see yet another pattern. Fear is associated with increased alcohol consumption. This is beneficial to health at moderate levels but becomes damaging at higher levels (ignoring, for the time being, that the impact of alcohol on different organ systems may differ at different levels). However, when it comes to health care seeking, more fear is better. And finally, for adherence, fear is most beneficial at moderately high levels but decreases at very high levels. This point corresponds with the level at which fear induces denial that is unhealthy shown in the middle graph of Figure 12.2 (presumably because the denial begins to have negative effects on several health behaviors). Thus, the optimal level of fear for health behaviors is higher than for physiological arousal or cognition. At the same time, the relationship between fear, health behaviors, and health depend to some degree on fear-associated cognitions and arousal.

Looking across emotions produces an even more complex picture. The relationships between distress-related physiological arousal (HPAC) and individual organ systems are likely to be quite different than they are for fear. Furthermore, fear and distress are not orthogonal but to some degree may potentiate each other, producing an emotional mix. Moreover, in this example we have looked at emotional arousal monolithically—it is quite possible that intensity, duration, and frequency are only loosely related. One individual may experience intense fear, but the episodes are short and infrequent. There is no reason to believe that this pattern of responding will produce the same results as those of someone who has ongoing low-level fear, despite the fact that these may somehow average to an equal level of fear over time.

How, then, do we define "healthy fear"? The first step may be to move beyond defining fear unidimensionally. Perhaps we need to deconstruct emotion and measure emotion-associated cognition, behavior, and physiological arousal on separate channels, examining their impact on specific organ systems separately. Alternatively, we could move to a dynamic model, where fear is measured by the strength of the correlation between behavior, physiology, and cognition. Another path would be to measure *patterns* of fear. Nonlinear dynamic theory suggests that there are not an infinite number of patterns by which systems organize themselves (Nicolis & Prigogine, 1989). Storms organize by forming cyclonic eddies. Thunderstorms organize into distinct cells. There may be relatively few patterns, or fear phenotypes, whose impact on health over time is consistent.

All of these suggestions entail examining emotion and health on an aggregate, population level. An alternative model, recently proposed by Howard Leventhal (1999), suggests taking an individual differences approach: "Every affect is responsive to a broad range of events and will have different effects on health and behavior as a function of situational context" (p. 7). The following subsection briefly explores individual differences in the relationship between emotion and health.

Individual Differences

Though there may be population norms defining the relationship between aspects of emotion and aspects of health, within that range individual differences play a defining role. Perhaps the first and most important individual difference is physical pathology. For individuals with advanced cardiovascular disease, a single intense episode of anger can produce myocardial infarct and result in death. As posited in the *stress–diathesis model,* underlying physiological vulnerabilities could make someone susceptible to emotion-associated illness at significantly lower levels. In the same vein, underlying strengths and hardiness could protect some individuals from health-damaging aspects of emotion. Thus, on a physiological level, there exist individual levels of affect tolerance, particular to specific emotions and specific organ systems.

As discussed previously, affect tolerance also exists in terms of an individual's ability to comfortably experience and express specific emotions, and likely extends to social networks. Emotions are "contagious" and spread within social systems, impacting those around us (Hatfield, Cacioppo, & Rapson, 1994). Regardless of our own comfort with an emotion, if the affect tolerance of those around us is low, there may well be negative consequences for experiencing and/or expressing an emotion. For example, moderate distress normally elicits help from close others. And there is a large literature indicating that social support is generally health promoting (Cohen & Wills, 1985; Uchino, Cacioppo, & Kiecolt-Glaser, 1996), though there are circumstances under which social support is not helpful (see Dakof & Taylor, 1990). But if those around us are intolerant of distress, then expression of this emotion is unlikely to elicit support and may even cause distance from close others. Therefore, regardless of the relationship between emotion and health in an individual, the greater social context must be taken into consideration in understanding how much of an emotion is optimal.

Finally, Leventhal (1999) has suggested that context is crucial for understanding the relationship between emotion and health: "Depressed mood in older women is a sign of involvement with older, ill husbands. Thus, older women are depressed and live longer. Depressed mood in older men is more tied to their somatic status, that is, whether or not they are ill. In each of these contexts depression should and will predict different health outcomes" (p. 7). Does the meaning of an emotion and its relationship to health become so context bound and individualized that it is impossible to establish meaningful relationships between these variables on a broader, population level? The answers are, it would seem, both yes and no.

It is possible that for the women in the previous example depression may have positive effects on self-relevant health cognitions and may serve to elicit support from others. For the men, there may well be an underlying pathology that depression exacerbates, which outweighs any other cognitive and behavioral benefit the emotion might provide. Thus, at similar levels, depression may lead to very different outcomes in these men and women, but the difference in outcomes can be explained using the parameters (cognitive, behavioral, physiological, and affect tolerance) discussed in this chapter. On the other hand, there are likely to be cohort effects both in terms of underlying physiology and individual/network affect tolerance that redefine the range of healthy emotional functioning in several parameters. Understanding what variables alter the relationship between components of emotion and components of health, and whether these changes can be predictably quantified, is a job for future emotion and health researchers.

THE FUTURE OF EMOTION AND HEALTH RESEARCH

Each chapter of this volume ends with a discussion of the future of emotion research in each of the areas covered. There are several key areas that can and will help increase our understanding of the complex relationships between complex variables. These include modeling emotion, positive emotion, emotion regulation, and individual differences.

Modeling Emotion

In order to model the relationship between emotion and health, there need to be more sophisticated theoretical and mathematical models of emotion itself. As pointed out by Ekman (1997) and Feldman Barrett (1998), emotion researchers often measure emotion on a single channel (physiological arousal, self-report, facial affect, etc). But emotions are systems and, as proposed by Levenson (1994), "The essential function of emotion is organization" (p. 123). A hurricane is not simply barometric pressure and humidity and wind—it is the organization of several meteorological components that together, in concert, form a weather system. So, emotion is not physiological arousal or cognition or behavior but is the coordination of these systems in response to a precipitating event. To advance the field of emotion and health, we need first to refine our understanding and measure of each of these systems. This, then, allows us the option of examining fear as a single entity, as a pattern, or deconstructing it into component parts.

In addition, there is far more attention paid to pathologically high emotion and the way it can damage health than to either normal or low levels of emotion. Indeed, the most studied models of emotion and health are essentially disease models. As we move forward, it may be possible to extend our models so that they cover the full spectrum of emotional experience and not focus as much on the 10th and 90th percentiles.

Positive Emotions

In general, much more is known about negative emotions than about positive emotions. Even our nomenclature for positive emotions is stunted when compared to negative emotions, as is our understanding of the physiology of positive affect. It is no surprise, then, that less is known about positive emotions and health. As proposed in the previous paragraph, we need a significantly clearer understanding of positive emotions as a construct in order to understand how it relates to health. As proposed by Frederickson and Branigan in Chapter 4, this volume, positive emotions may have a different purpose, organization, and time course than negative emotions and may affect health in different ways. As much as this chapter looked to address the misstatement that "negative emotions are bad for you," we also need to reexamine the premise that "positive emotions are good for you." With antidepressant and anxiolytic medications leading the nation in pharmacological sales, it would behoove us to understand the health ramifications of tipping the scales in favor of positive affect on a national scale.

Regulation

A significant portion of this chapter has dealt with emotion regulation—how regulating emotions up and down may affect health, and how regulating health can influence emotion. The emotion regulation literature, however, overwhelmingly focuses on *down*-regulating negative emotions. There are far less theory and far fewer data on how one would up-regulate a negative emotion like fear or anger, or techniques for inducing these emotions when they are overregulated or underexperienced. Conversely, there is a large literature for up-regulating positive emotions—everything from relaxation techniques to pharmacological treatment. Outside of the use of lithium carbonate to lessen the mood swings of manic depression, however, there is little consideration given to how one might down-regulate positive affect and the ramifications of doing so. As we better understand what the optimal levels of different affects are for health, we will need to better conceptualize and influence emotion regulation, and one day even propose a "recommended daily allowance" of love, fear, and disgust,

Individual Differences

There are clearly individual differences that affect the relationship between emotions and health. It is important to understand which variables do so systematically, and the direction in which they reliably influence those relationships. As indicated by Leventhal (1999), age, gender, and marital status are likely to be important variables that systematically affect both emotion and health. Other variables like socioeconomic status, education, and culture are likely to play significant roles. Exploring their impact on health in the context of a sophisticated model of affect is likely to only add to our overall understanding of health.

ACKNOWLEDGMENTS

I would like to thank Drs. Timothy Ambrose and David Vlahov for their helpful feedback and thoughts on the components and organization of this chapter.

NOTE

1. Though the theory has not yet been extended, one can imagine that this "undoing" strategy may be used to regulate emotions more generally. For example, individuals may up-regulate anger in an attempt to down-regulate depression or anxiety.

REFERENCES

Ader, R. (1970). The effects of early experience on adrenocortical response to different magnitudes of stimulation. *Physiology and Behavior, 5*, 837–839.
Amkraut, C., & Solomon, C. F. (1972). Stress and murine sarcoma virus (Maloney)-induced tumors. *Cancer Research, 32*, 1428–1433.

Arnold, M. B. (1970). Perennial problems in the field of emotion. In M. B. Arnold (Ed.), *Feelings and emotions*. New York: Academic Press.

Arnow, B., Kenardy, J., & Agras W. S. (1995). The Emotional Eating Scale: The development of a measure to assess coping with negative affect by eating. *International Journal of Eating Disorders, 18*, 79–90.

Ashby, F. G., Isen, A. M., & Turken, A. U. (1999). A neuropsychological theory of positive affect and its influence on cognition. *Psychological Review, 106*, 529–550.

Asnis, G. M., Halbreich, U., Ryan, N. D., Rabinowicz, H., Puig-Antich, J., Nelson, B., Novacenko, H., & Harkavy-Friedman, J. (1987). The relationship of the dexamethasone suppression test to basal plasma cortisol levels in endogenous depression. *Psychoneuroendocrinology, 12*, 295–301.

Barlow, D. H. (1988). *Anxiety and its disorders: The nature and treatment of anxiety and panic*. New York: Guilford Press.

Barlow, D. M., Sakhaira, D. K., & Beck, J. G. (1983). Anxiety increases sexual arousal. *Journal of Abnormal Psychology, 92*, 49–54.

Barsky, A. J., Cleary, P. D., Barnett, M. C., Christiansen, C. L., & Ruskin, J. N. (1994). The accuracy of symptom report by patients complaining of palpitations. *American Journal of Medicine, 97*, 214–221.

Barsky, A. J., Cleary, P. D., Brener, J., & Ruskin, J. N. (1993). The perception of cardiac activity in medical outpatients. *Cardiology, 83*, 304–315.

Beck, A. T., Rush, A. J., Shaw, B. F., & Emery, G. (1979). *Cognitive therapy of depression*. New York: Guilford Press.

Betrus, P. A., Elmore, S. K., & Hamilton, P. A. (1995). Women and somatization: Unrecognized depression. *Health Care for Women International, 16*, 287–297.

Bolger, N., & Schilling, E. A. (1991). Personality and the problems of everyday life: The role of neuroticism in exposure and reactivity to daily stressors. *Journal of Personality, 59*, 355–386.

Boulet, L. P., Turcotte, H., & Brochu, A. (1994). Persistence of airway obstruction and hyperresponsiveness in subjects with asthma remission. *Chest, 105*, 1024–1031.

Bower, G. H. (1981). Mood and memory. *American Psychologist, 36*, 129–148.

Boyce, T. W., Chesney, M., Alkon, A., Tschann, J. M., Adams, S., Chesterman, B., Cohen, F., Kaiser, P., Folkman, S., & Wara, D. (1995). Psychobiologic reactivity to stress and childhood respiratory illnesses: Results of two prospective studies. *Psychosomatic Medicine, 57*, 411–422.

Buunk, B. P., & Bakkov, A. B. (1997). Commit to the relationship, extradyadic sex and AIDS preventative behavior. *Journal of Applied Social Psychology, 27*, 1241–1257.

Bybee, J., Leckman, J. F., Mersica, R., & Miller, P. (1997, April). *Guilt and depression: Relationships to diabetic adherence and metabolic control in two high-risk samples*. Paper presented at the annual meeting of the Eastern Psychological Association, Washington, DC.

Callahan, C. M., Hui, S. L., Nienaber, N. A., & Musick, B. S. (1994). Longitudinal study of depression and health services use among elderly primary care patients. *Journal of the American Geriatrics Society, 42*, 833–838.

Cannon, W. B. (1911). Emotional stimulation of adrenal gland secretion. *American Journal of Physiology, 28*, 64–70.

Carney, R. M., Freedland, K. E., Eisen, S. A., Rich, M. W., & Jaffe, A. S. (1995). Major depression and medication adherence in elderly patients with coronary artery disease. *Health Psychology, 14*, 88–90.

Carney, R. M., Freedland, K. E., Rich, M. W., & Jaffe, A. S. (1995). Depression as a risk factor for cardiac events in established coronary heart disease: A review of possible mechanisms. *Annals of Behavioral Medicine, 17*, 142–149.

Christensen, A. J., & Smith, T. W. (1993). Cynical hostility and cardiovascular reactivity during self-disclosure. *Psychosomatic Medicine, 55*, 193–202.

Clark, M. S., Ouelette, R., Powell, M. C., & Milberg, S. (1987). Recipient's mood, relationship type, and helping. *Journal of Personality and Social Psychology, 53*, 94–103.

Cohen, S., Doyle, W., Skoner, D. P., Fireman, P., Gwaltney, J. M. Jr., & Newsom, J. T. (1995). State and trait negative affect as predictors of objective and subjective symptoms of respiratory viral infections. *Journal of Personality and Social Psychology, 68*, 159–169.

Cohen, S., & Wills, T. A. (1985). Stress, social support, and the buffering hypothesis. *Psychological Bulletin, 98*, 310–357.

Coleman, E. (1992). Is your patient suffering from compulsive sexual behavior? *Psychiatric Annals, 22*, 320–325.

Cooper, M. L., Frone, M. R., Russell, M., & Mudar, P. (1995). Drinking to regulate positive and negative emotions: A motivational model of alcohol use. *Journal of Personality and Social Psychology, 69*, 990–1005.

Cox, B. J., Norton, G. R., Dorward, J., & Fergusson, P. A. (1989). The relationship between panic attacks and chemical dependencies. *Addictive Behaviors, 14*, 53–60.

Coyne, J. C., & Delongis, A. (1986). Going beyond social support: The role of social relationships in adaptation. *Journal of Consulting and Clinical Psychology, 54*, 454–460.

Dakof, G. A., & Taylor, S. E. (1990). Victims' perceptions of social support: What is helpful from whom? *Journal of Personality and Social Psychology, 58*, 80–89.

Dielman, T. E., Leech, S. L., Miller, M. V., & Moss, G. E. (1991). Sex and age interactions with the structured interview global Type A behavior pattern and hostility in the prediction of health behaviors. *Multivariate Experimental Clinical Research, 10*, 67–83.

Dienstbier, R. A. (1989). Arousal and physiological toughness: Implications for mental and physical health. *Psychological Review, 96*, 84–100.

Dienstbier, R. A. (1991). Behavioral correlates of sympathoadrenal reactivity: The toughness model. *Medicine and Science in Sports and Exercise, 23*, 846–852.

Ekman, P. (1992). An argument for basic emotions. *Cognition and Emotion, 6*, 169–200.

Ekman, P. (1997). The future of emotion research. *Affect Scientist, 11*, 4–5.

Ekman, P., Levenson, R. W., & Friesen, W. V. (1983). Autonomic nervous system activity distinguishes among emotions. *Science, 221*, 1208–1210.

Ellertsen, C., Johnsen, T. B., & Ursin, H. (1978). Relationship between the hormonal responses to activation and coping. In H. Ursin, E. Baade, & S. Levine (Eds.), *Psychobiology of stress: A study of coping in men* (pp. 105–121). New York: Academic Press.

Esterling, B. A., Antoni, M. H., Fletcher, M. A., Margulies, S., & Schneiderman, N. (1994). Emotional disclosure through writing or speaking modulates latent Epstein–Barr virus antibody titers. *Journal of Consulting and Clinical Psychology, 62*, 130–140.

Feldman Barrett, L. (1998). The future of emotion research. *Affect Scientist, 12,* 4–7.

Festinger, L. (1957). *A theory of cognitive dissonance.* Evanston, IL: Row, Peterson.

Faber, S. D., & Burns, J. W. (1996). Anger management style, degree of expressed anger, and gender influence cardiovascular recovery from interpersonal harassment. *Journal of Behavioral Medicine, 19,* 35–53.

Fishbein, M., & Ajzen, F. (1975). *Belief, attitude and behavior: An introduction to theory and research.* Reading, MA: Addison-Wesley.

Folkman, S., & Lazarus, R. S. (1980). An analysis of coping in a middle-aged community sample. *Journal of Health and Social Behavior, 21,* 219–239.

Frankenhaeuser, M. (1980). Psychoneuroendocrine approaches to the study of stressful person-environment transactions. In H. Selye (Ed.), *Selye's guide to stress research* (Vol. 1, pp. 46–70). New York: Van Nostrand.

Fredrickson, B. L., & Levenson, R. W. (1998). Positive emotions speed recovery from the cardiovascular sequelae of negative emotions. *Cognition and Emotion, 12,* 191–220.

Fride, E., Hilaviki, L. A., & Arora, P. K. (1990). Neonatal handling affects immune function and behavior in Porsolt's swim test. *Society for Neuroscience Abstracts, 20,* 494.13.

Green, S. M. (1997). Obesity: Prevalence, causes, health risks and treatment. *British Journal of Nursing, 6,* 1181–1185.

Greer, S., Morris, T., & Pettingale, K. W. (1979). Psychological responses to breast cancer. *Lancet, 13,* 785–787.

Groop, L. C., & Tuomi, T. (1997). Non-insulin-dependent diabetes mellitus: A collision between thrifty genes and an affluent society. *Annals of Medicine, 29,* 37–53.

Gross, J. J., & Levenson, R. W. (1993). Emotional suppression: Physiology, self-report, and expressive behavior. *Journal of Personality and Social Psychology, 64,* 970–986.

Hall, S. M., Muñoz, R. F., Reus, V. I., & Sees, K. L. (1993). Nicotine, negative affect, and depression. *Journal of Consulting and Clinical Psychology, 61,* 761–767.

Hatfield, E., Cacioppo, J. T., & Rapson, R. L. (1994). *Emotional contagion.* New York: Cambridge University Press.

Hellstrand, K., Hermodsson, S., & Strannegard, O. (1985). Evidence for an adrenergic–adrenoreceptor–mediator regulation of human NK cells. *Journal of Immunology, 134,* 4095–4099.

Higbee, K. L. (1969). Fifteen years of fear arousal: Research on threat appeals, 1953–1968. *Psychological Bulletin, 72,* 426–444.

Hilaviki-Clark, L., Rowland, J., Clark, R., & Lipman, M. E. (1993). Psychosocial factors in the development and progression of breast cancer. *Breast Cancer Research and Treatment, 29,* 141–160.

Hitsman, B., Pingitore, R., Spring, B., Mahableshwarkar, A., Mizes, J. S., Segraves, K. A., Kristeller, J. L., & Xu, W. (1999). Antidepressant pharmacotherapy helps some cigarette smokers more than others. *Journal of Consulting and Clinical Psychology, 67,* 547–554.

Hoffman, M. L. (1978). Psychological and biological perspectives on altruism. *International Journal of Behavioral Development, 1*, 323–339.

Hokanson, J., & Burgess, M. (1962a). The effects of three types of aggression on vascular processes. *Journal of Abnormal Social Psychology, 64*, 446–449.

Hokanson, J., & Burgess, M. (1962b). The effect of status, type of frustration, and aggression on vascular processes. *Journal of Abnormal Social Psychology, 65*, 232–237.

Hokansen, J., Burgess, M., & Cohen, M. (1963). The effects of displaced aggression on systolic blood pressure. *Journal of Abnormal Social Psychology, 67*, 214–218.

Houston, B. K., & Vavak, C. R. (1991). Cynical hostility: Developmental factors, psychosocial correlates, and health behaviors. *Health Psychology, 10*, 9–17.

Huber, H. P., Hauke, D., & Gramer, M. (1988). Frustration-related elevation in blood pressure and its reduction via aggressive reactions. *Zeitschrift für Experimentelle und Angewandte Psychologie, 35*, 427–440.

Janis, I. L. (1967). Effects of fear arousal on attitude change: Recent developments in theory and experimental research. *Advances in Experimental Social Psychology, 3*, 166–225.

Jenkins, C. D. (1971a). Psychologic and social precursors of coronary disease. *New England Journal of Medicine, 284*, 244–255.

Jenkins, C. D. (1971b). Psychologic and social precursors of coronary disease. *New England Journal of Medicine, 284*, 307–317.

Johansson, G., & Frankenhaeuser, M. (1973). Temporal factors in sympatho-adrenomedullary activity following acute behavioral activation. *Biological Psychology, 1*, 63–73.

Johansson, G., Frankenhaeuser, M., & Magnusson, D. (1973). Catecholamine output in school children as related to performance and adjustment. *Scandinavian Journal of Psychology, 14*, 20–28.

Jung, A. C., Staiger, T., & Sullivan, M. (1997). The efficacy of selective serotonin reuptake inhibitors for the management of chronic pain. *Journal of General Internal Medicine, 12*, 384–399.

Kalichman, S. C., Johnson, J. R., Adair, V., Rompa, D., Multhauf, K., & Kelly, J. A. (1994). Sexual sensation seeking: Scale development and predicting AIDS-risk behavior among homosexually active men. *Journal of Personality Assessment, 62*, 385–397.

Karlsson, H., Lehtinen, V., & Joukamaa, M. (1995). Psychiatric morbidity among frequent attender patients in primary care. *General Hospital Psychiatry, 17*, 19–25.

Kelly, J. A., Murphy, D. A., Bahr, G. R., Koob, J. J., Morgan, M. G., Kalichman, S. C., Stevenson, L. Y., Brasfield, T. L., Bernstein, B. M., & St. Lawrence, J. S. (1993). Factors associated with severity of depression and high-risk sexual behavior among persons diagnosed with human immunodeficiency virus (HIV) infection. *Health Psychology, 12*, 215–219.

Kiecolt-Glaser, J. K., & Glaser, R. (1999). Psychoneuroimmunology and cancer: Fact or fiction? *European Journal of Cancer, 35*, 1603–1607.

King, A. C., Taylor, C. B., Albright, C. A., & Haskell, W. L. (1990). The relationship between repressive and defensive coping styles and blood pressure responses in healthy, middle-aged men and women. *Journal of Psychosomatic Research, 34,* 461–471.

Kirschbaum, C., Prussner, J. C., Stone, A. A., Federenko, I., Gaab, J., Lintz, D., Schommer, N., & Heilhammer, D. H. (1995). Persistent high cortisol responses to repeated psychological stress in a subpopulation of healthy men. *Psychosomatic Medicine, 57,* 468–474.

Knutson, B., Wolkowitz, O. M., Cole, S. W., Chan, T., Moore, E. A., Johnson, R. C., Terpstra, J., Turner, R. A., & Reus, V. I. (1998). Selective alteration of personality and social behavior by serotonergic intervention. *American Journal of Psychiatry, 155,* 373–379.

Lazarus, R. S., & Folkman, S. (1984). *Stress, appraisal, and coping.* New York: Springer.

LeDoux, J. (1998). *The emotional brain.* New York. Simon & Schuster.

Lehrer, P. M., Isenberg, S., & Hochron, S. M. (1993). Asthma and emotion: A review. *Journal of Asthma, 30,* 5–21.

Levenson, R. W. (1994). Human emotion: A functional view. In P. Ekman & R. J. Davidson (Eds.), *The nature of emotions* (pp. 123–126). New York: Oxford University Press.

Leventhal, H. (1970). Findings and theory in the study of health communications. *Advances in Experimental Social Psychology, 5,* 119–186.

Leventhal, H. (1999). The future of emotion research. *Emotion Researcher, 13,* 4–7.

Leventhal, H., Safer, M. A., & Panagis, D. M. (1983). The impact of communications on the self-regulation of health beliefs, decisions, and behavior. *Health Education Quarterly, 10,* 3–29.

Lewinsohn, P. M., Mischel, W., Chaplin, W., & Barton, R. (1980). Social competence and depression: The role of illusiory self-perceptions. *Journal of Abnormal Psychology, 89,* 203–212.

Lutz, C. A., & White, G. (1986). The anthropology of emotion. *Annual Review of Anthropology, 15,* 405–436.

Manuck, S. B., Marsland, A. L., Kaplan, J. R., & Williams, J. K. (1995). The pathogenicity of behavior and its neuroendocrine mediation: An example from coronary artery disease. *Psychosomatic Medicine, 57,* 275–283.

Mayne, T. J. (2000). Negative affect and health: The importance of being earnest. *Cognition and Emotion, 13,* 601–635.

Mayne, T. J., & Buck, R. W. (1997). Sex, emotion, and the triune brain. *Health Psychologist, 19,* 8–23.

Mayne, T. J., O'Leary, A., McCrady, B., Contrada, R., & Labouvie, E. (1997). The differential effects of acute marital distress on emotional, physiological, and immune functions in maritally distressed men and women. *Psychology and Health, 12,* 1–12.

Mayne, T. J., Vittinghoff, E., Chesney, M., Barrett, D., & Coates, T. (1996). Depressive affect and survival among gay and bisexual men infected with the human immunodeficiency virus. *Archives of Internal Medicine, 156,* 2233–2238.

McKenna, M. C., Zevon, M. A., Corn, B., & Rounds, J. (1999). Psychosocial factors and the development of breast cancer: A meta-analysis. *Health Psychology, 18,* 520–531.

McKinlay, J. B., & McKinlay, S. M. (1986). Medical measures and the decline of mortality. In P. Conrad & R. Kern (Eds.), *The sociology of health and illness: Critical perspectives*. (2nd ed., pp. 10–23). New York: St. Martin's Press.

Melamed, S., Kushnir, T., Strauss, E., & Vigiser, D. (1997). Negative association between reported life events and cardiovascular disease risk factors in employed men: The CORDIS Study—Cardiovascular Occupational Risk Factors Determination in Israel. *Journal of Psychosomatic Research, 43,* 247–258.

Merikangas, K. R., & Angst, J. (1995). Comorbidity and social phobia: Evidence from clinical, epidemiologic, and genetic studies. *European Archives of Psychiatry and Clinical Neuroscience, 244,* 197–303.

Mills, P. J., Berry, C. C., Dimsdale, J. E., Nelesen, R. A., & Ziegler, M. G. (1993). Temporal stability of task-induced cardiovascular, adrenergic, and psychological responses: The effects of race and hypertension. *Psychophysiology, 30,* 197–204.

Morgan, M. J., & Franklin, K. B. (1991). Dopamine receptor subtypes and formalin test analgesia. *Pharmacology, Biochemistry and Behavior, 40,* 317–22.

Newton, T. L., & Contrada, R. J. (1992). Repressive coping and verbal–autonomic response dissociation: The influence of social context. *Journal of Personality and Social Psychology, 62,* 159–167.

Nicolis, G., & Prigogine, I. (1989). *Exploring complexity.* New York: Freeman.

Nieburgs, H. E., Weiss, J., Navarrette, M., Strax, P., Teirstein, A., Grillme, G., & Siedlecki, B. (1979). The role of stress in human and experimental oncogenesis. *Cancer Detection and Prevention, 2,* 307–336.

Nisbett, R., & Ross, L. (1980). *Human inference: Strategies and shortcomings of social judgment.* Englewood Cliffs, NJ: Prentice-Hall.

Obrist, P. A. (1981). *Cardiovascular psychophysiology: A perspective.* New York: Plenum Press.

O'Leary, A., Temoshok, L., Sweet, D. M., & Jenkins, S. (1989). Autonomic reactivity and immune function in men with AIDS. *Psychophysiology, 26,* S47.

Paalzow, G. H. (1992). L-Dopa induces opposing effects on pain in intact rats: (−)-Sulpiride, SCH 23390 or alpha-methyl-DL-*p*-tyrosine methylester hydrochloride, reveals profound hyperalgesia in large antinociceptive doses. *Journal of Pharmacology and Experimental Therapeutics, 263,* 470–479.

Panksepp, J. (1988). Brain emotional circuits and psychopathology. In M. Clynes & J. Panksepp (Eds.), *Emotions and psychopathology* (pp. 37–76). New York: Plenum Press.

Pennebaker, J. W. (1982). *The psychology of physical symptoms.* New York: Springer-Verlag.

Pennebaker, J. W., Colder, M., & Sharp, L. K. (1990). Accelerating the coping process. *Journal of Personality and Social Psychology, 58,* 528–537.

Pennebaker, J. W., Hughes, C. F., & O'Heeron, R. C. (1987). The psychophysiology of confession: Linking inhibitory and psychosomatic processes. *Journal of Personality and Social Psychology, 52,* 781–793.

Pennebaker, J. W., Kiecolt-Glaser, J. K., & Glaser, R. (1988). Disclosure of traumas and immune function: Health implications for psychotherapy. *Journal of Consulting and Clinical Psychology, 56,* 239–245.

Pennebaker, J. W., & Susman, J. R. (1988). Disclosure of traumas and psychosomatic processes [Special issue: Stress and coping in relation to health and disease]. *Social Science and Medicine, 26,* 322–332.

Penninx, B. W., Guralnik, J. M., Pahor, M., Ferrucci, L., Cerhan, J. R., Wallace, R. B., & Havlik, R. J. (1998). Chronically depressed mood and cancer risk in older persons. *Journal of the National Cancer Institute, 90,* 1888–1893.

Petrie, K. J., Booth, R. J., & Pennebaker, J. W. (1998). The immunological effects of thought suppression. *Journal of Personality and Social Psychology, 75,* 1264–1272.

Petrie, K. J., Booth, R. J., Pennebaker, J. W., Davison, K. P., & Thomas, M. G. (1995). Disclosure of trauma and immune response to a hepatitis B vaccination program. *Journal of Consulting and Clinical Psychology, 63,* 787–792.

Rauste–von Wright, M., von Wright, J., & Frankenhaeuser, M. (1981). Relationships between sex-related psychological characteristics during adolescence and catecholamine excretion during achievement stress. *Psychophysiology, 18,* 362–370.

Richards, J. M., Pennebaker, J. W., & Beall, W. E. (1995, April). *The effects of criminal offense and disclosure of trauma on anxiety and illness in prison inmates.* Paper presented at the annual meeting of the Midwest Psychological Association, Chicago.

Rietveld, S., Prins, P. J., & Kolk, A. M. (1996). The capability of children with and without asthma to detect external resistive loads on breathing. *Journal of Asthma, 33,* 221–230.

Rosenstock, I. M. (1974). Historical origins of the health beliefs model. *Health Education Monographs, 2,* 328–335.

Safer, M. A., Thamps, Q. J., Jackson, T. C., & Leventhal, H. (1979). Determinants of three stages of delay in seeking care at a medical clinic. *Medical Care, 17,* 11–29.

Salovey, P. (1992). Mood-induced self-focused attention. *Journal of Personality and Social Psychology, 62,* 699–707.

Salovey, P., & Birnbaum, D. (1989). Influence of mood on health-relevant cognitions. *Journal of Personality and Social Psychology, 57,* 539–551.

Schandry, R., Leopold, C., & Vogt, M. (1996). Symptom reporting in asthma patients and insulin-dependent diabetics. *Biological Psychology, 42,* 231–244.

Scourfield, J., Stevens, D. E., & Merikangas, K. R. (1996). Substance abuse, comorbidity, and sensation seeking: Gender differences. *Comprehensive Psychiatry, 37,* 384–892.

Shapiro, D., Goldstein, I. B., & Jamner, L. D. (1996). Effects of cynical hostility, anger out, anxiety, and defensiveness on ambulatory blood pressure in black and white college students. *Psychosomatic Medicine, 58,* 354–364.

Sherbourne, C. D., Hays, R. D., Ordway. L., DiMatteo, M. R., & Kravitz, R. L. (1992). Antecedents of adherence to medical recommendations: Results from the Medical Outcomes Study. *Journal of Behavioral Medicine, 15,* 447–468.

Sklar, L. S., & Anisman, H. (1979). Stress and coping factors influence tumor growth. *Science, 205,* 347–365.

Sklar, L. S., & Anisman, H. (1981). Stress and cancer. *Psychological Bulletin, 89,* 369–406.

Smith, T. W. (1992). Hostility and health: Current status of a psychosomatic hypothesis. *Health Psychology, 11,* 139–150.

Solomon, G. F., Temoshok, L., O'Leary, A., & Zich, J. (1989). An intensive psychoimmunologic study of long-surviving persons with AIDS. *Annals of the New York Academy of Sciences, 496,* 647–655.

Stiff, J. B., Dillard, J. P., Somera, L., Kim, H., & Sleight, C. (1988). Empathy, communication, and prosocial behavior. *Communication Monographs, 55,* 198–213.

Targan, S. M., Britvan, L., & Dorey, F. (1981). Activation of human NKCC by moderate exercise: Increased frequency of NK cells with enhanced capability of effector target lytic interactions. *Clinical and Experimental Immunology, 45,* 352–360.

Taylor, D. N. (1995). Effects of a behavioral stress-management program on anxiety, mood, self-esteem, and T-cell count in HIV-positive men. *Psychological Reports, 76,* 451–457.

Taylor, S. E., & Brown, J. D. (1988). Illusion and well-being: A social psychological perspective on mental health. *Psychological Bulletin, 103,* 193–210.

Tejwani, G. A., Gudehithlu, K. P., Hanissian, S. H., Gienapp, I. E., Whitacre, C. C., & Malarkey, W. B. (1991). Facilitation of dimethylbenz[a]anthracene-induced rat mammary tumorigenesis by restraint stress: Role of -endorphin, prolactin, and naltrexone. *Carcinogenesis, 12,* 637–641.

Temoshok, L., O'Leary, A., & Jenkins, S. R. (1990, June). Survival time in men with AIDS: Relationships with psychological coping and autonomic arousal. *Proceedings of the Sixth International Conference on AIDS,* 435.

Tomkins, S. S. (1963). *Affect, imagery, consciousness: Vol. 2. The negative affects.* New York: Springer.

Tonnesen, E., Christensen, N. J., & Brinklov, M. M. (1987). NK cell activity during cortisol and adrenaline infusion in healthy volunteers. *European Journal of Clinical Investigation, 17,* 497–503.

Tonnessen, E., Tonnessen, J., & Christensen, N. J. (1984). Augmentation of cytotoxicity by natural killer (NK) cells after adrenaline administration in man. *Acta Pathologica Microbiologica Scandanavia, 92,* 81–83.

Tooby, J., & Cosmides, L. (1990). The past explains the present: Emotional adaptations and the structure of ancestral environments. *Ethology and Sociobiology, 11,* 375–424.

Uchino, B. N., Cacioppo, J. T., & Kiecolt-Glaser, J. K. (1996). The relationship between social support and physiological processes: A review with emphasis on underlying mechanisms and implications for health. *Psychological Bulletin, 119,* 488–531.

Ursin, H., Baade, E., & Levine, S. (1978). *Psychobiology of stress: A study of coping in men.* New York: Academic Press.

Watson, M., Haviland, J. S., Greer, S., Davidson, J., & Bliss, J. M. (1999). Influence of psychological response on survival in breast cancer: A population-based cohort study. *Lancet, 354,* 1331–1336.

Weinger, K., Jacobson, A. M., Draelos, M. T., Finkelstein, D. M., & Simonson, D. C. (1995). Blood glucose estimates and symptoms during hyperglycemia and hypoglycemia in patients with insulin-dependent diabetes mellitus. *American Journal of Medicine, 98,* 22–31.

Weinstein, N. D. (1984). Why it won't happen to me: Perceptions of risk factors and susceptibility. *Health Psychology, 3,* 431–457.

Weinstein, N. D. (1987). Unrealistic optimism about susceptibility to health problems: Conclusions from a community-wide sample. *Journal of Behavioral Medicine, 10,* 481–500.

Weinstein, N. D., & Klein, W. M. (1995). Resistance of personal risk perceptions to debiasing interventions. *Health Psychology, 14,* 132–140.

Weiss, J. M., Glazer, H. I., Pohorecky, L. A., Brink, T., & Miller, N. E. (1975). Effects of chronic exposure to stressors on avoidance–escape behavior and on brain norepinephrine. *Psychosomatic Medicine, 37,* 522–534.

Wiedenfeld, S. A., O'Leary, A., Bandura, A., Brown, S., Levine, S., & Raska, K. (1990). Impact of perceived self-efficacy in coping with stressors on components of the immune system. *Journal of Personality and Social Psychology, 59,* 1082–1094.

Wood, J. V., Saltzberg, J. A., & Goldsamt, L. A. (1990). Does affect induce self-focused attention? *Journal of Personality and Social Psychology, 58,* 899–908.

Zuckerman, M., Bone, R. N., Neary, R., Mangelsdorff, D., & Brustman, B. (1972). What is the sensation seeker?: Personality trait and experience correlates of the Sensation-Seeking Scales. *Journal of Consulting and Clinical Psychology, 39,* 308–321.

13

The Future of Emotion Research

GEORGE A. BONANNO
TRACY J. MAYNE

It is tempting at this dawn of a new millennium to prophesize. The modern study of emotion has reached a crucial juncture in its history. The dust has settled on several crucial debates and, although there are still myriad controversies, the study of emotion is now firmly established as a seminal area of inquiry. But just as the study of emotion has ripened, predictably it has also become time for challenges to many existing assumptions and approaches. The chapters in this volume have scrutinized contemporary emotion theory and research and presented a number of new ideas and approaches. In this concluding chapter, we review several common threads woven throughout the chapters and in doing so take a quick glimpse at the future of emotion research.

A BRIEF HISTORY OF RESEARCH AND THEORY ON EMOTION

Speculation about possible new directions in emotion research cannot be fully understood without at least a cursory history of where the field has been. One of the most notable features of the history of emotion is that there are in fact two histories. Initial theorizing about emotion was dominated by the role of the face. Most scholars can now agree that the scientific understanding of emotion was inaugurated in the 19th century with the publication of G. B. Duchenne de Bologne's (1862/1990) *The Mechanism of Human Facial Expression* and Charles Darwin's (1872/1999) *The Expression of the Emotions in Man and Animals*. These works concentrated on the crucial role played by facial displays in the emotional life of humans and animals, and introduced the seminal idea that emotions are best understood as inherited, reflex-like behaviors that had served adaptive functions in our ancestral past.

Although highly influential on contemporary emotion theory and in fact still widely cited, this initial scholarship was soon countered and to a large extent replaced by a second, competing track. Most notably, William James (1890/1981) proposed that our intuitive or "natural way" (p. 449) of understanding emotions was in fact wrong. When we reflect on our emotional life, he argued, we assume that "the mental perception of some fact excites the mental affection called the emotion" (p. 1065) and that this internal state then gives rise to some form of bodily expression or action. To cite the classic examples, we come face to face with a bear in the woods, experience fear, and run. In contrast to this intuitive view, James argued that a more correct sequence leading to emotion is that the perception of an "exciting fact" (p. 1065) or piece of information causes a bodily change which we then perceive and interpret as an emotion. Thus, we are confronted by a bear and we tremble or run, and as a result experience fear. James's theory of emotion, commonly merged in psychology textbooks with a similar view published independently a few years later in Denmark by Carl Lange as the James–Lange theory, rapidly became the dominant psychological theory of emotions.

Although the James–Lange theory has been controversial almost from its inception, it has been a remarkably generative theory. For much of the next century, while little attention was given to the face, the James–Lange approach shaped theory and research on emotion around the role of physiological reactivity. The sequence has been often repeated in introductory psychology courses. The first major critique of the James–Lange theory came from Walter B. Cannon (1932/1960), who argued that sympathetic reactions to arousing stimuli are relatively homogeneous and by themselves would be unable to produce the variety of subjective experiences we call emotions. Extending this line of reasoning, Schacter and Singer (1962) posited a cognitive theory of emotions in which the perception of arousal is shaped by a person's attributions about the situational context. Subsequent evidence, however, has shown that autonomic patterns are not as homogeneous as Cannon had originally believed (see, e.g., Marshall & Zimbardo, 1979). Indeed, there is now compelling evidence for emotion-specific autonomic activity concordant with anger, fear, sadness, and disgust (Ekman, Levenson, & Friesen, 1983). These findings have been replicated in older adults (Levenson, Carstensen, Friesen, & Ekman, 1991) and cross-culturally (Levenson, Ekman, Heider, & Friesen, 1992).

In conjunction with the increasingly sophisticated understanding of the complex relationship between autonomic arousal and the experience of emotion, the past 30 years has witnessed a renewed appreciation of the contributions of Darwin and Duchenne and of the important role of facial displays in emotion. By the midpoint of the 20th century, the expression of emotion in the face had been all but dismissed as a mere expressive by-product of the complex machinery of emotion generation. With the publication of Tomkins's (1962, 1963) two-volume work *Affect, Imagery, Consciousness*, the tide was turned. In contrast to the then-prevailing drive and wish-fulfillment theories of motivation, Tomkins argued for the importance of conscious experience, and for the primary role of emotion in motivating and organizing cognition, decision making, and action. Tomkins also argued that psychological theories had too easily neglected the full range of human behaviors and had paid little attention to positive emotional experiences and expressions. Even more importantly, Tomkins saw facial expression as a central component of the emotion system and initiated some of the first systematic research into the nuances of facial displays as they pertain to a small set of discrete emotions.

If there is a larger aspect of Tomkins's contribution, it is his role as mentor to a subsequent generation of emotion researchers, most notably Paul Ekman and Carroll E. Izard, whose contributions to the development of new methods for coding and cataloging basic human facial expressions of emotion have been highly influential (see, e.g., Ekman, 1993).

In many important ways, the chapters in this volume represent the extension and evolution of the work of these seminal researchers. And in addition to age-old themes (the structure and function of positive affect; the role of emotional in pathology; nature vs. nurture—or, in the current vernacular, genes vs. culture), we add a few timely additions: emotion regulation, and affective neuroscience. We discuss each below.

POSITIVE EMOTION

Perhaps the most exciting topic of study to emerge in recent years, and one with great promise for the coming decade, is the structure and function of positive emotion. Despite Tomkins's straightforward arguments that psychology had neglected positive aspects of emotional experience, there have been remarkably few empirical advances in our understanding of positive emotions. Barbara L. Fredrickson and Christine Branigan (Chapter 4, this volume) describe a number of factors that might explain this deficit, including psychology's more general tendency to focus on emotional problems and their treatment, and the fact that positive emotions are fewer in number and tend to be less differentiated than negative emotions.

Fredrickson (1998; see also Chapter 4) has argued persuasively that emotion theory must accommodate positive emotions. To this end, she has proposed a broaden-and-build approach to positive emotions. Emotion theory has thus far in its development given primacy to the *action tendencies* associated with specific emotions (see Frijda, 1986; Lazarus, 1991). The idea that emotions carry with them specific response patterns honed by evolution to prepare us for a variety of environmental threats is compelling. However, as Fredrickson and Branigan astutely note, the construct becomes awkward when applied to positive emotions. In place of action tendencies, they introduce the term *thought–action tendencies* so as to incorporate the way that positive emotions promote changes in cognitive activity. Negative emotions typically occur during environmental threat and tend to narrow the possible thought–action response patterns toward those time-tested behavioral responses that have proved effective to our ancestors (e.g., anger mobilizes resources and communicates the willingness to defend the self). In contrast, positive emotions are more likely to occur in nonthreatening or relaxed situations, and tend to momentarily broaden a person's thought–action responses so as to promote cognitive flexibility and build resources for future adaptive needs. As negative emotions are to threat, positive emotions are to opportunity. Although there is considerable indirect support for the broaden-and-build approach, owing to its relative recency direct empirical substantiation of its basic tenets is only in the beginning stages (Fredrickson & Branigan, 2000). Nonetheless, its is hard to imagine a more promising avenue for emotion research to pursue.

In addition to the role of positive emotions in benign situations, several authors in the present volume (Chapters 8, 10, and 12) note that there is still much to learn about the unique utility of positive emotions in the context of negative or threatening situations. Some two decades ago, Lazarus, Kanner, and Folkman (1980) argued for the functional value of positive emotions as breathers, sustainers, and restorers that foster efforts to cope with stress. As Judith Tedlie Moskowitz documents in Chapter 10, researchers have recently demonstrated the role of positive emotions in speeding recovery for such difficulties as the death of a spouse (Bonanno & Keltner, 1997) and cardiovascular disease (Fredrickson & Levenson, 1998). It would be a grave error, however, to swing the pendulum too strongly. As Tracy J. Mayne cautions in Chapter 12, there can also be a downside to positive affect—it may undercut perceiving, identifying, and acting on symptoms of illness. Further research in this context will greatly enhance the literature on coping and health promoting behaviors.

EMOTION REGULATION: DOWN AND UP

Another exciting topic promising to bear fruit in the coming decades pertains to the question of how people regulate both negative and positive emotions across situations. Traditionally, psychology has taken a rather narrow view of this question, emphasizing primarily the down-regulation of negative emotions, either by direct control (i.e., suppressing the emotion) or by venting and thereby gaining control and closure. Only recently has theorizing in this area become more ambitious, gravitating toward more complex modeling of the ways in which different emotions and different regulatory processes interact under different circumstances. This newer, broader approach to emotion regulation was necessitated in part by a growing appreciation of the unique adaptive functions thought to underlay different individual emotions (as discussed in Chapter 6). It was also necessitated by the growing accumulation of new empirical evidence on the variety of ways that emotion regulatory processes might enhance or detract from physical, mental, and social adjustment (see Chapters 8–12).

Also in the present volume, Lisa Feldman Barrett and James J. Gross (Chapter 9) have addressed the role of emotional processes in intelligent behavior (i.e., emotional intelligence) by integrating the concept of individual variations in emotional differentiation with the taxonomy of emotion regulatory processes. Their analysis includes both antecedent-focused regulatory processes (i.e., processes that short-circuit or enhance the likelihood that specific types of emotion will be instigated) and response-focused regulatory processes (i.e., processes that diminish or enhance the experience, expression, or physiological manifestation of emotion). From a different perspective, George A. Bonanno (Chapter 8) has addressed many of the same questions by applying a more generalized model of psychological self-regulation based on the concept of emotional homeostasis. Crucial to this approach is the idea that emotion regulatory processes are organized sequentially, proceeding from (1) *basic control processes* that modulate immediate emotional responses; to (2) *anticipatory processes,* such as instrumental behaviors that prepare for future emotional control needs; to (3) *exploratory processes* that lead to the development of new skills, knowledge, or resources that incidentally enhance emotion self-regulation efforts. Kevin N. Ochsner and Lisa Feldman Barrett (Chapter 2) discuss the neurological substrates that process information at these various levels (considered further in the next section) and are sensitive to different forms of regulatory behavior.

Although each of these approaches to some extent serves as a vehicle to integrate the traditional literature, each also extends emotion regulation beyond its traditional limits by including instances in which emotional experience might be up-regulated (augmented or enhanced) as well as down-regulated or controlled. As we noted above, there are advantages to enhancing positive emotions. For instance, positive emotions promote creativity in problem solving and increase the efficiency of decision making (Isen, 1993; Isen, Daubman, & Nowicki, 1987). However, there are also myriad ways in which the amplified experience or expression of negative emotions might foster adaptation. For example, rape victims are viewed more favorably by observers, and by extension are more likely to garner social support, when they display anger (Vrij & Fischer, 1997). Mayne (Chapter 12) has noted ways in which the up-regulation of negative emotions can be of particular relevance to health and health-promoting behaviors. For example, the increased experience of guilt has been associated with adherence to positive health behaviors (Bybee, Leckman, Mersica & Miller, 1997). Future research will need to address the clinical and ethical issues involved in up-regulating negative affect and down-regulating positive affect.

EMOTIONAL PATHOLOGY

The normal regulation of emotion and its role in adjustment is contrasted with important new evidence about the ways in which disturbances in emotional processing have been implicated in various forms of psychopathology. Ann M. Kring (Chapter 11) has emphasized that the functions of emotions in disordered and nondisordered individuals are essentially the same. The difference appears to be that individuals suffering from some form of psychopathology are impaired in one or more components of emotional processing and thus are unable to achieve normal emotion-related functions. In embracing this complex literature, Kring has adopted Barnett and Gotlib's (1988) tripartite distinction between the antecedents, concomitants, and consequences of a disorder, and she has applied the distinction to schizophrenia, depression, and social phobia.

Although the preliminary research has been extremely promising, there remain a number of important challenges for research in this area in the decades to come. In her analysis, Kring highlights two particularly important directions for future research: one is to map the specificity of emotional disturbances with greater detail and clarity; the other is to more clearly locate emotional disturbances within the temporal course of a particular disorder. In either case, the challenges of these endeavors are compounded by the myriad difficulties that generally plague research on psychopathology (e.g., confounding variance associated with medication regimes, lack of compliance, and participant dropout). Thus, this enterprise will require the full repertoire of methods and measures available to emotion researchers, including both laboratory and naturalistic methods, self-report and facial expression studies, and narrative-based approaches (see, e.g., Capps & Ochs, 1995). As research in this area progresses, it may be fruitful to forge links with research in emotion regulation as a means of developing emotion-based modes of treatment.

Mayne (Chapter 12) discusses emotion regulation and physical pathology in much the same terms, arguing for the need to identify the specific components of emotion that influence specific facets of health and to understand how these unfold over time in terms of intensity, duration, and frequency. In this model, behaviors used to regulate emotion (particularly substance use, eating, and sex) have both immediate and long-term consequences for physical health and pathology. By extending the psychophysiological model from arousal to behavior, emotion-associated change in any parameter can occur within a healthy range (promoting health) or pathological range (damaging health). Here again, the application of emotion regulation models from Chapters 8, 9, and 10 may provide a basis for designing and testing emotion-based primary and secondary disease prevention interventions.

NATURE VERSUS NURTURE:
UNTANGLING THE ROLE OF CULTURE AND SELFISH GENES

We noted at the beginning of this chapter that the earliest and currently dominant contributions to emotion research and theory have been rooted in the idea that emotions represent organized patterns of responding that developed gradually over the course of human evolution to provide effective solutions to specific environmental threats. Although not all emotion theorists subscribe to this view (see Averill, 1980, 1996), the bulk of the research and theory in this area has focused almost exclusively on documenting and affirming the original evolutionary view (Ekman, 1992, 1993, 1994; Izard, 1992, 1994; Lazarus, 1991; Panksepp, 1992).

As we have seen, the failure of such a model to accommodate positive emotions has pointed up the need for a broader approach. An even stronger revisionist argument comes from the field of evolutionary psychology itself. As Michael J. Owren and Jo-Anne Bachorowski (Chapter 5) note, much of the current theorizing on the evolutionary role of emotion is based on Darwin's original speculations. However, contemporary emotion theories have tended to ignore the considerable advances in biological conceptions of evolution, in particular those advances with profound implications about the possible roles and functions of positive emotion. Central to Owren and Bachorowski's analysis is the selfish-gene framework, which now dominates evolutionary biology.

The emphasis on gene-based (rather than individual-based) evolution carries with it several crucial implications for emotion theory. Primary among these is that the traditional emphasis on communication of information to others fails to account for the coevolutionary processes that encompass the interests of both senders and receivers (Hauser, 1996). Again, this concern is of particular importance for positive emotions. From the purely competitive viewpoint of the selfish gene, expressing positive emotions provides the receiver with vital information about the sender's internal state and thus places the sender at a distinct disadvantage. Thus, from a selfish-gene perspective, honest expression can be less adaptive than dishonest or deceptive signaling.

How these considerations actually pan out in human exchanges has only just begun to receive empirical attention. For instance, genuine (Duchenne) laughter has been found to evoke different types of responses in observers than volitional or polite laughter (Keltner & Bonanno, 1997). It is imperative that emotion researchers accommodate these concerns in the coming decades and attend to the cost-and-benefit trade-off that might be associated with expressing various emotions across different types of situations.

Additional avenues for research in this vein are suggested by Dacher Keltner and Jonathan Haidt (Chapter 6). They attempt to broaden the scope of the evolutionary psychology of emotion by incorporating the insights of social constructivist theorists, who have traditionally emphasized culturally specific influences on emotion (see, e.g., Averill, 1980; Lutz & White, 1986). Consistent with Owren and Bachorowski's emphasis on the coevolution of communication between sender and receiver, Keltner and Haidt underscore the ways that emotional expressions structure social interactions by evoking complementary emotional responses in others or by reinforcing social behavior in others over the course of repeated interchanges.

In addition, Keltner and Haidt note that cultural influences can loosen the evolutionary link between emotions and the social problems they were originally designed to solve. For instance, cultures may develop alternative solutions to ancient problems or find new uses for emotions that have little to do with their original function; these are areas ripe for cross-cultural comparative research. Indeed, Keltner and Haidt argue that, although significant headway has been made by examining individual research participants' response to controlled emotional stimuli, there is a need for more ambitious investigations of the role of emotion in the context of ongoing social interactions and practices. Such an approach necessarily will shift the units of analysis from the individual to the dyad or larger social group, from emotion as an outcome to emotion as a mediator of outcome, and from emotion in isolated settings to emotion in the context of specific social interactions and cultural practices.

The impact of culture on the experience and expression of our inherited emotional repertoire is spelled out even more clearly by Batja Mesquita (Chapter 7). In contrast to traditional universalist theories of emotion, which have aimed to demonstrate cross-cultural similarity in emotions, Mesquita elucidated two alternative approaches to culture, each with important implications for the future of emotion research. One approach, referred to as *componential theories*, emphasizes the multidimensional nature of emotional phenomena (e.g., antecedent events, appraisal processes, action readiness, expressive behaviors, and regulatory processes; see Frijda, 1986, and Lazarus, 1991). From a research perspective, componential theories carry with them the implication that cross-cultural variability needs to be examined at the level of each individual component. Further, this increased potential for variability suggests that emotions are less likely to be simply similar or different but rather to vary to different degrees across cultures. The second, more radical approach, referred to as the *cultural theories* of emotion, takes as its starting point the idea that emotions cannot be understood without consideration of the cultural frame within which they are experienced. At their most extreme, cultural theories are constructivist and thus dismissive of the evolutionary view of emotion in its entirety. However, at a more moderate level, cultural theories suggest the need to balance the traditional focus of emotion research, which has been dominated by the quest for pancultural similarities and universals, with a greater emphasis on cultural specificity or cultural differences.

Together, these different approaches highlight the complexities that must be accommodated by a new evolutionary psychology of emotion. There are time-tested, inherited emotional solutions to enduring social problems. There are the nuances of communication between senders and receivers motivated by the selfish concerns of gene-based survival. And there are multiple components of emotional phenomena that vary across individuals, dyads, groups, and cultures. It would be clearly impossible if not foolhardy to attempt to address each of these concerns fully in a single study. However, it is equally clear that future research and theorizing on emotion must at least consider each of these concerns as they pertain to the larger evolutionary and functional picture.

AFFECTIVE NEUROSCIENCE

As we have just completed what has been termed the decade of the brain, it is not surprising that major advances in neuroscience have shed significant light on the structure, function, and process of emotion. Many of the issues raised in the previous sections, issues that will define the future of emotion research, are beginning to be elucidated and examined through a more sophisticated understanding of the neural substrates and cognitive processes that give rise to emotion.

Kevin N. Ochsner and Lisa Feldman Barrett (Chapter 2) and Pierre Philippot and Alexandre Schaefer (Chapter 3) each tackle the concept that emotions involve multiple—independent yet often interdependent—levels of processing. Are there fundamental differences between positive and negative emotion? One would expect such differences in light of the finding that primitive processing for emotions like fear takes place in the amygdala via adrenergic neurons, whereas the processing of reward and positive valence takes place in the basal ganglia via dopaminergic neurons. With different underlying structures and functions, the expectation that positive and negative emotions must be processed or organized in an exclusively parallel manner makes little sense. Could this support and explain the positive–negative dimensional structure of self-reported emotion? Yes—but that does not preclude the presence of discrete emotion within these two realms.

The "nature versus nurture" or "genes versus culture" debate can also be resolved if one allows for multiple levels of emotional processing. Clearly, there is strong evidence for universal and basic emotions (Ekman, 1992). These are driven by automatic processing in lower cortical structures like the amygdala and basal ganglia. However, human evolution has also produced higher cortical structures that allow for learning and adaptation, a highly defined level of self-consciousness, and a high degree of abstraction and imagination. MacLean (1973) first posited that the evolutionary advances in brain structure (resulting from random mutations) were not a "planned" architectural design. As a result, communication and coordination between these structures is less then perfect but have become more intertwined with learning and experience. In other words, newborn infants may have only basic affects, processed predominantly in lower brain structures. As Leventhal and Scherer (1987) argue, cognitive development allows for schematization of emotion—we develop beliefs, expectations, and reactions to our emotions. New emotions develop over time (like shame and embarrassment) that do not appear until we have reached certain cognitive milestones (Lewis & Michalson, 1983). Given these multilevel structures and processes, one would be hard pressed to argue against either basic/universal or culturally determined emotions. In fact, neuroscience would predict the development of cultural specificity over time. The questions we turn our attention to now, like the J. LeDoux versus A. R. Damasio debate concerning whether or not the amygdala performs schematic processing, would have been unthinkable 10 years ago.

It is interesting, as pointed out by Philippot and Schaefer (Chapter 3), that from a different methodological tradition, cognitive psychologists have also concluded that emotional processing takes place on anywhere from two to five levels. The sense is overwhelming that we are rapidly approaching an integrated theory of neuroscience structure and cognitive functioning of emotion, which informs much of our empirical work. We do not have to argue over whether emotions are discrete or dimensional, but under what circumstances they manifest as one or the other. The question of nature versus nurture becomes pedantic if automatic programs in the brain can be influenced by learning and active cognition. Indeed, as Mayne points out (in Chapter 12), we must avoid the pitfall of trying to impose a simplistic organized structure on emotion that does not exist. Both affective neuroscience and cognitive theory suggest that we should observe complex and even paradoxical outcomes given the multiple layers of processing involved in emotion.

Where, then, is the future of emotion research? It will most certainly involve advances in neuropsychology that will inform all other areas of research. It will entail understanding positive emotions with the same clarity with which we now understand negative emotions, and perhaps revising our understanding of both in the process. It will involve advancing our understanding of emotional regulatory strategies to allow for up- *and* down-regulation of positive *and* negative emotion. This includes modeling the limits of adaptive regulation and an understanding of the pathology (both physical and mental) that results when emotions fall outside of a healthy range. It will also conceptualize the bounds and limits of genetically and culturally determined contributions to emotion. And it will involve the application of this knowledge to programs that foster health and prevent and treat pathology—at the physical, mental, social, and cultural levels.

REFERENCES

Averill, J. R. (1980). A constructivist view of emotion. In R. Plutchik & H. Kellerman (Eds.), *Emotion: Theory, research, and experience* (pp. 305–339). New York: Academic Press.

Averill, J. R. (1996). An analysis of psychophysiological symbolism and its influence on theories of emotion. In R. Harré & W. G. Parrott (Eds.), *The emotions: Social, cultural, and biological dimensions* (pp. 204–228). London: Sage.

Barnett, P. A., & Gotlib, I. H. (1988). Psychosocial functioning and depression: Distinguishing among antecedents, concomitants, and consequences. *Psychological Bulletin, 104,* 97–126.

Bonanno, G. A., & Keltner, D. (1997). Facial expressions of emotion and the course of bereavement. *Journal of Abnormal Psychology, 106,* 126–137.

Bybee, J., Leckman, J. F., Mersica, R., & Miller, P. (1997, April). *Guilt and depression: Relationships to diabetic adherence and metabolic control in two high-risk samples.* Paper presented at the annual meeting of the Eastern Psychological Association, Washington, DC.

Cannon, W. B. (1960). *The wisdom of the body.* New York: Norton. (Original work published 1932)

Capps, L., & Ochs, E. (1995). *Constructing panic: The discourse of agoraphobia.* Cambridge, MA: Harvard University Press.

Darwin, C. (1999). *The expression of the emotions in man and animals* (Introduction and commentary by P. Ekman). London: HarperCollins. (Original work published 1872)

Duchenne de Bologne, G. B. (1990). *The mechanism of human facial expression* (R. A. Cuthbertson, Trans.). New York: Cambridge University Press. (Original work published 1862)

Ekman, P. (1992). An argument for basic emotions. *Cognition and Emotion, 6*, 169–200.

Ekman, P. (1993). Facial expression and emotion. *American Psychologist, 48*, 384–392.

Ekman, P. (1994). Strong evidence for universals in facial expressions: A reply to Russell's mistaken critique. *Psychological Bulletin, 115*, 268–287.

Ekman, P., Levenson, R. W., & Friesen, W. V. (1983). Autonomic nervous system activity distinguishes between emotions. *Science, 221*, 1208–1210.

Fredrickson, B. L. (1998). What good are positive emotions? *Review of General Psychology, 2*, 300–319.

Fredrickson, B. L., & Branigan, C. (2000). *Positive emotions broaden thought–action repertoires: Evidence for the broaden-and-build model.* Manuscript in preparation.

Fredrickson, B. L., & Levenson, R. W. (1998). Positive emotions speed recovery from the cardiovascular sequelae of negative emotions. *Cognition and Emotion, 12*, 191–220.

Frijda, N. H. (1986). *The emotions.* Cambridge, UK: Cambridge University Press.

Hauser, M. D. (1996). *The evolution of communication.* Cambridge, MA: MIT Press.

Isen, A. M. (1993). Positive affect and decision making. In M. Lewis & J. M. Haviland (Eds.), *Handbook of emotions* (pp. 261–277). New York: Guilford Press.

Isen, A. M., Daubman, K. A., & Nowicki, G. P. (1987). Positive affect facilitates creative problem solving. *Journal of Personality and Social Psychology, 47*, 1206–1217.

Izard, C. (1992). Basic emotions, relations among emotions, and emotion–cognition relations. *Psychological Review, 99*, 561–564.

Izard, C. E. (1994). Innate and universal facial expressions: Evidence from developmental and cross-cultural research. *Psychological Bulletin, 115*, 288–299.

James, W. (1884). What is an emotion? *Mind, 9*, 188–205.

James, W. (1981). *The principles of psychology, Vol. II.* Cambridge, MA: Harvard University Press. (Original work published 1890)

Keltner, D., & Bonanno, G. A. (1997). A study of laughter and dissociation: Distinct correlates of laughter and smiling during bereavement. *Journal of Personality and Social Psychology, 73*, 687–702.

Lazarus, R. S. (1991). *Emotion and adaptation.* New York: Oxford University Press.

Lazarus, R. S., Kanner, A. D., & Folkman, S. (1980). Emotions: A cognitive–phenomenological analysis. In R. Plutchik & H. Kellerman (Eds.), *Theories of emotion* (pp. 189–217). New York: Academic Press.

Levenson, R. W., Carstensen, L. L., Friesen, W. V., & Ekman, P. (1991). Emotion, physiology, and expression in old age. *Physiology and Aging, 6*, 28–35.

Levenson, R. W., Ekman, P., Heider, K., & Friesen, W. V. (1992). Emotion and autonomic nervous system activity in the Minangkabau of West Sumatra. *Journal of Personality and Social Psychology, 62*, 972–988.

Leventhal, H., & Scherer, K. (1987). The relationship of emotion to cognition: A functional approach to a semantic controversy. *Cognition and Emotion, 1*, 3–28.

Lewis, M., & Michalson, L. (1983). *Children's emotions and moods: Developmental theory and measurement*. New York: Plenum Press.

Lutz, C. A., & White, G. (1986). The anthropology of emotion. *Annual Review of Anthropology*, pp.

MacLean, P. D. (1973). *A triune concept of the brain and behavior: Hincks Memorial Lectures*. Toronto, Ontario, Canada: University of Toronto Press.

Marshall, G. D., & Zimbardo, P. G. (1979). Affective consequences of inadequately explained physiological arousal. *Journal of Personality and Social Psychology, 37*, 970–988.

Panksepp, J. (1992). A critical role for "affective neuroscience" in resolving what is basic about basic emotions. *Psychological Review, 99*, 554–560.

Schachter, S., & Singer, J. (1962). Cognitive, social and physiological determinants of emotional state. *Psychological Review, 69*, 379–399.

Tomkins, S. S. (1962). *Affect, imagery, consciousness: Vol. 1. The positive affects*. New York: Springer.

Tomkins, S. S. (1963). *Affect, imagery, consciousness: Vol. 2. The negative affects*. New York: Springer.

Vrij, A., & Fischer, A. (1997). The role of displays of emotion and ethnicity in judgments of rape victims. *International Review of Victimology, 4*, 255–265.

Index

Affect, 338
    as the central organizing principle of
        individuals/society, 31
    core affect, 338
    "Affect programs" concept (Tomkins),
        200
Affective science
    need for paradigm shift, 33–34
    neurosciences and concept of emotions
        as organizing systems, 18
Amae. See Contentment
Amnesia and emotion, 98–99
    and affective valence learning, 99
    emotional memory system and
        declarative memory system
        study, 98
    and mere exposure effect, 98
Anger, 126, 363
    and bereavement, 267
    as a "best guess," 286
    and Type A construct, 364–365
    See also Emotion and physical health
Animal communication theory
    competitive coevolution and honest
        signaling, 163
    historical trends, 161–163
        "communication" not for signaling,
            162–163
        influence vs. information from
            selfish-gene perspective, 162
        "ritualization" of inadvertent cues
            theory, 162
    honesty and cheating interplay, 163–
        164
ANS (automatic nervous system) arousal

and emotional processing theory
    (Mandler), 84
Appraisal
    appraisal patterns–emotions linkage
        theory, 38
    and automatic emotion processing, 40
    as a core element of emotional
        experience, 228
    positive reappraisal in stress and
        coping theory, 323–324
Arnold. *See* Excitatory theory of emotion
Associative semantic network model
    (Bower), 85–87, 110
    application to emotional disorders, 86
    critiques, 87
    "mood-congruent memory," 85–86
    "mood-dependent memory," 85–86
"Attentional narrowing" hypothesis, 104
Autobiographical memory and emotion,
    102, 112
    activation, 107–110
    generic/"overgeneral" memories (g-
        ABM), 108
    and "hot" cognition, 110
    memory for emotional events, 102–
        103, 106–107
    eyewitness studies, 103–104
    flashbulb memory (FBM), 105–106
    and "repression," 103
    parallel between emotional memory
        systems and emotional
        autobiographical memories,
        107–108
    specific memories (s-ABM), 108
    study limitations, 104, 106

411